The Routledge Handbook of Religion, Spirituality and Social Work

This international volume provides a comprehensive account of contemporary research, new perspectives and cutting-edge issues surrounding religion and spirituality in social work. The introduction introduces key themes and conceptual issues such as understandings of religion and spirituality as well as definitions of social work, which can vary between countries. The main body of the book is divided up into sections on regional perspectives; religious and spiritual traditions; faith-based service provision; religion and spirituality across the lifespan; and social work practice. The final chapter identifies key challenges and opportunities for developing both social work scholarship and practice in this area.

Including a wide range of international perspectives from Australia, Canada, Hong Kong, India, Ireland, Israel, Malta, New Zealand, South Africa, Sweden, the UK and the USA, this *Handbook* succeeds in extending the dominant paradigms and comprises a mix of authors including major names, significant contributors and emerging scholars in the field, as well as leading contributors in other fields of social work who have an interest in religion and spirituality.

The Routledge Handbook of Religion, Spirituality and Social Work is an authoritative and comprehensive reference for academics and researchers as well as for organisations and practitioners committed to exploring why, and how, religion and spirituality should be integral to social work practice.

Beth R. Crisp is a professor in the School of Health and Social Development at Deakin University, Australia, where she is the discipline leader for social work. She has extensive experience in the international social work arena, having previously been Senior Lecturer in Social Work at the University of Glasgow, and more recently was the Australian lead of a consortium of eight Australian and European universities that explored curriculum development in social work at an international level. In addition to her PhD from La Trobe University, she has undergraduate degrees in social work (La Trobe University), political science (University of Melbourne) and theology (Melbourne College of Divinity). Beth has contributed around 100 major articles in peer-reviewed journals, as well as having written numerous research reports, book chapters and a number of books including *Social Work and Faith-based Organizations* (2014) and *Spirituality and Social Work* (2010).

The Routledge Handbook of Religion, Spirituality and Social Work

Edited by Beth R. Crisp

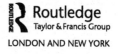

Routledge
Taylor & Francis Group

LONDON AND NEW YORK

First published 2017
by Routledge
2 Park Square, Milton Park, Abingdon, Oxon OX14 4RN

and by Routledge
711 Third Avenue, New York, NY 10017

Routledge is an imprint of the Taylor & Francis Group, an informa business

British Library Cataloguing in Publication Data
A catalogue record for this book is available from the British Library

Library of Congress Cataloging in Publication Data
A catalog record for this book has been requested

ISBN: 978-1-138-93122-0 (hbk)
ISBN: 978-1-315-67985-3 (ebk)

Typeset in Bembo and ITC Stone Sans by
Servis Filmsetting Ltd, Stockport, Cheshire

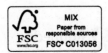

Printed and bound in Great Britain by
TJ International Ltd, Padstow, Cornwall

Contents

Contents

Tables

Contributors

Alean Al-Krenawi is the President of Ben-Gurion University of the Negev, Israel.

Sara Ashencaen Crabtree is Professor of Social and Cultural Diversity in the Department of Social Sciences and Social Work, University of Bournemouth, UK.

Nehami Baum is a professor in The Louis and Gabi Weisfeld School of Social Work, Bar Ilan University, Israel.

Linda Benavides is an assistant professor in the Center for Social Work Education, Widener University, USA.

Laura Béres is an associate professor in the School of Social Work, King's University College at Western University, Canada.

Fred H. Besthorn is a professor in the School of Social Work, Wichita State University, USA.

Raisuyah Bhagwan is a professor in the Child and Youth Care Program at Durban University of Technology, South Africa.

Heather Marie Boynton completed a PhD in social work at the University of Calgary, and is a lecturer at both Lakehead University and the Northern Ontario School of Medicine, Canada.

Edward R. Canda is a professor and Director of the Spiritual Diversity Initiative in the School of Social Welfare, University of Kansas, USA.

Patricia Carlisle completed her PhD in social work at the University of Stirling, UK.

Ann M. Carrington is a lecturer in social work in the College of Arts, Society and Education, James Cook University, Australia.

Cecilia Lai Wan Chan is Chair Professor in the Department of Social Work and Social Administration, University of Hong Kong, Hong Kong.

Celia Hoi Yan Chan is an assistant professor in the Department of Social Work and Social Administration, University of Hong Kong, Hong Kong.

Diana Coholic is an associate professor and Director of the School of Social Work at Laurentian University, Canada.

Beth R. Crisp is professor and discipline leader for social work in the School of Health and Social Development, Deakin University, Australia.

Malabika Das is an integrative social worker who recently completed a PhD in social work at the University of Hong Kong where she also serves as an honorary lecturer.

Adam Dinham is Professor of Faith and Public Policy and Director of the Faiths and Civil Society Unit, Goldsmiths, University of London, UK, and Professor of Religious Literacy at VID University, Oslo, Norway.

Linda Plitt Donaldson is an associate professor in the National Catholic School of Social Service, Catholic University of America, USA, and is the Editor of the *Journal of Religion and Spirituality in Social Work: Social Thought.*

Michael Dudley works as a psychiatrist at Prince of Wales and Sydney Children's Hospitals, and is a conjoint senior lecturer in psychiatry at University of New South Wales, Australia.

Arielle Dylan is an associate professor in the School of Social Work, St Thomas University, Canada.

John G. Fox is a lecturer in social work in the College of Health and Biomedicine, Victoria University, Australia.

Fran Gale is a senior lecturer in social work and community welfare, School of Social Sciences and Psychology, Western Sydney University, Australia.

Fiona Gardner is an associate professor in social work in the School of Rural Health, La Trobe University, Australia.

Philip Gilligan, formerly Senior Lecturer in Social Work, is now an honorary visiting research fellow in the Department of Social Work and Social Care, University of Bradford, UK.

Mark Henrickson is an associate professor in the School of Social Work, Massey University, New Zealand.

Katie Hirtz Bingaman is a forensic social worker in Harrisburg, Pennsylvania, USA.

David R. Hodge is a professor in the School of Social Work, Arizona State University, USA, and a senior nonresident fellow in the Program for Research on Religion and Urban Civil Society, University of Pennsylvania, USA.

Jon Hudson is an assistant professor in the Department of Social Work, University of Wisconsin-Oshkosh, USA.

Caroline Humphrey is a senior lecturer in social work in the Faculty of Health and Social Care, University of Hull, UK.

Eva Jeppsson Grassman is an emeritus professor at the Institute for the Study of Ageing and Later Life, Linköping University, Sweden.

Xiao-Wen Ji is from the Department of Social Work and Social Administration, University of Hong Kong, Hong Kong.

Kyung Mee Kim is an associate professor in the Department of Social Welfare, Soongsil University, South Korea.

James Lucas is a lecturer in social work at the Institute of Koorie Education, Deakin University, Australia.

Mishka Lysack is an associate professor in the Faculty of Social Work, University of Calgary, Canada.

Janet Melville-Wiseman is a principal lecturer in social work in the School of Public Health, Midwifery and Social Work, Canterbury Christ Church University, UK.

Jungrim Moon is a PhD student in the School of Social Welfare, University of Kansas, USA.

Samta P. Pandya is an assistant professor in the School of Social Work, Tata Institute of Social Sciences, India.

Claudia Psaila is a lecturer in the Department of Social Policy and Social Work, University of Malta, Malta.

Irene Renzenbrink is a social worker and expressive arts therapist in Melbourne, Australia.

Michael J. Sheridan is Special Advisor for Diversity and Wellness Programs, Office of Intramural Training and Education, National Institutes of Health, USA.

Bartholemew Smallboy is a PhD student studying the revitalization of Indigenous economic institutions at the University of New Brunswick, Canada.

Mark Smith is a senior lecturer in social work in the School of Social and Political Science, University of Edinburgh, UK.

Jo-Ann Vis is an associate professor in the Department of Social Work, Lakehead University, Canada.

Russell Whiting is a senior lecturer in social work in the School of Education and Social Work, University of Sussex, UK.

Martha Wiebe is associated with the School of Social Work at Carleton University, Canada.

Michael Wolf-Branigin is Professor of Social Work in the College of Health and Human Services, George Mason University, USA.

Yao Hong is a PhD student in the Department of Social Work and Social Administration, University of Hong Kong, Hong Kong.

Part I
Introduction

Religion and spirituality in social work

Creating an international dialogue

Beth R. Crisp

Introduction

The last two decades have witnessed a growing interest in the role of religion and spirituality in social work practice in many countries, including places where for much of the twentieth century, social work sought to distance itself from its religious roots. Indeed, all 40 chapters in this volume were authored or co-authored by social workers, enabling the expression of explicitly social work perspectives on religion and spirituality. This includes chapters contributed by authors whose professional legacy included having made a significant contribution to this growing recognition of the legitimate place that religion and spirituality have in professional social work, including Alean Al-Krenawi, Sara Ashencaen Crabtree, Ed Canda, Philip Gilligan, David Hodge and Michael Sheridan. However, readers with a keen knowledge of this field may also have observed some significant omissions from the author list, which reflects that several of those who have pioneered this work over the last two decades are reaching the age of retirement from professional work and were, for various reasons, unable to be part of this project. Nevertheless, the impact of their work is evident in both explicit discussions of the work of John Coates by Mishka Lysack, and also by Fred Besthorn and Jon Hudson, and also in the lists of references of many chapters, where readers will find evidence of the influence of scholars such as John Graham and Margaret Holloway.

There is always the possibility that once a group of prominent scholars who have been passionate about a field of research move on, that work in this field falls away. This volume includes several contributions from emerging social work researchers, many of whom have only recently completed doctoral studies, and whose contributions are expanding the dimensions of our understandings as to the relationship between social work and religion and spirituality. Contributions by early career researchers include chapters by Linda Benavides, Heather Boynton, Patricia Carlisle, Malabika Das, John Fox, James Lucas and Claudia Psaila. It should be noted there were other early career researchers who indicated a desire to be involved in this international project but were told by their employers that any publishing efforts should only be in journals, even if these were aimed at a national, rather than international, readership. Thankfully, this only applied to a few potential contributors, but contributes to the difficulty in creating international dialogue among social workers researching religion and spirituality.

Despite there now being a much wider recognition that religion and spirituality can make a very positive contribution to wellbeing for individuals and communities, the professional imagination as to what this might involve has frequently been confined by the known worlds of those social workers engaged in this quest to legitimise the place of religion and spirituality within the profession. Hence, much of the professional literature on religion, spirituality and social work has focussed on particular situations, stages of life or fields of practice:

- end of life care and bereavement
- treatment for substance misuse
- issues in migration, including issues for refugee and asylum seekers
- religion as problematic particularly in respect of mental health, providing care to children and hindering health promotion efforts associated with sexuality and sexual behaviours
- attitudes of religious social workers/social work students, which are conservative, judgmental or oppressive.

To a large extent, these emphases reflect the concerns of social workers in North America and the United Kingdom, whose voices dominate the international social work literature more generally (McDonald *et al.* 2003) and where, perhaps unsurprisingly, much of the readily available writing on religion, spirituality and social work to date has originated. While we have to thank authors in these countries for what many consider some of the seminal books and articles in this field, the extent to which their writings apply to ethnic and religious minorities in their own countries has been questioned (Regan *et al.* 2013).

Once implicit expectations of the homogeneity of social work practice between countries (Healy 2007) are increasingly acknowledged as unrealistic (Hugman *et al.* 2010). Furthermore, in many countries, social workers now accept that uncritical adoption of ideas about social work from North America and the United Kingdom can readily result in the privileging of Western values concerning social work (Mwansa 2011; Singh *et al.* 2011), even though this may be unintentional. This is most apparent when these values clash with those of another society in which the dominant religious culture is not Christianity (Holtzhausen 2011).

In seeking to provide an overview of the literature on religion, spirituality and social work, this volume seeks to challenge and extend the dominant paradigms by including authors from a broader range of countries rather than 'replicating a familiar process of colonial and post-colonial transfer of policy knowledge, processes, and practices' (McDonald *et al.* 2003: 193). Notwithstanding the need for social workers to take account of culturally-specific factors that impact on practice in their local context (Gray and Fook 2004), by offering an examination and discussion of new perspectives, it is envisaged that this volume will stimulate and provoke the social work community to further develop its thinking and practice regarding religion and spirituality. However, for this hope to be realised, readers may need to engage with ideas that may be unfamiliar, and even uncomfortable:

> To accept and incorporate other worldviews into one's frame of reference is difficult. It is necessary to move beyond "sensitivity" to the cultural views of others. This relates to an introductory comment concerning my own efforts to grapple with the question of the extent to which social work values can be held to be universal. A central challenge is in seeking to identify those aspects of social work that are universal and those which can be accepted as indigenous, including indigenous to the Western world. There may be defining characteristics of social work that hold true in most contexts and there may be defining features of social work that only hold true in a specific context. For example, social work, universally, has concern for those in society who are marginalized, but the ways in which

society and social work respond to need varies according to contextual factors including time, history, place and stage of development.

(Brydon 2012: 160–1).

Nevertheless, social workers often readily assume that their local experiences of how social work is practiced are universal (Brydon 2012; McCallum 2001). Consequently, despite not being in the original aims for this volume, inclusion of contributions from diverse countries, probably inevitably, results in the question emerging as to what is social work *per se*, and not just in relation to religion and spirituality. The various perspectives reflect 'a growing lack of agreement around the world about what social work is' (Gray and Fook 2004: 627). For example, readers may observe differences as to the involvement of social workers in different types of work, including different roles and involvements of social workers (Norman and Hintze 2005) and which issues or fields of practice are considered the domain of professional social work (Weber and Bugarszski 2007). The varying role of the state versus other providers in welfare provision (Liedgren 2015) is also apparent. Moreover, although the details may vary between countries, a not uncommon situation is that there are fields of social work practice that are typically regarded as 'secular' and others where a place for religion is considered legitimate.

Despite English being the most widely used language in the academic community (Obst and Kuder 2009) and frequently, the language in which non-Anglophones who speak different languages communicate with each other (Harrison 2006), language tends to be 'the forgotten dimension' (Ruzzene 1998: 17) in international social work projects. For example, Edward Canda, Jungrim Moon and Kyung Mee Kim note spirituality is a foreign concept and not well understood in Korea.

Many of the key concepts in social work have been framed in English, but adoption in other languages has not always been straightforward (Harrison 2006). It is quite plausible that an even broader range of perspectives could have been presented had there been the resources available to translate contributions from authors who were not able to write in English. Among social workers, there are also some English words that have acquired meanings or connotations that are country-specific (Gray and Fook 2004; Heron and Pilkington 2009). Moreover, there are differences between countries as to what is deemed acceptable or appropriate terminology by social workers (Norman and Hintze 2005; Simpson 2009), and although standardised terms could have been adopted throughout this volume, this becomes another form of colonialisation, which projects such as this are striving to overcome. Moreover, local differences are more apparent when indigenised vocabularies are given voice. This is particularly relevant when it comes to definitions of religion and spirituality.

As Fran Gale and Michael Dudley note, how social workers construct religion and spirituality is a significant factor as to whether religion and spirituality are able to be incorporated into emancipatory forms of social work. While editors can propose definitions that all authors are required to comply with, one of the drawbacks of this approach is that it can lead readers to assume a false homogeneity of understanding about these concepts, by prioritising a viewpoint from a particular country (e.g. Miller 2012). But while more messy for the reader who must engage with multiple understandings, this approach is arguably more meaningful in opening up an international dialogue (Cobb *et al.* 2012).

Regional perspectives

In their chapter, Arielle Dylan and Bartholemew Smallboy refer to a comment by Edward Said (1993: 7) in which he reflected that 'none of us is outside or beyond geography'. Collectively, the four chapters in Part II of this volume demonstrate some very different regional contexts in which social workers are grappling with issues of religion and spirituality. The first of these chapters provides a perspective on the complicated relationship between social work, religion and spirituality in Australia, which is the context in which the proposal for this volume was conceived and where much of the work to bring this volume to completion was undertaken. Although a particularly Australian form of social work has developed in response to contextual factors, remnants of the ideologies and models of welfare imported by the early British colonists linger:

> most contemporary accounts of welfare tend to privilege the role of the nation state in shaping welfare systems rather than pointing to the role of colonial expansion and other transnational influences. … processes of colonization and decolonization are still prominent in the lives of many people around the world.
>
> (Harrison and Melville 2010: 5)

In Australia, religion was intimately associated with the establishment and maintenance of social and political elites for much of the first two centuries of European colonisation. However, whereas Protestantism was associated with the ruling classes in Australia, its influence in Korea grew as nationalist movements opposed the occupation by Japan and the influx of Christian missionaries after the Korean War. Although religion can be linked with the return to peaceful society after conflict, the division of society and decades of civil unrest and violence in Northern Ireland was marked by religious identification, as Patricia Carlisle discusses in Chapter 4. Then in the final chapter of Part II, Claudia Psaila considers the impact on religious experience on Malta, and how the role of the Roman Catholic Church has seemingly diminished since Malta's accession into the European Union.

As each of the authors in Part II demonstrate, the local religious culture has implications for social work practice, and comparisons between Australia and Korea demonstrate this. In both Australia and Korea, a majority of individuals acknowledge an affinity with one of a range of religious groups, with no one form of religious belief and expression dominating, and there also being a substantial minority of the population who do not associate with any formal religion, some of whom may nevertheless be partial to forms of spirituality. Furthermore, in both countries, religious organisations play a substantial role in the provision of social welfare services in the broader community and not just to their own members. Reflecting the religious characteristics of the population, in Korea, both Buddhist and Christian welfare organisations are actively involved in welfare provision, whereas in Australia, most welfare provision associated with organised religion has a Christian auspice. Scholarship around spirituality and social work is also developing in both Australia and Korea, but whereas in Korea this tends to be associated with a religion and there are a number of schools of social work that are teaching social work aligned with particular religious viewpoints, Australian social work scholars are almost all located in secular institutions and many are interested in spirituality that transcends or is outside formal religions. Interestingly, the Australian *Code of Ethics* is much more explicit in its inclusion of religion and spirituality than its Korean counterpart.

Despite religious and spiritual diversity in both Australia and Korea, over the last two decades there has been a growing acceptance as to the legitimacy of religion and spirituality in social work practice. In contrast to these two countries, in which Christianity has become a dominant force only in the last two centuries, Malta and Northern Ireland are both places where Christianity became entrenched early in the Common Era, and both countries in which there is remarkably little social work literature about religion and spirituality. Marginalisation of matters religious or spiritual is common practice in social work in both of these countries, though for very different reasons. In Malta, as was previously the case in Australia, separation from its religious and spiritual roots has been part of the quest for the recognition of social work as a profession. Consequently, religion and spirituality are considered to be private, and religious and spiritual needs as not relevant to social work practice. By way of contrast, social workers in Northern Ireland may well recognise the impact of religion on wellbeing, but the close association between conflict and religion in that country has resulted in social workers considering issues of religion and spirituality too sensitive to raise with service users.

Many other chapters also provide glimpses as to why local concerns and the role of religion and spirituality in the culture must be taken into account by social workers. These include Alean Al-Krenawi's consideration of social work among Palestinians, Eva Jeppsson Grassman's discussions of the implications for social worker practice of the Church of Sweden ceasing to be a state church as well as chapters from a number of authors from Hong Kong. Notwithstanding the specific local factors discussed in these chapters, many raise questions that have much wider relevance, such as how social workers respond to and work with religious and spiritual diversity, what is the role of religious organisations in providing social work services, and perhaps most importantly, what are the implications of social workers ignoring religion and spirituality when they work with individuals, families and communities.

Religious and spiritual traditions

In line with seeking to avoid a north Atlantic Anglophone imperialism, it has been important to include contributions from a wide range of religious and spiritual traditions. Hence, this volume includes contributions concerning a range of religious traditions including various forms of Buddhism, Christianity, Confucianism, Daoism, Hinduism, Islam and Judaism, as well as from a range of spiritual perspectives not aligned with formal religions. Several of these traditions are discussed by multiple authors from very different contexts and perspectives. Having practice knowledge about a particular religious or spiritual tradition is not the same as understanding how associated beliefs and/or practices manifest themselves in the lives of particular individuals (Clark 2006). For instance, the lived experiences of Judaism for the Haredi women who live in closed communities in Israel, about whom Nehami Baum writes, are very different from the Jewish holocaust survivors in Melbourne whom John Fox notes are actively seeking to engage people of other religions or none, in their community education programmes. These varying perspectives, which highlight the complexities, and even contradictions, that occur among the people of a religion, challenge the simplistic stereotypes associated with particular religions (Anderson-Nathe et al. 2013).

Part III begins with three chapters concerning very ancient spiritual and religious traditions. Arielle Dylan and Bartholemew Smallboy introduce the reader to the spirituality of indigenous peoples in Canada and demonstrate the continuing consequences of the disrespect of the early European settlers for Aboriginal Canadians and their spirituality. That this indigenous spirituality has survived despite colonisation is also an important message in Raisuyah Bhagwan's chapter on African spirituality. This desire to maintain long-held traditions and lifestyles, despite immense outside pressures to modernise, is also an issue for the Haredi women in Israel, who are the focus of Nehami Baum's chapter.

The next two chapters focus on two Asian religions, both of which date back approximately 500 years BCE. Whereas the chapters by Dylan and Smallboy, and Bhagwan, note the negative impacts on indigenous spiritual traditions as a result of Western colonisation, Caroline Humphrey reminds us that Buddhism, which originated in Asia, has exported itself back to many Western nations. However, as Humphrey notes, many more Westerners adopt some Buddhist practices than becoming Buddhists *per se*. Like Buddhism, Daoism, which originated in a similar period in China, also places a strong emphasis on body, mind and spirit and the need to achieve a balancing of these dimensions. Yet as Celia Chan and colleagues point out, as with some other religious and spiritual traditions, taking seriously the tenets of Daoism may require social workers to reconsider what is appropriate professional practice.

Although it is estimated that more than half the world's population are Christian (31.5 per cent) or Muslim (23.2 per cent) (Pew Research Center 2012), these religions represent the newest of the traditions in Part III. Several chapters throughout this volume provide just a glimpse of the many expressions of Christianity influenced by both socio-religious cultures and the differing spiritualities. Laura Béres provides an introduction to Celtic spirituality, which emerged as the result of the indigenisation of Christianity in Ireland, where paganism was widespread in the early medieval period. While Celtic Christianity remains distinctive to this day, interest in Celtic spirituality transcends the traditional bounds of religion, with many aspects also appealing to those with more affinity to new age thinking.

The early period of Christianity also saw the emergence of Gnosticism. As Russell Whiting notes, there is no consensus as to whether Gnosticism should be regarded as a form of Christianity, Christian heresy or a separate religion. For social workers, such debates may well be superfluous as service users are unlikely to identify themselves as Gnostics, and the term itself maybe unfamiliar. Nevertheless, as Whiting notes, aspects of Gnostic thinking are readily found today. In particular he suggests that an understanding of Gnosticism can assist practitioners to understand conditions, such as anorexia nervosa, in which the relationship between mind and body have become disordered.

Part III concludes with two chapters concerning Islam. Sara Ashencaen Crabtree considers the experience of being Muslim in Britain, where not only is Islam a minority religion but frequently problematised, producing stereotypes that are unhelpful and fail to recognise the diversity of Muslims in Britain. By way of contrast, Alean Al-Krenawi explores the experiences of Palestinians living in the Gaza Strip and the West Bank, most of whom are Muslim. Despite being the majority population in these regions, Palestinians experience the negative impact of Israeli (i.e. Jewish) occupation on a daily basis.

As social workers and the organisations in which they work may need to be able to work with individuals, families and communities from a broad range of religious and spiritual traditions, the chapters from David Hodge and Adam Dinham in the section about social work practice address the practicalities of engaging with religious and spiritual diversity in a meaningful way. However, as Arielle Dylan and Bartholemew Smallboy point out, reducing peoples to their religion or spirituality and ignoring other fundamental needs is problematic and must be avoided.

Faith-based service provision

Prior to the twentieth century, religious groups were the main providers of welfare services in many countries. Despite social work services now being closely, if not totally, aligned with state provided services in many countries (Crisp 2013), the emergence of welfare state models may have altered the roles and services provided by religious welfare organisations but did not completely supplant their work (Crisp 2014). Indeed, a number of chapters in Sections 2 and 3 discuss the provision of charitable or welfare services as one of the characteristics that many religious traditions share, and faith-based service provision is the focus of Part IV. Today, the scope of services provided by churches and other faith-based agencies is likely to vary depending on the model of welfare state (Bäckström and Davie 2010), and expectations as to what services are considered appropriate for such agencies to provide vary considerably between countries (Crisp 2013).

Linda Plitt Donaldson provides an introduction to Catholic Social Teaching, which has been regarded as 'the most systematic and thorough attempt by a religious faith to articulate its position on social policy' (Brenden 2007: 477), and has been influential in informing understandings of social responsibility and welfare provision in other Christian traditions (Campbell 2012). Yet, notwithstanding the extent of its influence, the articulation of Catholic Social Teaching has not in itself ensured Catholic welfare organisations have provided appropriate services, as Mark Smith reflects in his chapter about residential childcare services provided by Catholic orders in Britain. Yet, despite the fact that some organisations provided care that is now considered scandalous, Smith reminds the reader that much good also came from services provided by the Catholic orders, and often the alternative had been no service at all.

Like the Roman Catholic Church, The Salvation Army is also present as both a religious organisation and service provider in many countries across the globe. As Michael Wolf-Branigin and Katie Hirtz Bingaman note, The Salvation Army has also been accused of scandalous behaviour in recent times, particularly in respect of its stance towards gay, lesbian, bisexual and transsexual individuals in the United States. In terms of drug and alcohol treatment, Salvation Army services typically take an abstinence approach, adopting principles consistent with groups such as Alcoholics Anonymous. This approach considers addiction to be a disease for which the only way to recovery is to abstain completely. However, this is not the only way in which faith-based organisations respond to the needs of service users who engage in substance misuse. For example, in Australia, the first medically supervised injecting room was set up under the auspice of another Christian church (Crisp 2014).

A very different philosophy is outlined by Samta Pandya, who provides an overview concerning the role of social service delivery in guru-led movements, which have their roots in Hindu traditions. As she points out, much of this service provision is financially dependent on the philanthropy of adherents and supporters in contrast to some other countries where service delivery organisations, despite their religious auspice, receive much of their funding from the state (Crisp 2014).

Issues relating to funding are noted by several authors in respect to faith-based organisations. Historically, both Catholic orders and The Salvation Army were strongly reliant on their members who had dedicated themselves to a life of service and a life of poverty. In turn, low costs have resulted in some state instrumentalities recognising that it is cheaper to contract with faith-based organisations than provide services themselves. While such contracts may be fair to all parties, there are also numerous examples of states failing to adequately resource faith-based organisations and having no qualms about exploiting their goodwill (Crisp 2014).

In addition to direct service provision, faith-based organisations have played an active role in the development of professional social work in some countries, as noted in both my chapter about Australia and Linda Plitt Donaldson's contribution to this volume. John Fox in his chapter about the work of the Jewish Holocaust Museum and Research Centre in Melbourne gives an example of how an organisation that provides critical services to members of the local Jewish community also makes an important contribution to educating the wider community about the suffering that continues to this day as a result of the Jewish Holocaust during World War II.

The notion of change and needing to adapt to new circumstances emerges in several of the chapters in Part IV. The Jewish Holocaust Museum and Research Centre recognises that in the near future, the last of the Holocaust survivors will no longer be alive and able to provide personal testimony about their experiences. Although change can present dilemmas, it can also open up new opportunities, as Eva Jeppsson Grassman explores in her consideration of the options for the Church of Sweden since ceasing to be a state church. These include bidding for service provision contracts, which were not open to the Church of Sweden prior to disestablishment. This in turn raises questions that are being asked in faith-based organisations in many countries, as to how to balance religious identity with expectations that emerge with state funding.

Religion and spirituality across the lifespan

It would be fair to say that for some social workers, the only time when religion and/or spirituality have a legitimate place is when death is approaching or has recently occurred. In their contributions, Martha Wiebe and Irene Renzenbrink certainly emphasise the importance of social workers taking account of spiritual needs in the face of death. However, as the contributions in this volume attest, religion and spirituality can be of critical importance at any life stage, and social workers need to recognise this.

Heather Boynton and Jo-Ann Vis have contributed the opening chapter in Part V, in which they consider the need for spiritual requirements to be recognised by social workers at all stages of life, recognising that these may manifest themselves very differently as one moves from childhood to old age. This is particularly important in the aftermath of traumatic events, when the capacity to engage with and express one's spirituality may be critical in the process of moving on. As Linda Benavides reflects in the subsequent chapter, encouraging spiritual development among children and adolescents can act as a protective factor, which facilitates resilience. Despite religious teachings that promote the prevention of child abuse by emphasising the duties of both parents and the community in caring for children (Bunge 2014; Dorff 2014), unfortunately, as Philip Gilligan writes, such potential has too often been destroyed by the sexual abuse of children in religious settings.

When asked what they meant by 'spirituality', over half the residents of the English town of Kendal provided answers associated with relationships (Heelas and Woodhead 2005). Indeed, marrying, or living in a marriage-like relationship, and having children together, are the expectations of the majority of the world's population on becoming an adult (Crisp 2010). Yet, as Mark Henrickson reminds us, this includes many people who do not identify as heterosexual, who often find themselves having to navigate their relationships in the face of vehement religious disapproval. Yao Hong and Celia Chan also explore the pressure to conform to societal expectations and the spiritual dilemmas this raises in their chapter about the experiences of couples seeking treatment for infertility. However, the birth of a child can lead to religious or spiritual questions, particularly if the child is considered to have a disability:

> In Kuwaiti culture, the disability of a family member has a stigmatising effect on the immediate and extended family … There is also the common traditional belief that disability is related to (1) God's will that the parent should have a child with a disability, (2) God punishing the parent, (3) God testing the parent, or (4) God selecting the parent for an unknown reason.
>
> (Al-Kandari 2015: 66)

While the experience of the previous writer is extreme, it is not uncommon for religion and disability to form an interrelated system of oppression (Bjornsdottir and Traustadottir 2010). Consequently, despite claims to being concerned about the whole person, social work practice frequently focuses on discrete problem areas of pressing concern. Hence, religious or spiritual needs are readily disregarded. For example, Delich (2014) notes an absence of social work literature about religion or spirituality in the deaf community, a situation that could no doubt be made about many of the groups of service users whom social workers encounter.

Social work practice

Although national differences shape the local practice of social work (Weiss-Gal and Welbourne 2008), the various authors in Part VI provide a wealth of perspectives and suggestions for social workers and the organisations that employ them, as to how religion and spirituality could or should be taken into account. Holding religious beliefs, and fearing that religious practices associated with these may not be appropriately respected, may lead to people not seeking out services that may benefit them (Regan *et al.* 2013). Hence, this section commences with a series of three chapters concerning the management of services. Adam Dinham begins with a contribution about the need for service provider organisations to have policies and practices that respect and acknowledge the religious diversity of service users. Janet Melville-Wiseman then goes on to explore the responsibilities of service providers in ensuring that service users are protected from the religious viewpoints of employees, particularly those that are potentially harmful. However, employers also have a responsibility for the care of their staff as well as for service users, and James Lucas suggests how mindfulness, when incorporated into professional practice, might promote resilience among the professional workforce.

The next five chapters are concerned with approaches to direct practice with individual service users, which for some readers is synonymous with social work practice. David Hodge proposes that effective practitioners must be equipped to competently respond to service users from varying religious and spiritual traditions. Importantly, this requires social workers to identify their own assumptions concerning religion and spirituality and recognise the impact of their own experiences in forming their viewpoints. In the following chapter, Ann Carrington does what Hodge recommends and provides an example as to how the theoretical approaches that inform her practice can be informed by and do not have to be in competition with practice, which takes seriously the place of spirituality as an essential element in the human condition. Like Ann Carrington, Fiona Gardner also draws on critical theory and postmodern ideas and has developed a framework that she argues enables 'the integration of the critical, the reflective and the spiritual into a coherent approach to practice that is holistic, inclusive and addresses issues of social justice'.

Holistic practice for a number of contributors in this volume requires an approach that enables integration of body, mind and spirit. For example, Malabika Das establishes that for survivors of conflict-induced trauma, an inability to address spiritual concerns represents a failure to understand the relationship between spirituality and both physical and mental health. Addressing spiritual concerns can facilitate improved health outcomes and also enable service users to explain their objections to certain health treatments or interventions (Hughes *et al.* 2015).

An emphasis on social work values and concepts such as 'self-determination' or being 'client-centred' may assume a level of choice for service users, which is not equally present in different countries (Tunney 2002) or even for all service users within a country. While recognising that social workers everywhere are subject to organisational, legislative and policy constraints on the ways in which they practice, facilitating service users to express their needs remains a universal concern. Arts-based approaches are advocated by several authors in this volume as providing vulnerable individuals with a method for expressing their needs and desires, particularly concerning spiritual and religious needs. Chapters that discuss arts-based approaches include those by Linda Benavides, Irene Renzenbrink, Martha Wiebe and Diana Coholic.

In addition to working with individuals, families and small groups of people, social workers in many countries are involved in the development of social policy. However, incorporating religion or spiritual components in such work is far less common than in direct practice. Mishka Lysack identifies how social workers can utilise religious teachings in the development of ethical principles to guide policy work around climate change. Fred Besthorn and Jon Hudson take these ideas further and argue that for ecosocial workers, commitment to addressing climate change is integral to their spirituality.

The final two contributions to Part VI remind the reader that while incorporating religion and spirituality into social work practice can be beneficial, care must be taken to ensure that harm is not an unintended outcome. Fran Gale and Michael Dudley note that all too often 'the claim that religion and spirituality can challenge oppression and disadvantage arising from social processes including globalisation remains at the level of the romantic'. Finally, Michael Sheridan alerts readers to the possibility that for some service users, their religious and spiritual beliefs and commitments may act as a cocoon, which prevents them from confronting issues in their life and hence hinders their development. While Sheridan does not go as far as the authors of a recent paper, who advocated that service users undergo a six-week 'religious abstinence' as part of the process of ceasing alcohol or other drug use (Cogdell *et al.* 2014), she reminds us that there will be times when social workers have an ethical responsibility to challenge service users about their religious and spiritual beliefs and practices.

Conclusion

In recent years, handbooks on the state of religion and spirituality research have been building international dialogues in areas related to social work such as healthcare (Cobb *et al.* 2012) and policy studies (Haynes 2009). This volume seeks to do the same for social work, and the final chapter will identify key challenges and opportunities for developing both social work scholarship and practice that engages with religion and spirituality. There are many gaps in our knowledge and this volume will probably raise more questions than it answers. Rather than viewing this as a shortcoming, it is hoped that readers will feel challenged to continue the undertaking of this volume and either begin, or persist in, contributing to the ongoing development of an international dialogue on the place of religion and spirituality in social work.

References

Al-Kandari, H.Y. (2015) 'High school students' contact with and attitudes towards persons with intellectual and developmental disabilities in Kuwait', *Australian Social Work*, 68(1): 65–83.

Anderson-Nathe, B., Gringer, C. and Wahab, S. (2013) 'Nurturing "critical hope" in teaching feminist social work research', *Journal of Social Work Education*, 49(2): 277–91.

Bäckström, A. and G. Davie (2010) 'The WREP Project: genesis, structure and scope', in A. Bäckström, G. Davie, N. Ergardh and P. Pettersson (eds) *Welfare and Religion in 21st Century Europe: volume 1 configuring the connections*, Farnham: Ashgate.

Bjornsdottir, K. and Traustadottir, R. (2010) 'Stuck in the land of disability? The intersection of learning difficulties, class, gender and religion', *Disability and Society*, 25(1): 49–62.

Brenden, M.A. (2007) 'Social work for social justice: strengthening social work practice through the integration of Catholic Social Teaching', *Social Work and Christianity*, 34(4): 472–97.

Brydon, K. (2012) 'Promoting diversity or confirming hegemony? In search of new insights for social work', *International Social Work*, 55(2): 155–67.

Bunge, M.J. (2014) 'The positive role of religion and religious communities in child protection', *Child Abuse and Neglect*, 38(4): 562–6.

Campbell, S. (2012) 'Explosion of the Spirit: a spiritual journey into the 2010 Healthcare Reform Legislation', *Journal of Religion and Spirituality in Social Work*, 31(1–2): 85–104.

Clark, J.L. (2006) 'Listening for meaning: a research-based model for attending to spirituality, culture and worldview in social work practice', *Critical Social Work*, 7(1). Online. Available HTTP: www1.uwindsor.ca/criticalsocialwork/listening-for-meaning-a-research-based-model-for-attending-to-spirituality-culture-and-worldview-in- (accessed 31 July 2016).

Cobb, M., Puchaski, C.M. and Rumbold, B. (2012) *Oxford Textbook of Spirituality in Healthcare*, New York: Oxford University Press.

Cogdell, C., Jackson, M.S. and Adedoyin, C. (2014) 'The nexus of religion and addiction counseling: a reflective perspective', *Journal of Human Behavior in the Social Environment*, 24(5): 621–34.

Crisp, B.R. (2010) *Spirituality and Social Work*, Farnham: Ashgate.

Crisp, B.R. (2013) 'Social work and faith-based agencies in Sweden and Australia', *International Social Work*, 56(3): 343–55.

Crisp, B.R. (2014) *Social Work and Faith-Based Organizations*, London: Routledge.

Delich, N.A.M. (2014) 'Spiritual direction and deaf spirituality: implications for social work practice', *Journal of Religion and Spirituality in Social Work*, 33(3–4): 317–38.

Dorff, E.N. (2014) 'Jewish provisions for protecting children', *Child Abuse and Neglect*, 38(4): 567–75.

Gray, M. and Fook, J. (2004) 'The quest for a universal social work: some issues and implications', *Social Work Education*, 23(5): 625–44.

Harrison, G. (2006) 'Broadening the conceptual lens on language in social work: difference, diversity and English as a global language', *The British Journal of Social Work*, 36(3): 401–18.

Harrison, G. and Melville, R. (2010) *Rethinking Social Work in a Global World*, Basingstoke: Palgrave Macmillan.

Haynes, J. (2009) (ed) *Routledge Handbook of Religion and Politics*, London: Routledge.

Healy, L.M. (2007) 'Universalism and cultural relativism in social work ethics', *International Social Work*, 50(1): 11–26.

Heelas, P. and Woodhead, L. (2005) *The Spiritual Revolution: why religion is giving way to spirituality*, Oxford: Blackwell Publishing.

Heron, G. and Pilkington, K. (2009) 'Examining the terminology of race issues in assessments for international exchange students', *International Social Work*, 52(3): 387–99.

Holtzhausen, L. (2011) 'When values collide: finding common ground for social work education in the United Arab Emirates', *International Social Work*, 54(2): 191–208.

Hughes, C.R., van Heugten, K. and Keeling, S. (2015) 'Cultural meaning-making in the journey from diagnosis to end of life', *Australian Social Work*, 68(2): 169–83.

Hugman, R., Moosa-Mitha, M. and Moyo, O. (2010) 'Towards a borderless social work: reconsidering the notions of international social work', *International Social Work* 53(5): 629–43.

Liedgren, P. (2015) 'Transfer of teaching styles: teaching social work in Iraqi Kurdistan as a Swede', *International Social Work*, 58(1): 175–85.

McCallum, S. (2001) 'Editorial', *Australian Social Work*, 54(3): 2.

McDonald, C., Harris, J. and Wintersteen, R. (2003) 'Contingent on context? Social work and the state in Australia, Britain and the USA', *The British Journal of Social Work*, 33(2): 191–208.

Miller, L.J. (2012) (ed) *The Oxford Handbook of Psychology and Spirituality*, New York: Oxford University Press.

Mwansa, L-K. (2011) 'Social work education in Africa: whence or whither?', *Social Work Education*, 30(1): 4–16.

Norman, J. and Hintze, H. (2005) 'A sampling of international practice variations', *International Social Work*, 48(5): 553–67.

Obst, D. and Kuder, M. (2009) 'Joint and double degree programs in the Transatlantic context: a survey report', in D. Obst and M. Kuder (eds) *Joint and Double Degree Programs: an emerging model for Transatlantic exchange*, New York: Institute of International Education.

Pew Research Center (2012) *The Global Religious Landscape: a report on the size and distribution of the world's major religious groups as of 2010*, Washington DC: Pew Research Center. Online. Available HTTP: www.pewforum.org/files/2014/01/global-religion-full.pdf (accessed 18 April 2016).

Regan, J.L., Bhattacharyya, S., Kevern, P. and Rana, T. (2013) 'A systematic review of religion and dementia care pathways in black and minority ethnic populations', *Mental Health Religion and Culture*, 16(1): 1–15.

Ruzzene, N. (1998) 'Language experience: the forgotten dimension in cross-cultural social work?', *Australian Social Work*, 51(2): 17–23.

Said, E.W. (1993) *Culture and Imperialism*, New York: Vintage.

Simpson, G. (2009) 'Global and local issues in the training of overseas social workers', *Social Work Education*, 28(6): 655–67.

Singh, S., Gumz, E.J. and Crawley, B.C. (2011) 'Predicting India's future: does it justify the exportation of US social work education?', *Social Work Education*, 30(7): 861–73.

Tunney, K. (2002) 'Learning to teach abroad: reflections on the role of the visiting social work educator', *International Social Work*, 45(4): 435–46.

Weber, Z. and Bugarzski, Z. (2007) 'Some reflections on social workers' perspectives on mental health services in two cities: Sydney, Australia and Budapest, Hungary', *International Social Work*, 50(2): 145–55.

Weiss-Gal, I. and Welbourne, P. (2008) 'The professionalisation of social work: a cross-national exploration', *International Journal of Social Welfare*, 17(4): 281–90.

Part II
Regional perspectives

2

Australia

It's complicated

Beth R. Crisp

Introduction: religion and spirituality in the Australian context

Technically, Australia is 'a deliberately secular nation' (Breward 1988: 99) with no official state church or religion. In fact the only mention of religion in Australia's constitution is that:

> The Commonwealth shall not make any law for establishing any religion, or for impos-
> ing any religious observance, or for prohibiting the free exercise of any religion, and no
> religious test shall be required as a qualification for any public office or public trust under
> the Commonwealth.
>
> (Section 116 in Sawer 1988: 63)

Nevertheless, class differentiation on the basis of religion has been a feature of Australian society for much of the time since British settlement commenced in 1788 as a penal colony. Among the early settlers, the more prosperous military and free settlers tended to be Anglican or Presbyterian, whereas convicts and former convicts, who were far more likely to have experienced poverty, were disproportionately Roman Catholic. Assumptions that Protestantism was essentially the religion of the ruling class held through much of the twentieth century (Dempsey 1983; Greenwood 2005).

In terms of participation, fewer than 10 per cent of Australians report regular attendance at religious services (Bellamy and Castle 2004), down from 33 per cent in 1955 and 19 per cent in 1980 (Wilson 1983). Despite this, the majority of Australians identify with a religion. Almost two-thirds (61 per cent) of all Australians identified themselves with some form of Christianity in the 2011 national census, with the largest groups being Catholics (25 per cent), Anglicans (17 per cent) and Uniting Church (5 per cent). A further 5 per cent identified with a non-Christian religion and 22 per cent stated they had no religion (ABS 2011). While migration is resulting in a diversification of religion in the Australian community, occasional involvement in religious events may be more for cultural reasons rather than religious (Bouma 2006). Hence, Davie's (1994) concept of a 'vicarious religion', i.e. religion performed by an active minority but on behalf of a much larger number who are happy that a minority are committed to maintaining

17

religious practice in the culture, is an apt depiction of the place of religion in Australian society. In the Australian context, this vicarious religion presents itself such as:

> The people of Australia expect the Churches to be active in the care of people, whether they are members or not. This expectation has been formed, not only by the Churches delivering ministries of care over the centuries, but also by the imperatives contained within the teachings of the Christian tradition.
>
> (Challen 1996: 26)

Although participation in formal religion has never been lower, in recent years it has been argued that Australians are more likely to acknowledge that spirituality, if not religion, has a place in their lives (Boer 2008; Tacey 2003). At the same time, there has been a growing recognition that religion and spirituality are not just concerned with privatised beliefs but play a prominent role in civic life (Boer 2008). As such, in recent years there has also been growing recognition of the spiritual needs of indigenous Australians, for whom the legacy of colonisation by the British resulted in dispossession and loss of their land (Harrison and Melville 2010), leading to disconnectedness from ancestors and other members of their communities (Gray *et al*. 2010). Consequently, it has been claimed that there are some distinctive aspects of Australian spirituality that impinge on the domains in which social work practice occurs. For example,

> Australian spirituality differs from American spirituality in many critical ways. The landscape, the beliefs and practices of the Indigenous people, the history of conquest and subsequent migration, the misuse of natural resources, the development of the labour movement and welfare services, and the current fledgling process of reconciliation between Indigenous and non-Indigenous, all have forms unique to Australia and are significant factors in both Australian social work discourses and Australian spirituality.
>
> (Lindsay 2002: 160)

It has further been suggested that an Australian spirituality also reflects historical patterns of immigration that brought a predominantly European community to the Asia Pacific (Hamilton 2005). The early immigrants not only disregarded the rights of the indigenous people who had a spiritual relationship with their land, but believed it was their moral and religious duty to take over the land and turn it into an outpost of European agriculture (Pascoe 2014; Watson 2014).

As the place of religion and spirituality have developed in particular ways in the Australian context, so too has social work. While there is a long tradition of drawing on both British and American versions of social work (Miller 2016; Napier and George 2001), the ways these, along with other influences, have been combined has resulted in a distinctively Australian version of social work, which reflects the nation's history, health and welfare systems, economic and social policies, as well as the experiences and expectations of social workers (McCallum 2001).

Social work practice, religion and spirituality

As in many other countries, prospective social workers in Australia may be drawn to a profession they perceive provides a way of working congruent with their own religious beliefs (Crisp 2014). However, a survey of Australian social work educators in 1999 found two-thirds claiming no religious affiliation, compared to less than one-third of the wider Australian population at the time (Lindsay 2002). While social work educators are not necessarily representative of the wider profession, they are entrusted with the nurture of future generations of practitioners. Although there is anecdotal evidence that social work educators in Australia are now more open to incorporating relevant content, particularly in respect of spirituality, generations of social work students recall little mention of matters associated with religion or spirituality except as an exotic feature of a case study (Lindsay 2002; Crisp 2015). Furthermore, social work students in many Australian universities who have had a particular interest in religion or spirituality, have often not been able to take elective units on these from elsewhere in their universities, given many Australian universities do not have a religious studies programme from which they can select units of study as part of their social work degree (Boer 2008). Consequently, Australian social workers often have very limited, if any, knowledge of the key beliefs and practices of other religions, and sometimes even of the religions they nominally identify with (Crisp 2015).

In the twenty-first century, academic interest in religion and spirituality has grown considerably in Australia. Much of this has been concerned with spirituality, sometimes not differentiated from religion (Lindsay 2002) but increasingly recognising that people have spiritual needs whether or not they identify with a religion (Carrington 2010; Crisp 2010a; Gardner 2011; Gray 2008). Associated with this, there has been scholarly work conducted by social workers around mindfulness (Lynn and Mensinga 2015) and yoga (Mensinga 2011). Some of this work is reported in other chapters in this volume; by James Lucas (Chapter 30), Ann Carrington (Chapter 32) and Fiona Gardner (Chapter 33).

The extent to which Australian social work literature on spirituality is being produced that is not explicitly religious, certainly distinguishes it from much of what is being published in many other countries where there is much less differentiation between spirituality and religion. This not only reflects the disproportionate interest in spirituality over religion in the broader community as previously discussed, but also the challenges for social workers in broaching spiritual matters in an allegedly secular nation, in which most welfare funding is provided by government on the basis of secular service delivery.

In the welfare arena, the historical involvement of religious organisations in now discredited practices has also potentially alienated many potential service users from matters associated with religion. These include removal of indigenous children from their families and communities resulting in what has become known as the 'Stolen Generation', forcing unmarried mothers to relinquish babies for adoption, and the mistreatment of child migrants sent from residential care providers in the United Kingdom (Crisp 2014).

Expectations of secular service delivery can create conundrums for non-government service providers. Almost all of the largest 25 Australian charities are linked to organisations that also have a religious focus (Lake 2013). Hence, it is not surprising that given the prominence of faith-based agencies in service provision, Australian social work researchers have also been exploring the contribution of these organisations to the welfare sector (Camilleri and Winkworth 2004; Crisp 2014).

It is not just among academics that the places for religion and spirituality have been legitimated. The *Code of Ethics* of the Australian Association of Social Workers (AASW) was revised in 2010. Compared to its predecessor, which acknowledged requirements to prevent discrimination on the basis of religion, the need for social workers to remain aware of conflicts of interest on the basis of religion and the need to be aware of their own religious values (AASW 1999), the current code retained these points but added several new clauses. These include an expectation under the heading of 'Respect for human dignity and worth', that:

> Social workers will respect others' beliefs, religious or spiritual world views, values, culture, goals, needs and desires, as well as kinship and communal bonds, within a framework of social justice and human rights.
>
> (AASW 2010: 17)

The *Code of Ethics* also recognises the right for social workers to have their religious or spiritual beliefs respected within the workplace:

> In carrying out their professional practice responsibilities, social workers are entitled to reciprocal rights, which include the right to ... hold cultural, religious or spiritual world views and for these to be acknowledged in the workplace and professional contexts to the extent that they do not impinge on the other guidelines in this *Code*.
>
> (AASW 2010: 16)

A further requirement is an expectation that social workers be respectful of faith-based agencies:

> Social workers will recognise, acknowledge and remain sensitive to and respectful of the religious and spiritual world views of individuals, groups, communities and social networks, and the operations and missions of faith and spiritually-based organisations.
>
> (AASW 2010: 18)

Despite the multiple references to religion in the *Code of Ethics*, many social workers remain ambivalent, if not antagonistic, that they might now be required to consider religious or spiritual beliefs and practices as relevant in their work with service users (Crisp 2011). However, while the place of religion and spirituality may well have been legitimated within Australian social work practice, unless social workers have a personal interest, their professional knowledge about these important life domains tends to be extremely limited (Crisp 2015).

Faith-based organisations

In a supposedly secular country, Australians are highly dependent on the services provided by faith-based organisations, particularly in respect of services provided to children and families and in aged care, but not confined to these (Swain 2009), although there are some differences between states (Murphy 2006). Conversely, services for people with a mental illness and prisoners are more likely to be provided by the state, although some exceptions occur (Swain 2009).

The expansion of British settlement in the early nineteenth century saw religious groups seeking to respond to the needs of their members and established welfare organisations similar to those operating in Britain at the time. While in part this reflected a general need for services, religious groups that had experienced persecution, such as Catholics and Jews, were often wary of services provided by others (Jupp 2009). During the twentieth century, many of these services became partially, if not fully, funded by the Commonwealth and state governments, but operated by faith-based organisations. Indeed, it has been suggested that their expertise in running community services means faith-based organisations are frequently the preferred partner of governments seeking to extend the range of services available in local communities (Crisp 2014).

While the stated rational for faith-based organisations being preferred service providers is often concerned with having existing links into communities, it may also be a cost-cutting measure. Non-government organisations typically receive funding for staffing and programme costs but often rely on funded organisations subsidising these, sometimes quite considerably (Crisp 2014; Gardner 2011). Furthermore, there have been several occasions in recent decades when conservative governments have sought to reduce welfare expenditure by suggesting services be provided by organisations associated with the various religions (Lake 2013). At times, governments have even announced that particular services would be devolved to named faith-based organisations, without consulting them (Holden and Trembath 2008). However, despite the public announcements, some faith-based organisations have refused to become involved in programmes they regard as immoral, particularly those involving harsh sanctions for social security recipients (Davis *et al.* 2008).

Instead of being delegated by government to implement unpopular programmes, many faith-based organisations have regarded it as their role to initiate new services that meet the needs of the most disadvantaged members of the community (Winkworth and Camilleri 2004). For example, in the late nineteenth century, it was the Salvation Army in Australia which established the first labour bureau open to all unemployed Australians as well as the world's first programme for released prisoners (Salvation Army 2013). And at the end of the twentieth century, it was faith-based organisations that not only supported the development of, but auspiced the country's first medically-supervised injecting centre (Crisp 2014).

In order to undertake the work they identified as needing to be done, religious organisations have been pivotal in the development of professional social work in Australia. The Catholic Church in 1928 sponsored scholarships for two students to undertake social work training at the Catholic University of America, who on their return were credited as being Australia's first trained social workers (Gleeson 2000). Since then, faith-based organisations were the first non-government organisations in Australia to employ professional social workers (Holden and Trembath 2008), and in the 1950s were the first to insist that government-funded counselling programmes employed qualified social workers (Gleeson 2008). Faith-based organisations remain a major employer of qualified social workers into the twenty-first century (Camilleri and Winkworth 2004).

In addition to developing and implementing innovative services, some of the larger faith-based organisations are active in the social policy space. The Brotherhood of St Laurence, an Anglican welfare agency in Melbourne, was in 1943 the first non-government welfare organisation in Australia to employ a research officer and has continued to employ social researchers ever since. Many of these have been qualified social workers (Holden and Trembath 2008), and this reflects the Australian understanding that both research and social policy analysis and advocacy are core social work roles (AASW 2010). Having come to regard its research and advocacy function as integral to its service delivery to disadvantaged individuals and communities, the Brotherhood of St Laurence is widely known and respected internationally for its work in the areas of poverty and welfare reform (Davis *et al.* 2008).

It has not just been in what and how they deliver services that faith-based organisations have had to adapt. While there have always been some organisations that are independent or unaligned, most Australian faith-based welfare services are associated with major religious groupings that have strong regional, national or even international structures. In order to remain both competitive and compliant with the conditions of government funding, many of the welfare agencies of the major Christian churches in Australia have formed alliances with similar agencies in either the same or from other regions during the last decade of the twentieth century. This has led to the establishment of some large organisations, some under a common management structure and others retaining a local focus but sharing resources and a common name under a federated structure (Crisp 2014).

Although the ability to adapt and change has ensured that the work of many faith-based organisations founded in the nineteenth century continues today, questions of identity form a challenge in the twenty-first century, particularly for organisations substantially dependent on government funding. State funding typically requires services to be provided to all members of the community and without any requirement that service recipients engage in any religious activities (Crisp 2014).

While some small religious organisations choose to forego state funding, so that they are not required to separate their religious and welfare delivery functions, most Australian agencies in the faith-based sector align with Torry's (2005: 3) definition of being 'firmly related to a religious tradition but which do not have a religious activity as their primary aim'. Hence, many adopt the role of being 'the quiet voice of God' rather than the 'mouthpiece of God' (Pessi 2010: 88), or in other words consider their primary role to be a presence in the community through service provision rather than engaging in religious teaching. To this end, some faith-based organisations have sought to distance their public identity from their religious connections (Swain 2009). Despite being an issue generating considerable discussion within some faith-based organisations (Crisp 2010b), there is evidence to suggest such tensions date back to the nineteenth century (Swain 2009).

Royal Commission into Institutional Responses to Child Sexual Abuse

Tensions about the relationship between religion and welfare have arguably been most apparent concerning issues of sexual abuse in religious contexts. In late 2012, the Australian government announced a Royal Commission into Institutional Responses to Child Sexual Abuse. Ostensibly this was in response to growing community anger and frustration with the hierarchy of the Catholic Church, which it was alleged had fostered a culture where sexual abuse of minors was widespread. Moreover, the care and protection of clergy offenders was alleged to have frequently taken precedence over appropriate responses to those alleging abuse (Middleton et al. 2014). In fact, the Catholic Church in 2012 acknowledged cases of sexual abuse involving 620 children in the State of Victoria over the previous 80 years (Catholic Church 2012).

Unlike in Ireland where the Ryan Commission restricted its inquiries into cases of abuse in residential care in Catholic institutions, the Australian Royal Commission has been concerned with sexual abuse in all institutional environments, including those operated by religious organisations, other community groups and government (Middleton et al. 2014). Specific inquiries have been undertaken about abuse cultures and responses to abuse in settings including residential care settings, schools, churches, scouting organisations and sport. While some of these involve children who were in the care of the state, e.g. children in residential care, by not limiting itself to the welfare sector, the Royal Commission has also sought to uncover abuse in community settings that provide services to a broad cross-section of children in the community (Royal Commission into Institutional Responses to Child Sexual Abuse 2014).

Having commenced public inquiries in 2013, it was initially anticipated the Royal Commission would be completed by 2015; however, due to the sheer amount of material being dealt with, it is now anticipated that the work will not be completed until 2017. Rachel Lev's reflection about the need to provide opportunities within the American Jewish community to talk about experiences of abuse is equally important in the context of the Royal Commission:

> We bear witness in part by listening to survivor stories. Then we address the questions: How do we help people heal? What do we do to stop these abuses? Where do we start? Simple answers will not work. Blaming and shaming won't work even though they're tempting. Healing and prevention happen together when we listen to the stories that must be told, then share resources and a commitment to peaceful relationships.
>
> (Lev 2003: xxvii)

In addition to public hearings, a large research programme has been commissioned to support the work of the Royal Commission and to inform its findings and recommendations for changes in practices, policies and legislation. Despite being far from complete, it is already clear that there will be difficult truths to be faced by organisations that are, or have been, involved in the care of children. While the public emphasis had previously been overwhelmingly on the Catholic Church, many members of the Australian community have been shocked to discover the extent of child abuse in non-Catholic institutions. For those involved in religious or faith-based organisations, the following statement, although originally written about the place of women in the Church of Sweden, may well apply:

> Questions posed include how to deal with the shifts in perceptions of authority which challenge old, hierarchical patterns of governance. They also include how to deal with the fact that churches, in spite of their claim to be transmitters of justification and forgiveness, regularly fail in *their practice* to be just communities of equal and responsible citizens.
>
> (Edgardh Beckman 2001: 12)

There will be expectations that faith-based welfare organisations will address, if they have not already done so, procedures that did not safeguard against sexual abuse. It can also mean having to have difficult conversations both within the organisation and with community members, including former service users. While the following reflects the experience of one faith-based welfare organisation that dates back to the nineteenth century, it is likely that there are many other faith-based organisations that have yet to meaningfully acknowledge past wrongs:

> [Organization's] leadership has talked a lot about how we have failed people as an organiza-tion in the past, and some reference to some dark things which have happened in the name of the orders. And I think a genuine desire to want to do anything in our power to make right the wrongs of the past. ... The organization does a lot of work with past residents and acknowledging the abuse that has happened and the care practices of the past that wouldn't be acceptable today. And I think that's a credit to the organization that we've tried to be upfront and honest about that and taken responsibility for those sensitive things that have happened.
>
> (in Crisp 2014: 132)

Conclusion

One of the options Facebook users have to describe their relationship is 'it's complicated'. In many ways this depicts the relationship between social work, religion and spirituality in Australia. Australians have a strong sense of spirituality but in the main are somewhat ambivalent about formal religion. Nevertheless, social welfare delivery is highly dependent on the faith-based sector, and governments show great willing to fund this sector to provide community services, just as long as they do not have a religious element. This potentially places faith-based organisations in a state of ambiguity if they cannot resolve the question of how they express their religious identity without violating funding agreements.

The relationship between social work, religion and spirituality is further complicated by the fact that it is constantly changing and evolving. The outcomes of the Royal Commission into Institutional Responses to Child Sexual Abuse may well result in further changes to the relationship, although many faith-based organisations have already taken steps to ensure many past practices are no longer tolerated. The other change is that the profile of faith-based wel-fare organisations tends to reflect the religious profile of Australians in previous generations and it will be interesting to see in coming years whether increasing numbers of Australians who identify as Buddhist or Muslim leads to growth in faith-based organisations with these affiliations.

References

Australian Association of Social Workers [AASW] (1999) *Code of Ethics*, Canberra: Australian Association of Social Workers.

Australian Association of Social Workers [AASW] (2010) *Code of Ethics*, Canberra: Australian Association of Social Workers. Online. Available HTTP: www.aasw.asn.au/document/item/1201 (accessed 29 January 2016).

Australian Bureau of Statistics (ABS) (2011) *2011 Census of Population and Housing, Religious Affiliation by Sex*, Dataset B14. Online. Available HTTP: http://stat.abs.gov.au/Index.aspx?DataSetCode=ABS_CENSUS2011_B14 (accessed 29 January 2016).

Bellamy, J. and Castle, K. (2004) *2001 Church Attendance Estimates*, Sydney: NCLS Research.

Boer, R. (2008) 'The new secularism', *Arena Journal*, 29/30: 35–57.

Bouma, G. (2006) *Australia's Soul: religion and spirituality in the twenty-first century*, Melbourne: Cambridge University Press.

Breward. I. (1988) *Australia: 'the most godless place under heaven?'*, Melbourne: Beacon Hill Books.

Camilleri, P. and Winkworth, G. (2004) 'Mapping the Catholic social services', *The Australasian Catholic Record*, 81(2): 184–97.

Carrington, A.M. (2010) 'Spiritual paradigms: a response to concerns within social work in relation to the inclusion of spirituality', *Journal of Religion and Spirituality in Social Work*, 29(4): 300–20.

Catholic Church (2012) *Facing the truth. Learning from the past. How the Catholic Church in Victoria has responded to child abuse. A Submission by the Catholic Church in Victoria to the Parliamentary Inquiry into the Handling of Child Abuse by Religious and other Non-Government Organisations*. Online. Available HTTP: www.parliament.vic.gov.au/images/stories/committees/fcdc/inquiries/57th/Child_Abuse_Inquiry/Submissions/Catholic_Church_in_Victoria.pdf (accessed 29 January 2016).

Challen, M.B. (1996) 'The changing roles of church and state in Australian welfare provision', *Social Security Journal*, June: 26–31.

Crisp, B.R. (2010a) *Spirituality and Social Work*, Farnham: Ashgate.

Crisp, B.R. (2010b) 'Catholic agencies: making a distinct contribution to Australian social welfare provision?', *The Australasian Catholic Record*, 87(4): 440–51.

Crisp, B.R. (2011) 'If a holistic approach to social work requires acknowledgement of religion, what does this mean for social work education?', *Social Work Education*, 30(6): 657–68.

Crisp, B.R. (2014) *Social Work and Faith-Based Organizations*, London: Routledge.

Crisp, B.R. (2015) 'Religious literacy and social work: the view from Australia', in A. Dinham and M. Francis (eds) *Religious Literacy: enhancing understanding and cooperation*, Bristol: Policy Press.

Davie, G. (1994) *Religion in Britain since 1945: believing without belonging*, Oxford: Blackwell Publishing.

Davis, F., Paulhus, E. and Bradstock, A. (2008) *Moral, But No Compass: government, church and the future of welfare*, Chelmsford: Matthew James Publishing.

Dempsey, K. (1983) 'Country town religion', in A.W. Black and P.E. Glasner (eds) *Practice and Belief: studies in the sociology of Australian religion*, Sydney: George Allen and Unwin.

Edgardh Beckman, N. (2001) 'Mrs Murphy's arising from the pew: ecclesiological implications', *Ecumenical Review*, 5(1): 5–13.

Gardner, F. (2011) *Critical Spirituality: a holistic approach to community practice*, Farnham: Ashgate.

Gleeson, D.J. (2000) 'Professional social workers and welfare bureaus: the origins of Australian Catholic social work', *The Australasian Catholic Record*, 77(2): 185–202.

Gleeson, D.J. (2008) 'The foundation and first decade of the National Catholic Welfare Committee', *The Australasian Catholic Record*, 85(1): 15–36.

Gray, M. (2008) 'Viewing spirituality in social work through the lens of contemporary social theory', *The British Journal of Social Work*, 38(1): 175–96.

Gray, M., Coates, J. and Yellow Bird, M. (eds) (2010) *Indigenous Social Work Around the World: towards culturally relevant education and practice*, Farnham: Ashgate.

Greenwood, K (2005) *Death by Water*, Crows Nest, NSW: Allen and Unwin.

Hamilton, A. (2005) 'Australasian spirituality', in P. Sheldrake (ed) *The New Westminster Dictionary of Christian Spirituality*, Louisville: Westminster John Know Press.

Harrison, G. and Melville, R. (2010) *Rethinking Social Work in a Global World*, Basingstoke: Palgrave Macmillan.

Holden, C. and Trembath, R. (2008) *Divine Discontent. The Brotherhood of St Laurence: a history*, North Melbourne: Australian Scholarly Publishing.

Jupp, J. (2009) 'Religion, immigration and refugees', in J. Jupp (ed) *Encyclopaedia of Religion in Australia*, Melbourne: Cambridge University Press.

Lake, M. (2013) *Faith in Action: Hammond Care*, Sydney: University of New South Wales Press.

Lev R. (2003) *Shine the Light: sexual abuse and healing in the Jewish community*, Boston: Northeastern University Press.

Lindsay, R. (2002) *Recognizing Spirituality: the interface between faith and social work*, Crawley: University of Western Australia Press.

Lynn, R. and Mensinga, J. (2015) 'Social workers' narratives of integrating mindfulness into practice', *Journal of Social Work Practice*, 29(3): 255–70.

McCallum, S. (2001) 'Editorial', *Australian Social Work*, 54(3): 2.

Mensinga, J. (2011) 'The feeling of being a social worker: including yoga as an embodied practice in social work education', *Social Work Education*, 30(6): 650–62.

Middleton, W., Stavropoulos, P., Dorahy, M.J., Krüger, C., Lewis-Fernandez, R., Martínez-Taboas, A., Sar, V. and Brand, B. (2014) 'The Australian Royal Commission into Institutional Responses to Child Sexual Abuse', *Australian and New Zealand Journal of Psychiatry*, 48(1): 17–21.

Miller, J. (2016) *Leading Social Work: 75 years at the University of Melbourne*, North Melbourne: Australian Scholarly Publishing.

Murphy, J. (2006) 'The other welfare state: non-government agencies and the mixed economy of welfare in Australia', *History Australia*, 3(2): 44.1–15.

Napier, L. and George, J. (2001) 'Changing social work education in Australia', *Social Work Education*, 20(1): 75–87.

Pascoe, B. (2014) *Dark Emu: black seeds agriculture or accident?* Broome: Magabala Books.

Pessi, A.B. (2010) 'The church as a place of encounter: communality and the good life in Finland', in A. Bäckström, G. Davie, N. Edgardh and P. Pettersson (eds) *Welfare and Religion in 21st Century Europe: volume 1 configuring the connections*, Farnham: Ashgate.

Royal Commission into Institutional Responses to Child Sexual Abuse (2014) *Interim Report, vol. 1*. Online. Available HTTP: www.childabuseroyalcommission.gov.au/about-us (accessed 29 January 2016).

Salvation Army (2013) *Foundation of Salvation Army Social Services*. Online. Available HTTP: www.salvationarmy.org.au/en/Who-We-Are/History-and-heritage/Foundation-of-Salvation-Army-social-services/ (accessed 29 January 2016).

Sawer, G. (1988) *The Australian Constitution*, 2nd edn, Canberra: AGPS.

Swain, S. (2009) 'Welfare work and charitable organisations', in J. Jupp (ed) *Encyclopaedia of Religion in Australia*, Melbourne: Cambridge University Press.

Tacey, D. (2003) *The Spirituality Revolution: the emergence of contemporary spirituality*, Sydney: HarperCollins Publishers.

Torry, M. (2005) *Managing God's Business: religious and faith-based organizations and their management*, Aldershot: Ashgate.

Watson, D. (2014) *The Bush: travels in the heart of Australia*, Melbourne: Hamish Hamilton.

Wilson, B. (1983) *Can God Survive in Australia?* Sutherland, NSW: Albatross Books.

Winkworth, G. and Camilleri, P. (2004) 'Keeping the faith: the impact of human services restructuring on Catholic social welfare services', *Australian Journal of Social Issues*, 39(3): 315–28.

3

Korean social welfare's approach to spiritual diversity

Edward R. Canda, Jungrim Moon and Kyung Mee Kim

Introduction

This chapter presents an overview of ways that the profession of social work in the Republic of Korea[1] engages with spirituality in its diverse religious and philosophical forms. This includes three sections: explanation of key concepts and Korean context; main religions and spiritually oriented philosophies that shape social welfare (i.e. traditionally rooted Buddhism, Confucianism, shamanism and recently introduced Christianity); and a concluding summary with suggestions for innovation.

Key concepts and Korean context

Korean culture sets a distinctive context for understanding spirituality; therefore, some key concepts and features of diversity related to spirituality and social work are explained in this section. For the purpose of this chapter, we adopt the concise conceptualisation of spirituality provided by Canda and Furman (1999), because it has been widely used both in North America and in South Korea, where their book was translated and published in 2003 (Canda and Furman 1999/2003; see also Yoo 2003). In this conceptualisation, spirituality refers to the human search for a sense of meaning, purpose and morally fulfilling relationships with oneself, other people, the universe and ultimate reality (however understood). In this sense, spirituality is expressed in diverse religious and nonreligious forms.

As Park (2003) pointed out in his translation of Canda and Furman's book, the word 'spirituality' is difficult to translate exactly into Korean. The most common translation in social work publications is *yeongseong*, derived from Chinese characters that have the literal connotation of spirit or ghost plus nature or characteristic. In typical Korean usage, the word often implies something to do with spirits or ghosts or with ideas in Christian theology, such as 'the Holy Spirit'. This is much more limited than the professional social work usage advocated in the Canda and Furman definition. Korean social work scholars therefore sometimes offer explanations for use of this term to make it more broad and inclusive in meaning, or simply borrow the English word (Chun 2013; Park 2003; Yoon *et al.* 2015).

Park addressed this dilemma by creating a new Korean word for spirituality, *eol al*, compounded from two Korean native words, meaning 'spirit' and 'essence'. He explained the nuances of the Canda and Furman definition, emphasising the importance of addressing in social work all the religious and nonreligious forms of spirituality in a respectful manner, without imposing particular personal or religious beliefs upon clients.

In general, it is common in Korean social work literature to address spirituality by referring to particular religions, rather than considering nonreligious spiritual perspectives (Kim and Canda 2009); therefore, the term for religion (*jonggyo*) and specific religious terms are found more commonly than 'spirituality.' Further, the pervasive traditional spiritual worldviews and helping practices of Confucianism and shamanism, which are considered religions by some scholars, are often not considered formal religions in Korea, so they are often left out of discussions of religion and spirituality in social welfare. The word '*gyo*' is now typically included in the name for all the spiritual perspectives described here.

According to 2005 government statistics, 53 per cent of Koreans align themselves with a religion. Of those who claim a religious affiliation, about 43 per cent are Buddhist, 55.1 per cent are Christian (including 34.5 per cent Protestant and 20.6 percent Catholic) and 1.9 per cent adhere to other religions such as Confucianism, Won Buddhism, Islam and other indigenous religions (Korea.net 2015). It should be noted that survey statistics on religious affiliation are likely to be imprecise due to culturally incongruent ways of eliciting religious affiliation. For example, most people, especially adults, are strongly influenced by Confucian worldviews and ethics, but do not belong to a Confucian religious organisation. Many utilise shamanistic practices, especially at times of crisis or distress, such as healing rituals, divination and prayers for blessings. However, few Koreans would identify this as a formal religious affiliation. Furthermore, many people (especially those who are not Protestant) actually blend involvement with multiple religious and nonreligious spiritual perspectives. Over the past 15 years, there has also been a rapid influx of migrants with various spiritual perspectives and worldviews from North Korea, the Middle East, Southeast Asia and the Philippines (Yoon 2008). Such complexity is not reflected in surveys. Given this complexity, in agreement with Baker's (2008) recommendation, we use the term 'spirituality' to include the full variety of religious and nonreligious spiritual perspectives in Korea.

The Korean understanding of the English term 'social work' also varies from what is understood in some other countries. Professional social work is typically translated in Korean as *sahoebokji*, which more literally means 'social welfare', which emphasises social welfare policy (such as social insurance, public assistance and NGO provided social service). This is because the English term 'social work' (literally translated as *sahoesaeop*) usually refers to direct helping, often connoting volunteer or unprofessional service activity. Yet when native Korean speakers refer to the Western context in English, they will usually follow the convention of referring to professional 'social work' and social workers. We therefore often use the terms 'social welfare' or 'social work' interchangeably in an encompassing sense.

Korean social workers must be prepared to work with people who are nonreligious, with religiously affiliated people from religions that are long established, and with people affiliated with Islam and other religions not previously widespread in South Korea (Yoon 2008). Nevertheless, in this chapter we will focus on the spiritual perspectives that are most prevalent: Buddhism, Christianity, Confucianism and shamanism. Given that other spiritual perspectives influencing Koreans who do not identify as religious have not been addressed yet in the Korean social work literature, we will not consider them here, but recognise that they deserve greater attention in future research.

Spiritual perspectives and social welfare

Buddhism

Buddhism moved from India to China and then into Korea about 2,000 years ago (Lew 1988). The predominant branch of Buddhism in Korea is Mahayana (described in detail by Caroline Humphrey in Chapter 9), which is also common in China, Japan and Vietnam.

Buddhism became highly influential in Korea during the Three Kingdoms Period (especially from about 372 to 660 CE). It was the state sponsored religion during the Unified Silla Dynasty (661–918) and the Goryeo Dynasty (918–1392). Therefore, Buddhism had a pervasive influence on Korean society and human services for about 1,000 years (Lee 1993). It continued to have an influence, though somewhat marginalised, during the Joseon Dynasty (1392–1910). The largest denomination is named the Jogye Order, but there are several other denominations and many small nondenominational temples that may blend in elements of shamanism (Tedesco 2003). This section will focus on the Jogye Order as the largest denomination involved with social welfare.

Buddhism's emphasis on relief of human suffering naturally leads to a concern for social welfare (Canda *et al.* 1993). As of 2003, among 2,162 religiously affiliated social welfare agencies recognised by law (which is 53 per cent of all agencies), 21 per cent (n=402) were Buddhist (Koh 2006). A 2011 government report (Korean Ministry of Culture, Sports and Tourism), using different criteria, identified about 500 religiously operated agencies, of which 125 are Buddhist. Further, many temples provide informal social supports to their members, volunteer help such as day care for children, and 'temple visit' programmes of short retreats to encourage stress relief and spiritual cultivation for the general public.

A major way to help overcome suffering is by teaching people how to practice meditation and to live in a compassionate way that leads to clarity and eventually enlightenment. Traditionally, there was an emphasis on monastics living in temple communities to practice meditation, chanting and rituals extensively. When Buddhism was sponsored by the state, temples provided relief services for the public such as distributing grains and water, providing medical treatment, constructing bridges and roads, and giving shelter and support to orphans and isolated elders. In contemporary society, the monastic practices continue. For the general public, meditation and chanting techniques are taught for mental cultivation and rituals are provided for solace. Many contemporary lay Buddhists are concerned mainly to seek blessings and practical benefits for themselves and loved ones (Tedesco 2003).

Regarding professional social work, the Jogye Order's Korean Buddhist Welfare Foundation was established in 1995 to contribute to social welfare development in Korea through research, education and welfare activities (Jogye Order of Korean Buddhist Welfare Foundation 2015). Currently, there are 180 welfare agencies and projects operated by the foundation, including 24 general welfare agencies and numerous agencies for specific populations such as people with disabilities, families and youths, the elderly and the homeless. The foundation holds national conferences, various workshops and forums. Lately, the foundation is operating international aid projects in various countries. The Jogye Order also provides social work education at two universities. These include courses on professional social work as well as Buddhist philosophy in addition to supporting scholarship on Buddhist social work in Korea. There is a *Journal of Buddhist Social Welfare*, and Kim and Canda (2009) identified 11 articles and five books on Buddhist social work in the Korean context.

In addition to traditional mainline Buddhist denominations, there is an indigenous denomination named Won Buddhism (*wonbulgyo* or One Circle Buddhism), founded in Korea in

1916. Won Buddhist teachings draw on Buddhism, Confucianism, Daoism and shamanism, but Buddhism was taken as the primary guiding perspective. Won Buddhism emphasises an egalitarian and socially engaged approach (Bongkil 1988). Although membership is less than 1 per cent of the Korean population, it is disproportionately strongly involved in social welfare and human services. It has been providing social relief and educational services, especially for low income or vulnerable people in rural and suburban areas and education of social workers, since 1927 (Gupta 2014). The Won Buddhist Social Welfare Association was founded in November 1998, to facilitate collaboration among welfare agencies affiliated with Won Buddhism for research, curriculum development, professional and volunteer training, policy development, publication and resource development in collaboration with affiliated domestic and international agencies (Won-Buddhist Social Welfare Association 2015). Their social welfare practice is based on the ideal to repay the grace of Buddha by relating to every person and creature as Buddha. Their programmes in social welfare, education and health include insights from Eastern and Western traditions and spiritual practices. Government statistics variously report 75 (Koh 2006) or 16 (Korean Ministry 2011) Won Bulgyo-operated agencies, but there are known to be many more not included in these numbers. Wonkwang University Department of Social Welfare offers Bachelor of Social Welfare, MSW and PhD degrees that are promoting the ongoing involvement of Won Buddhism in welfare provision and social work scholarship. In their 2009 review, Kim and Canda identified 11 scholarly social work articles related to Won Buddhism.

Christianity

Korean language typically distinguishes between Christianity (*gidokgyo*, meaning Protestant Christian congregations) and Catholicism (*katollikgyo*), but in this chapter we use the term Christian to refer to both and distinguish where necessary.

Catholicism was introduced from China in the late Joseon Dynasty but it was marginalised and persecuted (Lee 1983). Protestantism was introduced in the latter 1880s. After the Joseon Dynasty, the influence of Christianity grew, including in nationalist movements against Japanese occupation. This influence grew further after the Korean War when Christian missionaries, educators and relief agencies made a major impact on the development of modern style health, educational and social welfare services (Canda and Canda 1996). By the 1980s, the increase of Christian adherents in Korea was growing at one of the fastest paces in the world.

The Christian commitment to charitable works has made a dramatic impact on Korean social welfare. This reflects the Christian virtue of *caritas*, a Latin word referring to love expressed in service, as a reflection of God's love for humanity (Dal Toso *et al.* 2015). According to the Korean Ministry of Culture (2011), there are at least 251 Protestant and 105 Catholic registered social welfare organisations, which is about 72 per cent of all religiously affiliated agencies. Koh's (2006) figures also indicate about 70 per cent of all religiously affiliated agencies are Christian based.

The Korean Christian Social Services Association is a joint body comprised of the members of eight Protestant denominations and the National Council of Churches. Since its inception in 1963, the association has been providing charity works, mainly focusing on providing monetary and material aids to the poor both domestically and internationally (Korean Christian Social Services Association 2015). Caritas Korea was established in 1975 as the official social work and international development committee of the Korean Catholic churches. Caritas Korea seeks to contribute to the development of a better society by carrying out relief projects and social services in Korea and internationally (Caritas Korea 2015). These various Christian affiliated agencies address many kinds of social welfare services, including disaster and poverty relief, international development, healthcare, migrant support programmes, child and family services, and gerontology.

Many social work education degree programmes are affiliated with Christian universities and these often imbue Christian perspective in a broad way within general education. Soongsil University (Protestant) has a course on spirituality and social work in an inclusive sense, established in 2015. It uses the Canda and Furman (1999/2003) book as a main text. Kkotdongnae University (Catholic) focuses on social welfare education and sometimes sponsors special lectures on theology and spirituality in relation to social work.

The academic journal *Church Social Work* has been published by the Korean Academy of Church Social Work since 2003 (Kim and Canda 2009). Initiatives such as this undoubtedly contribute to Kim and Canda's (2009) finding that Korean social work scholarship about spirituality is dominated by literature from a Christian perspective. They identified 63 social work articles with a Christian perspective, almost six times more than Buddhist and Won Buddhist. Given this emphasis in the literature and that many social welfare departments are located in Christian affiliated universities, it seems likely that Christian ideas about social welfare have the widest influence among spiritual perspectives. This view was shared by participants in Canda and Canda's (1996) field study.

Confucianism

Like Buddhism, Confucianism was introduced to the Korean region from China about 2,000 years ago (Lee 1993; Lew 1988). It influenced the formation of Korean culture during the Three Kingdoms period and afterward, especially as Confucianism was connected with the transmission of Chinese literature, art, educational materials and written characters. During the Silla and Goryeo dynasties, Confucianism also influenced social mores and governmental social welfare services (Canda *et al.* 1993; Lew 1988). The Joseon Dynasty adopted the Zhu Xi (*juhui*) school of Neo-Confucianism as the state ideology. Therefore, for about 500 years, Neo-Confucianism provided a comprehensive metaphysical, ethical and social organisation system. Korean Neo-Confucianism is known as 'the Learning of the Way' (*dohak*) and 'the Learning of the Sage' (*songhak*). It largely supplanted Buddhism in provision of formal social welfare services.

Confucius lived in China 551–470 BCE. He taught a small cadre of students and consulted with nobles, seeking to promote governance and interpersonal conduct based on virtues, the most central being 'benevolence' (*in*, Korean; *ren*, Chinese), which refers to humane interrelatedness and connotes unconditional love (Canda 2013; Lew 2003). Another virtue that became very influential in family-based care of elders and social ethics is filial piety, which refers to children honouring their parents, and by extension, younger honouring elder, and humans honouring Heaven and Earth as cosmic parents. Confucian social ethics are strongly concerned with promoting harmonious family and societal relationships.

Neo-Confucian approaches to social welfare included promoting individual mindfulness, sincerity and social concern through practices of quiet sitting; scholarly study to acquire wisdom and skill for social administration; teaching about insights from sages from Chinese classics in state and private schools; scholars' remonstrance with the king and nobles for just governance; collective protest; administration of formal social welfare programmes for relief of the poor; help for people considered vulnerable (such as widows, isolated elders, orphans, homeless and people with disabilities); and promotion of the village-based mutual support system of *hyangyak* (Canda *et al.* 1993; Canda and Canda 1996).

The periods of the Japanese imperialistic occupation of Korea (about 1910–1945), separation between North and South, and the Korean War (1950–1953) caused drastic disruptions of

Korean culture, including marginalisation of Confucianism as a basis for governance and social welfare. Further, many contemporary Koreans have come to identify Confucianism with abuses of feudalism and patriarchy, although there is a small movement of Confucian philosophers who advocate for the democratic and justice promoting features of the Way of the Sages, as opposed to the corrupted practices of former political rulers (Lew 1988, 2003).

Only about 0.4 per cent of Koreans identify as Confucian (Kim and Canda 2009). Nevertheless, there remains a pervasive indirect influence on social welfare policy and informal patterns of mutual support based on Confucian social ethics. However, there is very little utilisation of Confucian thought in professional social welfare education or institutions. Kim and Canda (2009) identified only four social work articles on Confucianism and of these, two mentioned that its communitarian approach might be more suitable to guide social welfare than Western individualistic views. For about the past 10 years, Sungkyunkwan University, which has Confucian roots, has been offering a course on spirituality and social work in an inclusive sense, drawing on many religious and philosophical perspectives. The instructor, Professor Park Seung-Hee, includes discussion of ways that Confucianism can promote respect for cultural and spiritual diversity (personal communications and Park 2006). Like the Soongsil University course, it uses the Canda and Furman book as a main text.

Shamanism

Shamanism (*musok* or *mugyo*) is the most ancient indigenous tradition of Korea (Canda *et al.* 1993; Kendall 2011). It is rooted in an animistic worldview that promotes harmony between humans, the spirit beings of the natural world (such as mountain spirits, *sansin*) and other spirit powers, such as the culture-founding hero Dangun, ancestors and spirits that affect health and fortune. Shamans (commonly referred to as *mudang*), most often women, are mediators between the human and spirit realms who are skilled in trance performance and rituals for divination and healing of personal, family and community maladies, misfortunes and disruptions of harmony (Canda and Canda 1996). Shamans often help people to release deeply ingrained emotional distress through cathartic rituals involving intense music and dance, evocative symbols and psychodrama-like enactments of communication with spirits and deceased relatives.

Korean shamanism is not organised according to formal bureaucratic organisations and membership, so it does not show up much in formal surveys of religious affiliation. Shamans tend to have an informal network of regular and occasional clients who request their services at times of crisis or life cycle transition. Although shamanism has had a pervasive influence on Korean traditional worldview and continues to be influential, it has rarely been addressed in social welfare education or research (Canda and Canda 1996; Chun 2013; Kim and Canda 2009).

Conclusion

The contemporary stance of the profession of Korean social work on spiritual diversity has several features. In scholarly publications, education and human service organisations, spirituality is mainly addressed in terms of religiously-based social welfare perspectives and religiously sponsored agencies, mostly Buddhist and Christian (i.e. Protestant and Catholic). Most often this includes religion-specific contexts and types of practice or policy (Kim and Canda 2009). Although Confucianism and shamanism have very long histories of social welfare and human service involvement, they are little addressed.

However, efforts toward an inclusive approach to spirituality are emerging. Some authors identify broad themes that are said to be common across Korean religions. For example, Yoo

(2004) made connections between Christianity and shamanism to reveal ideals for church social work characterised by freedom, unity and elegance. Ro (2010) suggests that the spiritual principle of love for human beings is universal across religions and that this principle should be central to social welfare practice. Ro also cautions against detrimental impacts of self-centredness and closed-mindedness that may contribute to conflict and competition between different religions. In this context, Ro promotes 'spiritual social work' and refers to the work of Canda and Furman (1999/2003). Yoo (2003) also advocated for spiritually-sensitive social work in both micro and macro practice, influenced by the work of Canda and Furman. Likewise, Chun (2013) promotes a client-centred approach to spiritual needs in social welfare, rather than inappropriate imposition of religious agendas.

These authors' positions are in accord with the Korean constitutional guarantee of freedom of religion and the *Korean National Social Work Code of Ethics*' requirement of respect for human diversity, including prohibition of discrimination based on religious affiliation (Korea Association of Social Workers n.d.). However, there is no consensus about the importance of spirituality, including religious and non-religious forms, in professional standards for education or practice, and the topic is rarely addressed in the professional preparation of social workers.

An inclusive approach is also offered in at least two universities that have recently offered social work courses on spirituality: Sungkyunkwan and Soongsil. Professor Park Seung-Hee of Sungkyunkwan University has recently been offering a popular seminar on insights from Confucianism and Daoism for the Association for Social Work Practice. Furthermore, in 2011, the Korean Association of Spirituality and Social Welfare was established in order to promote clarification of spiritual principles found in various religions for application to social work practice and to develop educational curricula for producing spiritually sensitive social workers (Korean Association of Spirituality and Social Welfare 2015). This organisation provides workshops, annual conferences and a journal.

These religious, inter-religious and spiritually-inclusive initiatives offer opportunity for further innovations. First, national professional standards for ethics and education could build on the prohibition of religious discrimination to develop proactive approaches to respecting and engaging spiritual diversity in religious and nonreligious forms. Second, prominent spiritual perspectives that have been most neglected, including Confucianism and shamanism, can be further examined for their potential to contribute to culturally appropriate social welfare. Third, currently growing religions with social welfare traditions, such as Islam, need to be examined, especially for relevance to work with clients among immigrant communities. Fourth, some Western paradigms for holistic social work that have drawn strongly on Indigenous and Eastern perspectives might be valuable to consider, such as deep ecological social work (Coates 2003) and transpersonal social work (Canda and Smith 2001). Fifth, since Korean religions and philosophies include many kinds of meditation, contemplative arts, prayer and ritual, these could be linked with evidence-based mindfulness practices and expressive arts therapies in social work (Canda and Warren 2013; Land 2015; Park 2013). As Yoo (2004) pointed out, Korean and Western social work scholars could learn from each other and foster innovations cross-culturally. A very pertinent example of this type of innovation is body-mind-spirit integrative social work as developed by Chinese and Chinese American social work scholars (Lee *et al.* 2009).

Korean society has been characterised by a plurality of spiritual perspectives for at least 2,000 years, and this diversity has grown in scale and complexity in the past 50 years. Further, Korean culture is noted for its relatively homogenous ethnic composition combined with mainly peaceful co-existence of multiple spiritual perspectives (Baker 2008). It may be fertile ground for further growth of both religion-specific and inclusive approaches to spiritual diversity in social welfare.

Note

1 The official English name of the country is Republic of Korea but is commonly referred to as South Korea. We will use these terms interchangeably. If we use the term Korea when discussing history prior to partition after the Korean War, we will specify the relevant time period and kingdoms.

References

Baker, D. (2008) *Korean Spirituality*, Honolulu: University of Hawai'i Press.

Bongkil, C. (1988) 'The position of Won Buddhism in the cultural history of Korea', *Korea Religion*, 13: 75–93.

Canda, E.R. (2013) 'Filial piety and care for elders: a contested Confucian virtue re-examined', *Journal of Ethnic and Cultural Diversity in Social Work,* 22(3–4): 213–34.

Canda E.R. and Canda, H. (1996) 'Korean spiritual philosophies of human service: current state and prospects', *Social Development Issues*, 18(3): 53–70.

Canda, E.R. and Furman, L.E. (1999) *Spiritual Diversity in Social Work Practice: the heart of helping*, New York: Free Press. Also published in Korean, translated by Seung-Hee Park (2003) as 종교사회복지 실천론: 사회복지 실천에서 얼알의 다양성, Seoul: Sungkyunkwan University Press.

Canda, E.R. and Smith, E. (2001) *Transpersonal Perspectives on Spirituality in Social Work*, Binghamton, NY: Haworth Press.

Canda, E.R. and Warren, S. (2013) 'Mindfulness', in C. Franklin (ed) *Encyclopedia of Social Work,* e-reference edition, New York: Oxford University Press. Online. Available HTTP: http://socialwork.oxfordre.com/ (accessed 23 December 2015).

Canda, E.R., Shin, S. and Canda, H. (1993) 'Traditional philosophies of human service in Korea and contemporary social work implications', *Social Development Issues*, 15(3): 84–104.

Caritas Korea (2015) *Caritas Korea.* Online. Available HTTP: www.caritas.or.kr/ (accessed 21 November 2015).

Coates, J. (2003) *Ecology and Social Work: toward a new paradigm*, Halifax, Nova Scotia: Fernwood Publishing.

Chun, M.S. (2013) 종교사회복지담론의 재고찰 ['Discourse of religious social welfare: a critical reflection and prospects'], 종교문화연구 *(Journal of Religion and Culture)*, 20: 279–311.

Dal Toso, G., Pompey, H. and Dolezel, J. (2015) *Caritas Church Ministry in the Perspective of Caritas-Theology and Catholic Social Teaching*, Olomouc, Czech Republic: Palacky University.

Gupta, S.K. (2014) *A Comparative Study of Socially Engaged Buddhism: Won-Buddhism in Korea and Neo-Buddhism in India*, Doctor of Philosophy thesis, The Academy of Korean Studies, Seongnam, Korea. Online. Available HTTP: www.riss.kr/link?id=T13738140 (accessed 8 January 2016).

Jogye Order of Korean Buddhist Welfare Foundation (2015) 대한불교조계종사회복지재단 *[Jogye Order of Korean Buddhist Welfare Foundation]*. Online. Available HTTP: www.mahayana.or.kr (accessed 21 November 2015).

Kendall, L. (2011) 'The contraction and expansion of shamanic landscapes in contemporary South Korea', *Cross Currents*, 61(3): 328–44.

Kim, K.M. and Canda, E.R. (2009) 'Spirituality and social work scholarship in Korea: a content analysis', *Korean Journal of Social Welfare Studies*, 40(2): 203–25.

Koh, K.H. (2006) 한국종교계의 사회복지시설 지원금 실태분석 ['Analysis of religious organizations' contribution to social welfare facilities in Korea: 2001–2003'], 보건복지포럼 *[Health Welfare Policy]*, 115: 65–73.

Korea.net (2015) *Religion.* Online. Available HTTP: www.korea.net/AboutKorea/Korean-Life/Religion (accessed 11 November 2015).

Korea Association of Social Workers (n.d.) *Korea Association of Social Workers Code of Ethics.* Online. Available HTTP: http://cdn.ifsw.org/assets/ifsw_12405-10.pdf (accessed 20 November 2015).

Korean Association of Spirituality and Social Welfare (2015) *Korean Association of Spirituality and Social Welfare.* Online. Available HTTP: http://www.kassw.net/ (accessed 17 November 2015).

Korean Christian Social Services Association (2015) 한국 기독교 사회봉사회 *[Korean Christian Social Services Association]*. Online. Available HTTP: www.charity.or.kr/ (accessed 21 November 2015).

Korean Ministry of Culture, Sports and Tourism (2011) 한국의 종교 현황 *[Current Statistics of Religions in Korea]*. Online. Available HTTP: http://mcst.go.kr/web/s_data/research/researchView.jsp?pSeq=1528 (accessed 17 December 2015).

Land, H. (2015) *Spirituality, Religion, and Faith in Psychotherapy: evidence-based expressive methods for mind, brain, and body*, Chicago: Lyceum Books.

Lee, J.Y. (1983) 'The American missionary movement in Korea, 1882–1945: its contributions and American diplomacy', *Missiology: an international review*, 11(4): 387–402.

Lee, M.Y., Ng, S.M., Leung, P.P.Y. and Chan, C.L.W. (2009) *Integrative Body-Mind-Spirit Social Work: an empirically based approach to assessment and treatment*, Oxford: Oxford University Press.

Lee, P.H. (1993) *Sourcebook of Korean Civilization, vol. 1*, New York: Columbia University Press.

Lew, S.K. (1988) *A Study of Oriental Philosophy*, Seoul: Institute of Eastern Studies.

Lew, S.K. (2003) 'Life, peace and mutual growth as the basic themes of Eastern Asia', paper presented at the International Conference on World Life Culture, Gyeonggi-Do, Republic of Korea, December 18–21.

Park, S.H. (2006) 'Insights from Confucian classics for respecting spiritual diversity in social work practice', paper presented at the International Conference on Health and Mental Health in Social Work, Hong Kong, December 13.

Park, S.K. (2013) 치유문화의 비전: 불교에 현대인의 치유를 묻다 ['Vision of healing culture: to inquire about the healing of modern people to Buddhism'], *Won-Buddhist Thought and Religious Culture*, 55: 75–106.

Park, S.T. (2003) 종교사회복지실천에서의 얼알 연구 ['Spirituality: a study of spirituality in religious social work practice'], *Theology and Ministry*, 20: 373–411.

Ro, K.M. (2010) 종교 사회복지의 성격과 과제 ['The Characteristics and Tasks of Religious Social Welfare in Korea'], 종교와사회, 1(1): 191–215.

Tedesco, F. (2003) 'Social engagement in South Korean Buddhism', in C. Queen, C. Prebish and D. Keown (eds) *Action Dharma: new studies in engaged Buddhism*, London: RoutledgeCurzon.

Won-Buddhist Social Welfare Association (2015) 원불교 사회복지 협의회 [*Won-Buddhist Social Welfare Association*]. Online. Available HTTP: www.wonwelfare.net/ (accessed 21 November 2015).

Yoo, J. (2003) 사회복지실천을 위한 영성적 접근 가능성에 대한 탐색 ['An exploration of the possibilities of a spirituality approach to social work practice'], 통합연구 [*Journal of Integration Studies*], 16(2): 9–44.

Yoo, J. (2004) 영성의 다양성과 한국인의 토착적 영성 그리고 교회사회사업적 과제 ['Diversity of spirituality, endemic spirituality of Korean people and the tasks of church social work'], 교회와 사회복지 (*Church Social Work*), 2: 221–45.

Yoon, H., Lim, Y., Koh, Y. and Beum, K. (2015) 노인의 영성, 사회적 지지, 우울이 죽음불안에 영향을 미치는 경로분석 ['A study on the effect of spirituality, social support, depression to death anxiety of the older adults'], 한국지역사회복지학 [*Journal of Community Welfare*], 53: 229–54.

Yoon, I. (2008) 'The development and characteristics of multiculturalism in South Korea', *Korean Journal of Sociology*, 42(2), 72–103.

4

The absent presence of religion and spirituality in mental health social work in Northern Ireland

Patricia Carlisle

Introduction

Northern Ireland (NI) has experienced thirty years of violent civil conflict, the boundaries of which are marked, although not entirely defined, by religious identification. In this way religion is an inherent part of social identification and community construction in NI. Although the violence has significantly decreased since the late 1990s, its legacy remains. Research evidences a complex relationship between religious and spiritual beliefs and mental wellbeing. However, there is a lack of research about how political conflict, in which religion plays a dominant role, may shape the impact of faith on mental health. Literature on religion, spirituality and social work practice suggests the need to examine the social and political processes that persist around this subject in social work practice (Henery 2003; O'Leary *et al.* 2013; Wong and Vinsky 2009). This examination is appropriate given the role of religion within the political conflict in NI (Brewer *et al.* 2010, 2011), the impact of the conflict upon social work practice (Campbell *et al.* 2013), the high incidence of mental ill health in NI (Ferry *et al.* 2011) and the apparent role of religion and spirituality within mental distress (Gilbert 2010; Koenig and Larson 2011).

An established body of research from the 1980s onwards demonstrates that spirituality, inclusive of religion, is generally associated with greater wellbeing, less depression and anxiety, greater social support and less substance abuse (Koenig and Larson 2001). Research within the United Kingdom (UK), and the Royal College of Psychiatry's special interest group on Spirituality (RCP 2010) is beginning to explore explanations for these relationships in the UK context (Awara and Fasey 2008; Cook and Powell 2013; King *et al.* 2013; Pearce *et al.* 2008; Sims and Cook 2009; Swinton 2001). These studies identify a need for exploring the complexities around this subject in recovery and the importance of engaging with a holistic approach to spirituality within mental health.

Drawing upon empirical research, carried out by the author, and upon other relevant literature, this chapter considers while religion and spirituality are woven into the cultural fabric of NI, and are acknowledged within recovery orientated approaches to mental health, their engagement in mental health social work practice appears to be uncertain, problematic or even absent. Discussion considers if, and in what ways, the conflict and secularisation have shaped how the profession has conceptualised religion and spirituality. Although the chapter focuses upon mental health social work practice in NI, it raises questions about how the social work profession engages with religion and spirituality, as an aspect of holistic care, in societies where religion has been a site of political conflict.

The 'troubles' and secularism

Mitchell (2005) explores the role of religion in social identification in NI and advocates deconstructing its meaning in individuals' lives and in the community. Religion, according to Mitchell, is more than an ethnic marker, and limiting one's understanding of religion to this overlooks its social and political significance. In particular, religion informs processes of social identification and community construction in NI in four main ways: where it acts as an identity marker; where religious rituals play a practical role; where religious ideas play a symbolic role in the construction of community; and where doctrine can legitimise oppositional social identifications.

Brewer (2011) examined the role of the churches in dealing with the legacy of violence, both for individual victims/survivors and society more generally. A key aspect of his study is the 'translation of people's private troubles into public issues' (Brewer 2011: 2). Brewer's analysis focuses on how, in the context of a society where religion is inextricably linked with political conflict, religion and beliefs (as he terms it) are brought out of people's private lives into the public realm. Both Brewer and Mitchell's work raises questions about whether religion and spirituality as aspects of a mental health service user's mental health are brought into the public area of social work practice in NI: if issues of spirituality and or religion are important for some people experiencing mental ill health in Northern Ireland, how does the social work profession engage with this in its work with service users?

A key feature of social work in NI, according to Heenan and Birrell (2011), is the impact of the political conflict and sectarianism on social work practice and service delivery. Literature suggests that as a consequence of practicing in a politically divided society, the profession has not addressed issues that have arisen out of the conflict such as sectarianism, the emotional impact of the conflict and aspects of conflict-based forms of oppression (Campbell and McCrystal 2005; Pinkerton and Campbell 2002). Campbell *et al.* (2013) state that greater understanding is needed surrounding how social work practice is affected by the historical trajectory of violent conflicts. Furthermore, there is a sense of inevitability that as social workers are socialised and then practice in these contexts, they, like other members of society, fit their conflict histories to meet their world view. Despite growing interest in religion and spirituality in the social work profession globally (Crisp 2010; Holloway and Moss 2010), there is a notable lack of literature and research about religion, spirituality and social work practice in NI. This raises questions about how, in a post-conflict situation and as an aspect of experiencing mental ill health, religion and spirituality were engaged with in the mental health social worker/service user relationship. This question points to the interface between the role of the social worker from the public sphere, and the role of religion and spirituality within the mental health service users' private experience of mental distress.

Not only is it necessary to consider the context of conflict, it is also important to recognise the impact of secularisation. Commentators of secularisation suggest that rather than proposing that interest in religion in Western societies is diminishing, it may be more appropriate to suggest that it is being reshaped (Hay and Nye 2006; Wood 20108). Hay and Nye (2006: 35) coined the term 'secularization of the intellect' following research by Hay and Morisy (1985) and Hay and Hunt (2000) on the spirituality of people who don't go to church. While the secularisation of British culture is occurring very rapidly, Hay (2002: 4) suggests it appears to be 'only skin deep', thus a religious understanding of spirituality is still normative for most British people. This may suggest that while there are large numbers of people who actively choose not to be associated with religious institutions, they may have a strong interest in spirituality. In a similar manner, Hayes and Dowds (2010) found that while there are some signs secularisation is occurring in NI, it appears that religion as a public institution is weakening, but retains a presence in people's private beliefs and day-to-day practices.

Thus it appears that the secularisation thesis offers a limited picture of dwindling church membership, which does not adequately account for how religion and spirituality are drawn upon within people's lives. Furthermore, secularisation fails to examine the social and political context surrounding religion and spirituality in contemporary society. The individualistic perspective fails to take account of the wider social context informing how religion and spirituality are understood and experienced: the impact relationships have upon the individual's spirituality (Wong and Vinsky 2009), the importance of environment and community (Zapf 2005) and the importance of history and tradition (Carrette and King 2005; Wong and Vinsky 2009).

The absent presence of religion and spirituality in mental health social work practice

The purpose of this chapter is to raise questions and encourage discussion about how the social work profession engages with religion and spirituality in a context of both secularism and, more significantly, where religion has been an historical site of civil conflict. The introduction referred to research carried out by the author, which has been discussed elsewhere (Carlisle 2015a, 2015b, 2016). The study was qualitative, small scale and drew upon, in specific ways, both narrative inquiry and grounded theory. Approval for the study was obtained from the author's university ethics board and the regional Research Ethics Committee (REC). Using a combination of purposive and snowball sampling (Denscombe 2010), 12 mental health service users were recruited from various centres of a voluntary mental health organisation, and 12 social workers were recruited from various integrated community mental health teams. All participants were recruited within various locations within the geographical boundaries of a Health and Social Care Trust (HSCT), which is the statutory provider of health care services. All of the participants took part in a one-to-one semi-structured interview and were invited to bring an object that signified what religion and/or spirituality meant to them to the interview. Half of the participants from each group were invited to a follow-up telephone interview.

This study offers insight into how the conflict dominates the way in which social worker participants engage with religion, spirituality and mental distress and the sensitive quality of the subject in NI. The interviews focused upon locating the participants' stories within the wider social context regarding religion, spirituality, mental distress and social work practice. Through analysis it became apparent that none of the service users had discussed religion, spirituality and mental distress with their mental health professional. Interestingly, social worker participants stated that the assessment forms used in their practice included a box about the service users' religious and/ or spiritual beliefs. However, social worker participants varied in whether they asked service users about their religious and/or spiritual beliefs. This question on the assessment form may be viewed simply as an equality monitoring exercise, used for statistical purposes in the HSCT.

Arguably, this is the acknowledgement of religion and spirituality at its most basic. It is basic because it simply acknowledges religion in a tick box manner but does not explore its meaning in any depth. Interestingly, the majority of social worker participants did not engage with religion and spirituality even in this most basic form. These social worker participants stated that they did not ask service users about their religion because it was too personal a question to ask at a first meeting, or perhaps it was too sensitive a question to ask at all. Others stated that they did not ask about religion but if the service user offered this information during the interview then they would fill it in on the assessment form.

Social worker participants cited the political conflict and the continued sensitive nature of talking about religion and its link with division, as the basis for not asking service users this question. Analysis suggested that social worker participants readily acknowledged religion on a cultural level in NI and were concerned about issues such as offending service users, revealing their own identity and causing tension within the relationship if they explored religion and spirituality. However, overall they appeared uncomfortable engaging with this as an aspect of meaning-making within their practice with mental health service users. Despite social workers acknowledging its relevance for some service users and although service users were articulate regarding its importance within their experience of mental distress, its exploration within the service user/social worker relationship was marked with questions of legitimacy.

Service user participants expressed concern about offending the mental health professional, and questioned whether the worker could relate to them if they were from a different denomination. Analysis of the mental health service user participants' stories suggested they placed high priority on knowing what denomination the mental health worker belonged to, and this would apparently enable them to determine whether the worker would understand their religion and/or spirituality within their experience of mental distress. However, despite knowing that the worker was from the same denomination, analysis suggested that the service user would not talk to their mental health worker about religion, spirituality and mental distress. While this cannot be linked exclusively to the political conflict, it appeared that this may be a significant factor within the context of how religion, spirituality and mental distress are conceptualised within contemporary Northern Irish society. It appeared that there is an ongoing sense of religion and spirituality being an absent presence within the mental health social worker/service user relationship and that the legacy of the conflict significantly hinders exploration of the subject.

Existing literature around sectarianism in NI and social work practice suggests that in a climate of conflict, practitioners have sought to be 'neutral', not seeming to align themselves with either community (Heenan and Birrell 2011; Pinkerton and Campbell 2002; Ramon et al. 2006; Traynor 1998). This was necessary not only to enable them to work with service users across community divisions but also to work alongside colleagues from 'opposite' denominations. Yet avoidance of addressing the impact of sectarianism upon social work practice in NI also presents particular challenges for individual social workers and the profession. This study suggests that the pervasiveness of sectarianism has led to the absent presence of religion and spirituality in practice.

By taking cognisance of the wider social context, analysis highlighted the absent presence of religion and spirituality in mental health social work practice in NI. Analysis suggested that the conflict and seeking to avoid any acknowledgement of it and its sectarian nature within practice, informed its lack of exploration, and purposefully choosing not to offer this choice to the service user, in the majority of the social worker participants' practice. This lack of choice is significant given that religion is a highly sensitive issue. While a service user may want to discuss religion, spirituality and mental distress with their social worker, they too must navigate this complex conflict terrain and may determine that raising this subject may be too fraught.

Coulter (2014), writing about reintroducing themes of religion and spirituality to professional social work training in NI, states that a practitioner's ability to practice in a culturally competent manner is based on the practitioner's self-awareness and both an appreciation and knowledge of the service user's culture. There appears to be a lack of debate about what religion and spirituality means in the North of Ireland; thus, our understanding of it continues to be restricted to these culturally divisive, political boundaries, and an exploration of it in terms of meaning-making is missing (Brewer 2011; Brewer *et al.* 2010, 2011; Hayes and Dowds 2010; Mitchell 2005). This study identifies a lack of permission-giving for service users to explore religion, spirituality and mental distress in their relationship with the mental health social worker and this significantly shapes its lack of exploration within mental health services.

Social workers do not ask: assumed privacy and individualism

Earlier I discussed the problem of individualism and the secularisation thesis, and the way in which they fail to take account of how religion and spirituality are drawn upon within an individual's life. The problem with individualism and privacy, argue Carrette and King (2005: 57), is that it constructs a person as a singular unit, 'a kind of hermetically sealed and isolated self' that does not recognise the 'relational and interdependent self'. This study develops this further and suggests that this may have contributed to how the mental health social worker participants engaged with religion and spirituality within their practice. The social worker participants stated that they were reluctant to ask service users about religion, spirituality and mental distress as they perceived this to be a very private topic and that they would wait for the service user to express this subject, rather than introduce it themselves. Furthermore, social worker participants described being willing to discuss the subject with service users, but because it is a private matter it rarely arose in practice.

Furness and Gilligan (2010) suggest that while social workers may recognise the potential significance of religion and spirituality in their own practice, there is an overwhelming perception of the subject being too personal an issue to discuss in practice. Furthermore, Starnino *et al.* (2014: 856) discussed professionals stating that service users may perceive exploring spirituality with the professional as 'too personal', especially if a trusting relationship has not developed. Similarly, in this study service user participants stated that the subject may be 'a private matter' for some individuals, and therefore they may not want to discuss it with a mental health professional. These various reasons highlight both the 'privatisation' of religion as an aspect of the secularisation thesis (Henery 2003; Wong and Vinsky 2009), and the idea of assumed privacy, that religion and spirituality within mental distress is a private matter for the service user, as some service user participants in this study expressed. However, that is not to say that it should not be acknowledged in social work practice. Again, the core issue here is service user choice to discuss these issues and the social workers' willingness to give the service user permission to discuss this culturally difficult subject.

Secularisation proposes a weakening of religion in modern societies where religion is not entirely 'abandoned', but is privatised. This perspective suggests that religion may weaken as a public institution, but retains a presence in people's private beliefs and day-to-day practices (Hayes and Dowds 2010). Hayes and Dowds (2010:4) suggest that while there are 'creeping signs' of secularisation in NI, it is only 'lukewarm' and points to the 'privatisation of religion' rather than a complete shift to secularisation. My study develops this further by examining whether religion and spirituality is understood as exclusively private within the social work profession, which therefore contributes to its lack of exploration within practice. The question of 'privatisation' of religion prompts consideration of the paradox that emerged in the study: as social workers employed and practicing in a secular profession, social workers also engage in people's private and personal lives. Thus, to what extent as social workers in the public sphere do social workers explore religion and spirituality as an aspect of the private sphere? Analysis suggested a separation between those areas of the service users' lives that were perceived relevant for the worker to explore, and those that were not. It appeared that social worker participants varied regarding their interpretation of religion and spirituality being a social work concern.

Some social worker participants were willing to explore religion, spirituality and mental distress, on the basis that they may be an aspect of the service user's identity. On the other hand, others stated that a service user's spiritual and/or religious needs will be addressed by the relevant religious leader or spiritual advisor. I suggest that this second approach is suggestive of the assumed privatisation of religion and the assumed lack of appropriateness for mental health social workers to explore this area of the service user's life.

Conclusion and looking forward

This study has raised questions, for the first time, within mental health social work practice in NI about if and how practitioners address religion, spirituality and mental distress in practice. This discussion readily acknowledges the difficult emotions this complex and multifaceted subject evokes for mental health service users and mental health social workers alike. It is not offered as a criticism of service users and social workers, but drawing upon participants' diverse views and experiences, this discussion has sought to offer insight about this area of service user experience and social worker professional practice. It is hoped that these issues will be critiqued and developed by further research in the field of social work practice, other helping professions and in mental health. The study is also relevant within peace and conflict studies regarding how religion and spirituality are engaged with in post conflict societies.

The study suggests that the lack of exploration within social work discourse about this subject may be associated with the legacy of conflict and the pervasive nature of sectarianism. While mental health social workers acknowledge the importance of religion and spirituality for some people experiencing mental distress, it appears that its translation into mental health social work practice is marked with uncertainty. This uncertainty was multifaceted and included both the workers' own sense of spirituality coupled with their navigating of the social context in which religion is a sensitive subject. While the social context included issues of secularisation, it was dominated by the 'Northern Ireland context' in which religion has become linked with sectarianism. It appears that the conceptualisation of religion within the conflict and the impact of the conflict upon the social work profession have produced an ambivalent approach to religion, spirituality and mental distress within social work practice in NI. When carrying out the research it became apparent that this subject was highly emotive for both service users and social workers. There is a need to create legitimacy around this subject for both mental health service users and social workers. I suggest the overarching idea of developing 'safe places' for social workers to explore this subject and for mental health service users to 'give voice to' this aspect of their lives, should they wish to do so.

Analysis indicates that many social worker participants continued to associate talking about religion with being sectarian while seemingly under acknowledging its value as a site of meaning-making and recovery. This study highlighted that religion and spirituality evoked various responses among social worker participants. It appeared that this sensitivity significantly contributed to the subject not being explored with mental health service users in practice. Thus, the study builds upon O'Leary et al.'s (2013: 147) call for a more 'connected, inclusive, reflective and participatory approach' to the social worker/service user relationship that addresses the particular contexts of the relationship. I suggest that while a more connected approach in relation to religion, spirituality and mental distress might challenge existing approaches to the subject, it is only by addressing the particular contexts of the relationship that mental health service users and social workers are enabled to explore it in practice. These explorations may be difficult for service users and mental health social workers alike. However, these explorations may be needful in this post-conflict transition.

As the interviews progressed and through the telephone interviews, it became apparent that social worker participants valued having time and space to critically explore this subject both in terms of their own spirituality, or lack thereof, and of how they engage with this subject in practice. A key message from this study is the importance and value of encouraging social workers to critically reflect upon their own values and experiences in relation to religion and spirituality, and to consider their own practice around this subject. The Northern Ireland Social Care Council (NISCC), the social care regulatory body in NI, recently updated the standards of conduct and practice for social workers (NISCC 2015). These new regulations are based on six standards of conduct and nine standards of practice. Standard of conduct number one states the importance of protecting the rights and promoting the interests and wellbeing of service users and carers (NISCC 2015: 5). This standard details the importance, when working with service users, of promoting their right to control their own lives, respecting and maintaining their dignity and privacy, promoting equal opportunities and respecting diversity and different culture and values (NISCC 2015: 7). This standard of conduct may be understood as promoting an anti-oppressive practice agenda where diversity is acknowledged and responded to positively. The importance of addressing the role of spirituality and religion within some mental health service users' lives is supported in these standards.

References

Awara, M. and Fasey, C. (2008) 'Is spirituality worth exploring in psychiatric out-patient clinics?', *Journal of Mental Health*, 17(2): 183–91.

Brewer, J. (2011) 'Spiritual capital and the role of religion in the public domain', Paper presented at Trauma & Spirituality: An International Dialogue, Belfast 9–13 March 2011. Online. Available HTTP: www.journeytowardshealing.org/links/pdfs/John_Brewer_11March2011.pdf (accessed 31 August 2012).

Brewer, J., Higgins, G. and Teeney, F. (2010) 'Religion and peacemaking: a conceptualisation', *Sociology*, 44(6): 1019–37.

Brewer, J., Higgins, G. and Teeney, F. (2011) *Religion, Civil Society and Peace in Northern Ireland,* Oxford: Oxford University Press.

Campbell, J. and McCrystal, P. (2005) 'Mental health social work and the Troubles in Northern Ireland: a study of practitioner experiences', *Journal of Social Work*, 5(2): 173–90.

Campbell, J., Duffy, J., Traynor, C., Reilly, I. and Pinkerton, J. (2013) 'Social work education and political conflict: preparing students to address the needs of victims and survivors of the Troubles in Northern Ireland', *European Journal of Social Work*, 16(4): 506–20.

Carlisle, P. (2015a) 'A tricky question: spirituality and mental health social work practice in Northern Ireland', *Journal of Religion and Spirituality in Social Work*, 34(2): 117–39.

Carlisle, P. (2015b) 'We don't talk about that around here: religion, spirituality and mental health in Northern Ireland', *Mental Health, Religion and Culture*, 18(5): 396–407.

Carlisle, P. (2016) 'Religion and spirituality as troublesome knowledge: the views and experiences of mental health social workers in Northern Ireland', *The British Journal of Social Work*, 46(3): 583–98.

Carrette, J.R. and King, R. (2005) *Selling Spirituality: the silent takeover of religion,* London: Routledge.

Cook, C.H. and Powell, A. (2013) 'Spirituality is not bad for your health', *The British Journal of Psychiatry*, 202(5): 385–6.

Coulter, S. (2014) '(Re)-introducing themes of religion and spirituality to professional social work training in the land of "saints and scholars"', in C. Readdick (ed) *Irish Families and Globalization: conversations about belonging and identity across space and time,* Ann Arbor, Michigan: Michigan Publishing, University of Michigan Library.

Crisp, B.R (2010) *Spirituality and Social Work,* Farnham: Ashgate.

Denscombe, M. (2010) *The Good Research Guide: for small-scale social research projects,* 4th edn, Maidenhead: Open University Press.

Ferry, F., Bolton, D., Bunting, B., O'Neill, S., Murphy, S. and Devine, B. (2011) *The Economic Impact of Post-Traumatic Stress Disorder in Northern Ireland,* The Lupina Foundation, The Northern Ireland Centre for Trauma and Transformation and University of Ulster.

Furness, S. and Gilligan, P. (2010) *Religion, Belief and Social Work: making a difference*, Bristol: Policy Press.

Gilbert, P. (2010) 'Spirituality: the "forgotten" dimension?', in P. Bates and P. Gilbert (eds) *Social Work and Mental Health: the value of everything*, 2nd edn, Lyme Regis: Russell House.

Hay, D. (2002) 'The spirituality of adults in Britain: recent research', *Scottish Journal of Healthcare Chaplaincy*, 5(1): 4–9.

Hay, D. and Hunt, K. (2000) *Understanding the Spirituality of People Who Don't Go to Church: final report of the Adult Spirituality Project*, Nottingham: Nottingham University.

Hay, D. and Morisy, A. (1985) 'Secular society/religious meanings: a contemporary paradox', *Review of Religious Research*, 26(3): 213–77.

Hay, D. and Nye, R. (2006) *The Spirit of the Child*, London: Jessica Kingsley Publishers.

Hayes, B.C. and Dowds, L. (2010) 'Vacant seats and empty pews', *Research Update, Access Research Knowledge (ARK)*, 65 (February): 1–4.

Heenan, D. and Birrell, D. (2011) *Social Work in Northern Ireland: conflict and change*, Bristol: Policy Press.

Henery, N. (2003) 'The reality of visions: contemporary theories of spirituality in social work', *The British Journal of Social Work*, 33(8): 1105–13.

Holloway, M. and Moss, B. (2010) *Spirituality and Social Work*, Basingstoke: Palgrave Macmillan.

King, M., Marston, L., McManus, S., Brugha, T., Meltzer, H. and Bebbington, P. (2013) 'Religion, spirituality and mental health: results from a national study of English households', *The British Journal of Psychiatry*, 202(1): 68–73.

Koenig, H. G. and Larson, D.B. (2001) 'Religion and mental health: evidence for an association', *International Review of Psychiatry*, 13(2): 67–78.

Mitchell, C. (2005) 'Behind the ethnic marker: religion and social identification in Northern Ireland', *Sociology of Religion*, 66(1): 3–21.

Northern Ireland Social Care Council [NISCC] (2015) *Standards of Conduct and Practice for Social Workers*, Belfast: NISCC. Online. Available HTTP: www.niscc.info/files/Standards%20of%20Conduct%20 and%20Practice/WEB_OPTIMISED_91740_NISCC_Standards_of_Conduct_and_Practice_ BluePurple.pdf (accessed 7 October 2015).

O'Leary, P., Tsui, M.S. and Ruch, G. (2013) 'The boundaries of the social work relationship revisited: towards a connected, inclusive and dynamic conceptualisation', *The British Journal of Social Work*, 43(1): 135–53.

Pearce, M. J., Rivinoja, C.M. and Koenig, H.G. (2008) 'Spirituality and health: empirically based reflections on recovery', in M. Galanter and L.A. Kaskutas (eds) *Recent Developments in Alcoholism: vol. 18 research on Alcoholics Anonymous and spirituality in addiction recovery*, New York: Springer-Verlag.

Pinkerton, J. and Campbell, J. (2002) 'Social work and social justice in Northern Ireland: towards a new occupational space', *The British Journal of Social Work*, 32(6): 723–37.

Ramon, S., Campbell, J., Lindsay, J., McCrystal, P. and Baidoun, N. (2006) 'The impact of political conflict on social work: experiences from Northern Ireland, Israel and Palestine', *The British Journal of Social Work*, 36(3): 435–50.

Royal College of Psychiatrists [RCP] (2010) *Spirituality and Mental Health*, London: Royal College of Psychiatrists.

Sims, A. and Cook, C.H. (2009) 'Spirituality in psychiatry', in C. Cook, A., Powell and A. Sims (eds) *Spirituality and Psychiatry*, London: Royal College of Psychiatrists.

Starnino, V.R., Gomi, S. and Canda, E.R. (2014) 'Spiritual strengths assessment in mental health practice', *The British Journal of Social Work*, 44(3): 849–67.

Swinton, J. (2001) *Spirituality and Mental Health Care: rediscovering a 'forgotten' dimension*, London: Jessica Kingsley Publishers.

Traynor, C. (1998) 'Social work in a sectarian society', in M. Anderson, S. Bogues, J. Campbell, H. Douglas and M. McColgan (eds) *Social Work and Social Change in Northern Ireland: issues for contemporary practice*, London: Central Council for Education and Training in Social Work.

Wong, Y.L.R. and Vinsky, J. (2009) 'Speaking from the margins: a critical reflection on the "spiritual-but-not-religious" discourse in social work', *The British Journal of Social Work*, 39(7): 1343–59.

Wood, M. (2010) 'The sociology of spirituality: reflections on a problematic endeavour', in B.S. Turner (ed) *The New Blackwell Companion to the Sociology of Religion*, Oxford: Wiley-Blackwell.

Zapf, M.K. (2005) 'The spiritual dimension of person and environment', *International Social Work*, 48(5): 633–42.

5

Spirituality and religion in Maltese social work practice

A taboo?

Claudia Psaila

Introduction

The Maltese Islands have experienced rapid change in the past few years, mainly as a consequence of their accession into the European Union and the phenomenon of globalisation. This socio-political-cultural change has contributed to a more open, secular and diverse society that is in constant flux. These changes have contributed to the diminishing role of the Roman Catholic Church, which, until this time, was dominant in most facets of Maltese life (Psaila 2014). It is my contention that such a context has also impacted helping professions such as social work particularly as a result of the secularisation of the profession.

As is the case in many other countries (Canda and Furman 2010; Crisp 2013; Holloway and Moss 2010), social work in Malta is rooted in the dominant religion of our Islands, that is, Roman Catholicism (Schembri 2002). Much of social welfare provision was initially delivered by religious organisations with the 'help of the lay person/professional'. With the birth of the welfare state in the 1950s, these services became more centralised and diverse such that these religious institutions were then seen as partners in statutory service provision. The service being provided, while having strong links to these religious entities, became more professionalised and secular.

In its efforts to be perceived as a profession, Maltese social work may have divorced itself from its religious (and perhaps spiritual) roots. This seems to parallel similar developments abroad (Mathews 2009). In this process, while Christian values such as compassion and solidarity, and beliefs such as 'helping those in need' remain strong, 'religion' and 'spirituality' have all but disappeared in social work education, training, research and provision. It seems to me that these have become taboo subjects for many social workers in most fields. The exception to this rule may be in service provision in faith-based organisations and in the areas of health (terminal illness and palliative care) and some work in the addictions field. In these areas, religion and/or spirituality seem to be not only acceptable but important dimensions of care. Within these contexts, meaning making, values, beliefs and the use of religion and spirituality as a resource, may be particularly pertinent, although this may still be done from a mainly Christian, religious perspective.

Furthermore, the marginalisation of the spiritual dimension in social work practice may parallel the same phenomenon in psychotherapy and psychology that were affected by: the past tensions between religion, spirituality, and psychology and psychotherapy; the fear of inflicting one's values onto the client; being trained to consider the spiritual/religious dimension to be outside one's area of competence; having a negative attitude towards religion; lack of training and education in spiritually-sensitive practice; and pathologising and/or minimising a client's spiritual/religious issues (Aten and Leach 2009; Psaila 2012; Richards and Bergin 2005).

The changing context described above and the spiritual dimension of professional helping, particularly psychotherapy, were the subject of a recent qualitative exploratory study with Maltese mental health practitioners: psychotherapists and psychologists (Psaila 2012). The findings may highlight potentially similar trends in the field of Maltese social work practice. However, before this discussion, I will briefly describe the methodology adopted for the study.

Methodology

A qualitative methodology was adopted since the aims of the study were to describe, explore and explain the spiritual dimension of psychotherapy from the perspective of Maltese mental health practitioners practicing in Malta. Due to the contested, and at times ambiguous, nature of understanding spirituality and religion, as well as the spiritual dimension to psychotherapy, adopting a qualitative approach was considered essential. Qualitative methodologies allow for the study of such complex, multidimensional and diverse phenomena (Denzin and Lincoln 2011). Phenomenological and social constructionist perspectives were utilised in the research design. This allowed for the phenomenological exploration of the participants' understanding and meaning of the spiritual dimension of psychotherapy (Creswell 2007). A social constructionist approach was deemed important since 'there is a strong interplay between what is personal and public and what is individually and socially constructed' (Psaila 2012: 96) particularly in relation to spirituality and religion.

The focus group method was chosen as it incorporates the elements of individual meaning making as well as social construction (Barbour 2007; Linhorst 2002). However, this method was adapted to allow for an evolutionary process to develop in terms of safety and trust, reflection and co-construction. I therefore created the FOST group method, which 'is a blend of a focus and a study group such that both individual reflection and group discussion could take place over a period of time in an evolutionary and spiral manner' (Psaila 2012: 11). The FOST group participants met 'over a stipulated period of time to reflect and discuss a particular topic with the aim of generating and gathering data on that topic' (Psaila 2012: 100). Participants were recruited through purposive and snowball sampling. Two groups were formed with one group of five and the other of six Maltese counseling and clinical psychologists and psychotherapists having two years of clinical practice working with adults. The data that was gathered was analysed thematically. What follows is a discussion of some of the findings.

The spiritual dimension as integral to practice

The participants in the study perceived the spiritual dimension to be integral to psychotherapy. This was partly due to their understanding and experience of 'spirituality' and 'religion'. They described these as having different elements.

Spirituality, religion and practice

At times, the participants understood spirituality and religion to be distinct and opposite, with religion stunting people's spiritual and/or psychological growth as opposed to spirituality, which was linked to development. A religious person was described as not necessarily being spiritual and vice versa. Moreover, the participants claimed that spirituality is about 'being' since it involves meaning making, values and connection, and as such observed that we are 'spiritual beings'. Spirituality was described as 'private' (Jade) or as 'personal creative energy' (Mandy), while religion was described as impersonal, dogmatic, ideological, cultural and having to do with dogma, norms, legality and ritual. It is this oppositional differentiation that at times led the participants to view spirituality as inducing people to grow while religion was perceived as stifling a person's spiritual and psychological growth. They explained that, as spiritual beings, people's spirituality needs to be developed. Some saw this process as one where the person frees themselves from the 'shoulds' imposed by religion.

In perceiving spirituality and religion to be at opposing poles of the spectrum, the participants often appraised spirituality positively and religion negatively. At other moments, they understood spirituality and religion as overlapping with the relationship between them being portrayed as either one informing the other. Spirituality was also described as being 'bigger than' religion and subsuming it. When perceived as interrelated, religion was no longer simply described as normative, ritualistic and structural.

While meaning making, purpose and values were central to the participants' understanding of spirituality, the participants saw these as important to religion too. This was also true to the participants' understanding of spirituality and religion as being about connection and relationship. Central to their perception of these elements to spirituality was their understanding of it involving connectedness to self (including self-awareness and self-knowledge), others (including after death), God or a Higher Power, and nature. Connection also involved the elements of relating, sharing and loving. They perceived the need to connect as a spiritual need since it was universal and gave meaning to life. Apart from being central to their conceptualisation of spirituality while important to religion, the participants also described a communal or shared dimension to these elements in their understanding of religion.

Participants highlighted the following factors as idiosyncratic to spirituality: difficult to define; personal and unique; part of the self; about 'being'; that it 'relieves my soul' (Mandy) and involves containment, serenity and surrender; it involves 'going beyond'; is 'greater than us' and involves a transcendent dimension, 'whether that is a personal God or transcendence understood from a psychological perspective' (Alex); and that there are different ways of expressing spirituality, including being present to the other, such that it is pervasive and tacit.

As a result of their understanding of religion and spirituality, the participants perceived spirituality to be integral to psychotherapy. All persons make meaning and this affects their worldview, gives purpose and direction, helps them survive and be guided by their values. However, this is not necessarily the case for religion (particularly when they saw spirituality and religion to be distinct and opposite). Furthermore, spirituality was perceived as integral to psychotherapy because people need connection and people's problems often include a relationship dimension. Moreover, therapy is based on the rapport that is created between the therapist and the client. In fact, at times, the participants understood psychotherapy to be a spiritual journey since it involves meaning making, connection (to self and others, including the therapist), the therapist's way of being and presence, and transcendence – particularly in-depth psychotherapy that involves self-growth. This oppositional differentiation also led them to experience a degree of reluctance in including religion into the psychotherapy process. They claimed to be comfortable doing so if clearly indicated by the client as being important to them, if useful as a resource, or if they perceived religious issues to underlie their psychological problems; for example, excessive guilt stemming from their religious beliefs. This could also be experienced as spiritual distress that would need addressing.

The therapeutic relationship as sacred space

Another theme that emerged and highlighted the participants' experience of spirituality being integral to psychotherapy is that they viewed the therapeutic relationship as a sacred space. This was highly influenced by their understanding of spirituality *and* psychotherapy involving meaning making, connection and transcendence. The participants explained that spirituality is present in the relationship and is expressed through the relationship. They described therapy without connection as 'soul-less'. Furthermore, in-depth psychotherapy is based on this relationship, which is built over time, such that transformation is possible. The connection was described in terms of emotionally and psychologically 'touching' and 'being touched by' the other (both therapist and client). It involves a profundity of understanding at both cognitive and affective levels that would normally lead to increased insight and deeper rapport. This type of relating involves the therapist's way of being and not only employing skills and techniques.

The therapist

The therapeutic relationship as 'sacred space' requires that the therapist embody respect, empathy, presence, genuineness, trustworthiness, nurturance, a nonjudgmental attitude and acceptance. Furthermore, it requires that the therapist meet the client 'in our common humanity' (Maureen). It involves 'the spirit of two human beings actually meeting somewhere and connecting' (Mandy). The therapist's 'way of being' was emphasised by the participants in providing this type of relationship. They insisted that 'we bring who we are'. They described the therapist as a 'dance partner' (Sandra) and a 'wounded healer' (Bridget).

Participants also focused on the influence of the therapist's own spiritual and religious lives with the possible resultant countertransferential issues. Consequently, the therapist's openness, self-awareness and self-care were considered essential in this type of relating. The participants also stressed that for this to happen, the therapist must be committed to their own growth and be spiritually alive. Through this relationship, deep change is possible because the client feels seen and allows him/herself to be seen. Furthermore, the participants insisted that it is a relationship in which they are also touched, healed and transformed.

Apart from describing psychotherapy as a spiritual journey that occurs in and through the therapeutic relationship that is developed by the therapist's skills and way of being, the participants also discussed other dimensions to spiritually-sensitive practice.

Addressing the client's spiritual and religious needs and issues

Some of the participants claimed that they would assess and address a client's spiritual dimension in the same way that they would other aspects of a person's personality. A degree of readiness to engage with spiritual needs and issues contrasted with some of the participant's wariness in dealing with religious matters, unless these are 'specifically mentioned by my client' (Audrey) and/or the clients' religious beliefs were particularly pertinent to their problems. For example, helping a client 'make sense' of their concern 'religiously' (Maureen). The participants spoke about the clients' problem situation being processed through their religious beliefs or being fuelled by such beliefs (for example, excessive guilt in relation to psychological and/or relational issues). In such situations, their oppositional understanding of spirituality and religion seemed to influence their thinking. Moreover, the participants discussed the importance of not imposing their own beliefs and/or spirituality onto their clients. They also highlighted the difficulty of respecting the client's beliefs or spirituality when this was contrary to their own beliefs/

spirituality or when they understood the client's beliefs as underpinning their psychological problems.

Some of the participants seemed to equate spiritual needs with therapeutic needs. For example, Bridget explained that the following universal spiritual needs 'belongingness/love, meaning making and healing' are also, broadly, people's therapeutic needs. However, others claimed that while they agreed, addressing a client's spiritual needs was also dependent upon their assessment of the client's presenting problem. Furthermore, they identified the following client issues as those where spirituality is more tangible: anxiety, depression, anger, abuse, old age, existential questions and people having a near-death experience, among other factors.

Spirituality and religion as a resource

Apart from addressing a client's spiritual and/or religious needs in therapy, the participants also spoke about using spirituality and/or religion as an internal or external resource. As already noted, the therapist may utilise the client's religious and/or spiritual beliefs to make sense of their concerns or to place 'themselves in the world according to their value system' (Claire), therefore making meaning and deriving internal strength and support. It was also discussed as a resource in the shape of cognitive processing (for example, challenging introjects and dealing with transferential issues, such as *'God is punishing me'*). Furthermore, it was connected to deep introspection and reflection. Interestingly, the participants also discussed how their religion and/or spirituality could provide internal strength and support for themselves in their work with their clients. Moreover, the therapists identified external spiritual and/or religious sources of support, such as a parish priest, spiritual advisor, a religious support group, prayer group and so on. When discussing this, however, they were also aware of these networks as being problematic and possibly contributing to the client's problem. They discussed the complexity and difficulty of dealing with such issues.

The participants in the study seemed to suggest that psychotherapy is imbued with spirituality while also discussing spiritually-integrated psychotherapy that focuses on assessing and addressing the client's spiritual needs. In the next section, I will describe possible parallels that may be drawn to social work in Malta. These include the following implications: clinical, theoretical and those related to education, training and research.

Spirituality and social work in Malta: a question of reclamation?

Theoretical implications

As Canda and Furman (2010: 3) explain: 'Spirituality is the heart of helping. It is the heart of empathy and care, the pulse of compassion, the vital flow of practice wisdom, and the driving energy of service'. Furthermore, the findings reported in this chapter concur with earlier authors who found that

> many of the people we serve draw upon spirituality, by whatever names they call it, to help them thrive, to succeed at challenges, and to infuse the resources and relationships we assist them with to have meaning beyond mere survival value.
>
> (Canda and Furman 2010: 3).

A person's spirituality provides a lens with which to view and make meaning of one's life: identity, relationships, problems, resources etc. Therefore, this cannot be left out of the equation in practice, including in assessment and intervention. Moreover, as was evident in my study, the practitioners' spirituality may also be important to them as they live out their lives and help others, at times, whether consciously or unconsciously. This is an aspect of what I am referring to as 'reclamation'. So far, many social workers in Malta may be resistant to including spirituality and/or religion in their practice, even though, perhaps unbeknownst to them, they may be doing so. I believe that, as in the case of the participants in the study, this is partly due to the social worker's conceptualisations of 'spirituality', 'religion' and social work practice and the relationship between all three.

Similar to other helping professionals, social workers work with 'troubled people or people in trouble' (Kadushin and Kadushin 2013: 13). However, of particular importance to social workers are the person and his/her environment and how the latter may contribute to the person's problem and/or be utilised as a resource. Persons and their environments are intertwined such that they may influence their environment while also being impacted by the latter. As is evident in my study and also in the literature (Mathews 2009; McSherry 2006), the broader environment, whether it is cultural, societal or familial, influences the way a person conceptualises and experiences his/her spirituality, whether it is religiously-inspired or not.

Moreover, as we have seen, a person's spirituality may also be a resource or may underlie certain psychological and/or relational problems. Consequently, spirituality may be an important dimension in the 'person-in-the-environment' conceptual framework of the social worker. This may be particularly the case in the Maltese context due to the strong, although diminishing, influence of the Roman Catholic Church and the rapid change that is being experienced in Maltese society. From a rather insular society, it is becoming more diverse, multicultural and secular with a plurality of voices that claim different values, beliefs and worldviews. This may have an effect on the individual, family, community and society. Moreover, it may have further practice implications.

Practice implications

The secularisation of Maltese society may also create a 'push-pull dynamic' that was experienced by the participants in the study. For the participants, the 'push-pull dynamic' was highlighted in their acceptance of spirituality as being integral to psychotherapy while being hesitant of including religion in the therapeutic process. Furthermore, this dynamic was evident in their oscillation between perceiving spirituality and religion as separate and distinct while also as overlapping (Psaila 2012). This ambiguity may be the result of being immersed in a particular religion such that it remains the reference point, whether consciously or unconsciously and willingly or unwillingly. It may also stem from their disenchantment with the institutional aspects of religion such that some participants discarded any inclusion of religion in their experience and understanding of spirituality (Psaila 2012). They also experienced this 'push-pull dynamic' on affective levels including in their 'rejection' of religion having to do with spirituality. Other examples comprise their sense of frustration and, at times, pain, that was directed at the Church and its teachings as it affected them and their clients. This may be experienced by themselves and/or their clients intrapersonally, for example, feeling rejected, guilty, confused about one's identity and values, etc. However, it may also be experienced interpersonally, for example, in conflictual relationships with family members as a result of values and beliefs that have changed. Exline, Yali and Sanderson (2000) explain how 'religious rifts' (interpersonal) and 'religious strain' (intrapersonal) may lead to depression and suicidality. I therefore believe that social workers and service users could experience a similar, multifaceted 'push-pull dynamic'.

The 'push-pull dynamic' is also evident in understanding spirituality as a double-edged sword.

This was highlighted when the participants described spirituality and religion as resources while also underlying certain problems. It was also apparent at community levels, for example when they described priests, spiritual advisers and/or the client's parish group as being supportive or as contributing to the problem. Examples include promoting situations of injustice and/or oppression, such as telling a woman experiencing domestic violence, 'This is your cross and you must bear it'. Another example given by the participants was of a person being torn about his homosexuality as a result of the Church's teaching, and the crisis in faith and in his identity that this was creating. On the other hand, the participants mentioned that they have identified a network of 'gay-friendly' priests and a Catholic support group (Drachma 2015) with whom they work closely and refer clients. I therefore wonder whether Maltese social workers are practicing in the same way as the research participants and whether they identify this as spiritually-sensitive practice. Furthermore, I question whether they experience the same dynamic, both personally and in their practice at micro, meso and macro levels. This may be especially the case with social workers who are employed by faith-based organisations particularly when their values, spirituality, religious beliefs and worldview may be different to the policies, values, etc. of the Church-run institution.

Crisp (2015) describes how spirituality in faith-based organisations is expressed, among other things, in 'strategic directions' (Crisp 2015: 50) and philosophical underpinnings of service provision. She describes how religious communities may strongly influence strategic decisions at managerial levels that may be a way of ensuring that the service provision is congruent with the values and mission of the particular faith. This is often expressed in the mission and vision statements of such an organisation. This is clear, for example, in the mission statements of Caritas Malta (2015) and Hospice Malta (2012), where specific reference is made to the Christian faith and Gospel values. Both these organisations offer social work services. So far, no similar research has been carried out in Malta. However, it is my opinion that social workers working in such organisations may either experience a degree of congruence with regards to their personal spirituality or, perhaps, a degree of conflict if their spirituality is different to that of the faith-based organisation in which they work and if the policies and/or managerial decisions are incongruent to them. The latter can therefore create a push-pull dynamic on an organisational and/or personal level.

However, as the research participants described, it is also true that spirituality can be empowering and is linked to resilience, better mental and physical health, hope and coping (Bullis 1996; Coyte et al. 2007; Holloway and Moss 2010; Koenig 2004). Holloway and Moss (2010) draw a parallel between social work and spirituality as both being empowering. Furthermore, spirituality was also linked to transformation and transcendence by the participants as well as in social work literature (Canda and Furman 2010; Holloway and Moss 2010). The participants in the study identified transformation, particularly that which is a result of in-depth psychotherapy, as spiritual. This change involves increased self-awareness and self-knowledge, change in the self and becoming 'whole'.

Participants also perceived transcendence, including 'letting go', 'surrendering', dealing with suffering, finding meaning and purpose, and connection to a Higher Being or God, as dimensions of spirituality. However, this is also part of the reality of social work practice and both transcendence and transformation, as well as wholeness, hope and resilience are important elements to spiritual care (Payne 2014). Providing spiritual care in social work practice that includes assessing and addressing spiritual need and spiritual distress is perceived as essential to providing holistic, multicultural anti-oppressive care (Canda and Furman 2010; Holloway and Moss 2010; Payne 2014).

While so far, not much research has been carried out in Malta, it seems to me that social workers in Malta provide the same type of care to varying degrees. The latter may depend upon the setting in which they practice. For example, a social worker at Child Protection Services may feel restricted in providing such care due to their emphasis on investigative practice. However, other social workers in different settings may not necessarily label the service they provide as spiritually-sensitive practice or as providing spiritual care. Furthermore, I question whether they actively engage in assessment that involves the spiritual (including religious) dimensions as I have been presenting here.

Holloway and Moss (2010: 111) explain that in providing such care, attention is paid to the partnership model of practice, including paying particular attention to the therapeutic relationship. They describe a 'fellow traveller model' that focuses on accompaniment as well as reciprocity. This parallels the participants' description of the therapeutic relationship as sacred space as well as the emphasis on the 'being' of the therapist who was described as 'dance partner' and 'wounded healer'. It also focuses on the professional and service-user meeting in their humanity with both being on a spiritual journey. This model resonates with the humanistic model of practice (Payne 2014), which, as an academic member of staff in the Department of Social Policy and Social Work at the University of Malta, I have observed is a strong influence on student social workers in Malta.

Education, training and research

Earlier, I discussed how social workers might be resistant to including spirituality/religion in their practice. Their resistance may be a result of lack of training and feeling of incompetence, as well as the resultant perception that the spiritual and/or religion should not be part of secular social work practice. So far, the curriculum content on religion and spirituality as has been clarified in this chapter is rather weak and narrowly focused in the education programme of social workers in Malta. In the curriculum, emphasis is placed on the concept of the person-in-the-environment, multicultural and anti-oppressive practice, being user-centred, focusing on the relationship between the social worker and service-user, the centrality of values and ethics, reflexivity, and self-awareness and self-knowledge, which are all important to providing spiritually-sensitive practice. Yet, this is not adequately linked to providing spiritual care that includes spiritual assessment and sensitivity to the client's spiritual pain and distress. The student social worker is not encouraged to reflect enough on their understanding of spirituality and religion either in their lives or in their client's lives. Similarly to students in other countries (Payne 2014), this is also the case for many of those students in Malta who enter into social work motivated by their faith and values. It is, however, encouraging to note that over the years, a number of students are choosing to study the spiritual dimension of social work practice as part of their undergraduate research. This may be promising to the future provision of spiritually-sensitive social work practice, training and research.

Conclusion: from taboo to reclamation?

I believe that spirituality and religion in Maltese social work practice may be partly a question of making the invisible visible, and reclaiming spirituality and religion as important to practice. Additionally, more needs to be done in the fields of social work education, training and research. It may be a question of reclaiming part of our spiritual and cultural heritage and embracing who we are as spiritual beings in a society that is becoming more secular and multicultural. This process may involve a movement from a stance where spirituality/religion are perceived as 'taboo' and outside one's area of competence to a position of reclamation of spirituality as central to who we are as human beings. The latter would include providing holistic, multicultural practice where spirituality and religion may be important to either or both the social worker and service user.

References

Aten, J.D. and Leach, M.M. (2009) 'A primer on spirituality and mental health', in J.D. Aten and M.M. Leach (eds) *Spirituality and the Therapeutic Process: a comprehensive resource from intake to termination*, Washington DC: American Psychological Association.

Barbour, R. (2007) *Doing Focus Groups*, London: Sage.

Bullis, R.K. (1996) *Spirituality in Social Work Practice*, London: Taylor and Francis.

Canda, E.R. and Furman, L.D. (2010) *Spiritual Diversity in Social Work Practice: the heart of helping*, 2nd edn, New York: Oxford University Press.

Caritas Malta (2015) *About*. Online. Available HTTP: www.caritasmalta.org/about (accessed 15 December 2015).

Coyte, M.E., Gilbert, P. and Nicholls, V. (eds) (2007) *Spirituality, Values and Mental Health: jewels for the journey*, London: Jessica Kingsley Publishers.

Creswell, J.W. (2007) *Qualitative Inquiry and Research Design*. London: Sage.

Crisp, B.R. (2013) 'Social work and faith-based agencies in Sweden and Australia', *International Social Work*, 56(3): 343–55.

Crisp, B.R. (2015) 'Challenges to organizational spirituality as a result of state funding', *Journal for the Study of Spirituality*, 5(1): 47–59.

Denzin, N.K. and Lincoln Y.S. (2011) 'Introduction: the discipline and practice of qualitative research', in N.K. Denzin and Y.S. Lincoln (eds) *The Sage Handbook of Qualitative Research*, London: Sage.

Drachma (2015) *About Us*. Online. Available HTTP: http://drachmalgbt.blogspot.com.mt/p/about-us_22.html (accessed 15 December 2015).

Exline, J.J., Yali, A.M. and Sanderson, W.C. (2000) 'Guilt, discord, and alienation: the role of religious strain in depression and suicidality', *Journal of Clinical Psychology*, 26(12): 1481–96.

Holloway, M. and Moss B. (2010) *Spirituality and Social Work*, Basingstoke: Palgrave Macmillan.

Hospice Malta (2012) *Hospice Malta*. Online. Available HTTP: http://hospicemalta.org/about-us/mission-statement/ (accessed 15 December 2015).

Kadushin, A. and Kadushin, G. (2013) *The Social Work Interview*, 4th edn, New York: Columbia University Press.

Koenig, H.G. (2004) 'Religion, spirituality and medicine: research findings and implications for clinical practice', *The Southern Medical Association*, 97(12): 1194–200.

Linhorst, D.M. (2002) 'A review of the use and potential of focus groups in social work research', *Qualitative Social Work*, 1(2): 208–28.

Mathews, I. (2009) *Social Work and Spirituality*, Exeter: Learning Matters.

McSherry, W. (2006) 'The principal components model: a model for advancing spirituality and spiritual care within nursing and health care practice', *Journal of Clinical Nursing*, 15(7): 905–17.

Payne, M. (2014) *Modern Social Work Theory*, 4th edn, Basingstoke: Palgrave Macmillan.

Psaila, C. (2012) 'Spirituality in Psychotherapy: a hidden dimension. An Exploratory Study' unpublished PhD thesis, Open University, United Kingdom.

Psaila, C. (2014) 'Mental health practitioners' understanding and experience of spirituality and religion: implications for practice', *Journal for the Study of Spirituality*, 4(2): 189–203.

Richards, P.S. and Bergin, A.E. (2005) *A Spiritual Strategy for Counseling and Psychotherapy*, Washington DC: American Psychological Association.

Schembri, P. (2002) 'In Search of Our Roots: a historical review of early social work practice in Malta (1950s to 1970s)' unpublished dissertation, University of Malta, Malta.

Part III
Religious and spiritual traditions

6

The constructed 'Indian' and Indigenous sovereignty

Social work practice with Indigenous peoples

Arielle Dylan and Bartholemew Smallboy

Introduction

It is impossible to write a chapter on Aboriginal spirituality, for there is no pan-Aboriginal spirituality. Many First Nations authors, who recognise commonalities among the perspectives of various Aboriginal peoples in Canada, and Native American communities in the United States, have written of Aboriginal spirituality in the context of wellness and healing (e.g. McCabe 2008; Mawhiney and Nabigon 2011; Verniest 2006), being careful to articulate the diversity of spiritual understandings and practices across Aboriginal communities. Any discussion of Aboriginal spirituality that neglects to mention the distinctive expression of spirituality across Indigenous communities (e.g. Abbott 1989; Christ 1990; Ruether 2001), however well intended, is problematic. In the same way that Christie (in press) argues that it is necessary to know the particulars of a First Nation community to begin to understand its economic needs and how such a community might best negotiate an agreement with an industrial proponent, it is necessary to be well acquainted with the specificities of a First Nation in order to understand the spirituality of its people. Representations of pan-Aboriginal spirituality, even in their broadest, most generous articulation, run the risk of reinscribing the stereotype of the 'spiritual Indian'. This stereotype, of course, is an illusory, essentialised construct, which constrains possibilities for Indigenous expression, lived experiences and Indigenous-non-Indigenous understandings by engendering a discursive terrain that is too tightly scripted (Appiah 1994: 163). This chapter seeks to debunk and deconstruct the 'spiritual Indian', while also problematising the notion of pan-Aboriginality more generally, with the purpose of making the case for specificities, the need to attend to particularities and context not only when discussing but also when, in a helping role, engaging with Indigenous peoples and their communities.

This chapter will begin with an investigation of early constructions, from pre-confederate Canadian history, of the otherised Indian and then interrogate more recent surfacing of romantic Indian reifications occurring in the latter part of the twentieth century and persisting today. Having looked at these discursive formations and the way that they operate to limit and oppress, an examination of some historic social work practices with Indigenous peoples will be explored for the purpose of underscoring the professional failures that resulted from unexamined participation in colonisation and its attendant dyad, racism and cultural superiority. These areas will be examined with the express purpose of making an iterative case for the imperative of attending to context and particularities when considering Indigenous spirituality. In this manner this chapter, which is written from a critical Indigenous perspective, will serve as a respectful departure from earlier writings regarding Aboriginal spirituality in which various models are suggested for use.

First Nations refracted through Jesuit eyes

Social work scholars Baskin (2011), Blackstock (2007, 2009, 2011) and Sinclair (2004), among others, have written of the vexed relationship between First Peoples of Canada and the settler-colonialists, and the role of social work both in the colonial past and present, and in the context of the contemporary decolonisation project. Examples of the troubled Indigenous-settler-colonial relationship are found in Indigenous-French culture contact in the early seventeenth century in regions that are now the Atlantic Provinces, Quebec and Ontario, as captured in the *Jesuit Relations* (Thwaites 1898). The *Relations* are the journals kept by French missionaries to document their activities in 'New France'. These journals were sent annually to France, the colonial metropole, as a record of religious, social, cultural and linguistic – and political and economic – progress of the missionaries. In these documents the Jesuits constructed an Indian/'savage' who is 'innocent', 'childish', 'like beasts' and in need of Christian instruction to become fully human. Throughout the *Jesuit Relations*, the Jesuits promoted an understanding of First Nations that pivots on hierarchical dualisms, situating the Jesuits (and often French culture more broadly) as superior to First Nations. In this process, moments of cultural humility and respect demonstrated by Indigenous peoples toward the French are mistakenly (or deliberately) construed as inferiority, as illustrated by the following example of proselytising efforts among the Wendat:

> They are very diligent and attentive to the instructions we give them; I do not know whether it is through complaisance, for they have a great deal of this naturally, or through an instinct from above, that they listen to us so willingly concerning the mysteries of our Faith, and repeat after us, whether they understand it or not, all that we declare to them. They very willingly make the sign of the Cross, as they see us make it, raising their hands and eyes to Heaven and pronouncing the words, "Jesus, Mary", as we do,—so far that, having observed the honor we render to the Cross, these poor people paint it on their faces, chests, arms, and legs, without being asked to do so.
>
> (Thwaites 1898 vol. 10: 163)

The Jesuits interpreted this behavior as a Wendat disposition to comply or an instinctual response to Christian teachings. What has occurred in this interpretative process is a reduction of the Wendat to malleability and instinct, features often attributed to animals and women, who are to be ruled and contained according to Western patriarchal and anthropocentric values. Absent are the recognition of Wendat exquisite cultural and religious diplomacy, and the steps of reasoning undoubtedly employed to arrive at the collective Wendat handling of the Christian cross.

In an earlier *Relation*, the Jesuits reported 'on the belief, superstitions, and errors of the Montagnais savages' and, in so doing, reveal again not only a belief in their own cultural superiority but also a conviction that Indigenous peoples needed French intervention.

> I believe that souls are all made from the same stock, and that they do not materially differ; hence, these barbarians having well formed bodies, and organs well regulated and well

arranged, their minds ought to work with ease. Education and instruction alone are lacking. Their soul is a soil which is naturally good, but loaded down with all the evils that a land abandoned since the birth of the world can produce.

(Thwaites 1898 vol. 6: 229)

Here it is apparent that the construction of the 'barbarian' not only situates Indigenous peoples as inferior to the French and other so-called civilised peoples, but also eradicates the unique characteristics of distinct groups. The words 'savage' and 'barbarians' are used throughout the *Jesuit Relations* to define First Nations peoples, and the understanding for the inexperienced reader in France, as largely culturally homogeneous. This excerpt also reinforces the idea that Indigenous peoples needed to be Gallicised and Christianised to become fully human. Such a view served French imperialist and colonial aims, as possession of territory required observance of the 1095 papal bull, *Terra Nullius*, an international law allowing Western European Christian nations to appropriate lands deemed uninhabited. As Wolfe (2006: 388) cogently argues, 'access to territory' is the raison d'être of colonial practices, and toward this end '[s]ettler colonialism is inherently eliminatory but not invariably genocidal' (Wolfe 2006: 387). A final trope to be identified in this passage is that of Indigenous backwardness, the idea that, in this case, French society was considerably more advanced than Indigenous societies. Sadly, this false understanding persists today, in the belief that Western Europeans brought technological progress to Indigenous peoples and, in this misguided assumption, appreciation of Indigenous technologies is missed. Zemon-Davis (1996: 30) has provided a wonderful corrective to disabuse people of this notion: she puts forward the idea of 'absolute simultaneity' and 'radical contemporaneity' in which Indigenous and colonising societies are understood as sharing the same timeline, even if using different methods to achieve sometimes similar, sometimes different goals.

The 'ecological' and 'spiritual Indian'

Having looked briefly at the folly of negative stereotyping of Indigenous peoples in early Canadian history, this chapter will now turn to putative positive stereotyping or romantic ideals developed surrounding Indigenous peoples of this continent. In particular, the constructs of the 'ecological' and 'spiritual' Indian will be explored. The ideas of the ecological and spiritual Indian are inescapably intertwined in the non-Indigenous imaginary as Indigenous peoples are often misunderstood as being pagan (Riverwind 2006), so these misconceptions will be discussed here together. The precursor to the notion of the 'ecological Indian' developed in the pre-industrial era in Europe in response to dissatisfaction with the restrictions of Western society.

The Western imagination was ignited by thoughts of primitivism and galvanised by misconceptions gained through false representations of peoples in the 'New World' (Berkhofer 1976). This prompted a reworking of the utopian ideal and, in the process, posited a reified 'noble savage' as its hero, casting the excessively urbane, disconnected city dweller as the antihero, lacking in courage, liberty and vigour. Over the centuries, the 'noble savage' trope came to embody, for disenchanted Western Europeans, a resistance to all the perceived shortcomings of Western civilisation: disconnection from the natural world, primacy on reason over feeling, conformity instead of liberty and premeditation at the expense of spontaneity (Berkhofer 1976). Of note, the term 'noble savage' and all its romantic trappings are unrelated to Indigenous peoples and exists almost entirely in the minds, unhappy experiences and relentless strivings of non-Indigenous peoples. A further irony is that the romantic stereotype of the noble savage that holds such promise for dissatisfied white people has its roots in the violence of dispossession of

Indigenous peoples, the 'strategic deployment of violent sovereign power' that inevitably marks the colonial enterprise (Coulthard 2014: 36).

In keeping with the burgeoning environmental movement of the 1960s, the 'noble savage' construct conveniently transmogrified into the 'ecological Indian' to be used on billboards and in other forms of media to advance environmental aims (Krech 1999; Strickland 1997). Harding's (2005) content analysis investigating media portrayals of Aboriginal peoples in three Canadian newspapers, over three-quarters of a decade, found the 'noble environmentalist' to be among the stereotypes prominently recurring in the analysis. Not unlike the idealised and stereotypical association of Indigenous peoples with the environment, the New Age movement, which gained momentum in the 1980s, began to promulgate the idea of the 'spiritual Indian' by appropriating and profiting from Native American spiritual traditions (Aldred 2000; King 2012).

These romantic representations of Indigenous peoples serve the interests of non-Indigenous peoples, spiritually, sometimes economically as false medicine people charge exorbitant fees for retreats (King 2012), and anthropologically through a kind of cultural voyeurism. As a consequence of this social, cultural, discursive climate, individuals who have never met an Indigenous person will often ascribe to Indigenous peoples generally the characteristics of spirituality and ecological responsibility. Such ascription is not wrong for these are certainly fundamental dimensions of Indigenous ontology, axiology and praxis (McGregor 2009; Tallbear 2000).

However, the issues with this are several. First, the dominant culture is defining who and what an Indigenous person is and can be, and this is done in the interest of non-Indigenous, mostly white, objectives and gains. Second, when the dominant culture controls how Indigenous peoples are constructed, bizarre things happen. For example, Indigenous peoples typically become either one stereotype (lazy, drunken, social-problem riddled, etc., see for example, Proulx 2011) or another (that being discussed here), both being equally damning: damning because they do not reflect reality, damning because they do not include Indigenous authoring and circulation of their own representations, and damning because they do nothing to further the reconciliation project underway in this country and the sovereigntist aims of First Nations. In this way, the dominant culture through these purportedly positive ideals perversely 'allows' Indigenous peoples to be 'spiritual' and 'ecological' but does not create space for other understandings of Indigenous people to emerge or circulate. For example, in the dominant culture, discursive formations associated with Indigenous peoples do not typically include the words 'reason', 'intellect', 'political acumen', 'logic' and so on.

What has this line of investigation to do with Aboriginal spirituality? All these erroneous constructs of the Indigenous other limit possibilities for Indigenous peoples in very real ways, with respect to everyday practices, aspirational endeavours and future possibilities. Indeed, what can be described as nothing less than sanctioned quotidian violence perpetuates colonialism in the form of 'structured dispossession' (Coulthard 2014: 16), perhaps not of property in this iteration but dispossession nonetheless in the social, cultural and discursive terrain.

Discursive formations that include mostly caricatures of Indigenous peoples, usually negative, occasionally positive, create epistemic ignorance where there is a conviction of knowing but knowledge is absent. A social work course in group work in which a non-First Nation person drums and sings as a guest in the course, speaking of First Nation spirituality, but not mentioning Indigenous sovereignty, the Idle No More movement or the Indigenous intellectual tradition – all areas one would expect to be discussed in an academic discipline built around social justice and social transformation – is one example of this epistemic ignorance. An overwhelming number of applicants to a social work programme writing long tracts in their admission essays about their desire to help 'Canada's Aboriginals' (as if the state possesses First Nations peoples), to rescue them from poverty and a litany of social afflictions, is another. It is in response to these pernicious understandings that we have sought in this chapter to resist any broadly articulated notion of Indigenous spirituality and have instead argued for the particular, for specificities, for it is only through understanding on this level that space is created for a real relationship to occur, and help, professional social work help or otherwise, can only occur in a relationship.

Social work and First Nations

Jennissen and Lundy (2006: 1) assert that the historical arc of social work in Canada suggests social workers have an 'unremitting commitment ... to the dual roles of alleviating human suffering of the individual and promoting broader social, political, and economic change through social action'. While this is undoubtedly an accurate historical depiction of social work development and practice among certain sectors of the Canadian population, sadly this does not obtain in the context of social work among First Nations peoples. In fact, Indian welfare policy in Canada in both its initial religio-political and later secular-economic incarnations has been oppressive, marginalising and assimilationist, and social workers, despite various professional articulations of social justice objectives, have been agents in these culturally genocidal practices (Blackstock 2009; Miller 2003; Shewell 2004). Heron's (2007) observations about the raced, classed and gendered ways that self is constituted in helping relationships and the implicit need of a disadvantaged other in the construction of the 'white helper' is instructive here. A social welfare system that emerged in a colonialist state and has not sufficiently reformed or radical-ised, as is the case in Canada, inevitably serves the colonialist aims of the system from which it derives (Hart 2002; Mullaly 2007). In Canada, where the 'logic of elimination' that marks settler-colonialism (Wolfe 2006) is inarguably writ large, the appalling record of child welfare with Aboriginal peoples is unsurprising.

The overrepresentation of Aboriginal children in state care and the overwhelming evidence that this phenomenon results from a racist child welfare policy rather than true neglect or abuse, leads Blackstock (2007: 71) to question, with no intended irony, whether the institution of the residential school has 'just morph[ed] into child welfare'. This is a tremendously unsettling point that must be conceded: non-Indigenous helpers, trained social workers, have been enact-ing state-sanctioned harm, in the guise of child welfare, in Aboriginal communities throughout this country for decades, performing a form of cultural violence that runs roughshod over the unique Indigenous legal orders inherent to each Indigenous community in this country, legal traditions that would have mechanisms for addressing child neglect situations (Friedland and Napoleon 2015). These culturally constituted responses would not involve removing children from the community, but instead would see the situation in its broader context both in its origination and in its handling, often involving an ethic of community care (Blackstock 2009).

Child welfare is but one example of the way social work has participated in the cultural dis-location and assimilationist performances enacted by the Canadian state in a contemporary con-text. In a significant ruling by the Canadian Human Rights Tribunal, in response to the claim filed against the Federal government by the First Nations Child and Family Caring Society of Canada and the Assembly of First Nations, the Canadian government was found to racially dis-criminate against First Nations through service management and a funding model that 'resulted in denials of services and created various adverse impacts for many First Nations children and families living on reserves' (Canadian Human Rights Tribunal 2016: 161). It is hoped that the Federal government will not appeal this ruling and will instead begin implementing measures to redress this wrong.

Prime Minister Justin Trudeau, in his victory speech, evoked Wilfrid Laurier when uttering the phrase 'sunny ways', signaling how politics can be embraced as a force for positive social change. His father, former Prime Minister Pierre Trudeau, had before him imagined a 'just society', but this vision was trenchantly critiqued by Cardinal (1969) in his seminal work *The Unjust Society* in which the reach of racist Aboriginal policy is detailed, and a call for profound and extensive policy change was made. Almost half a century later, Cardinal's vision is still unfulfilled. However, this is an era of reconciliation, and there are many opportunities for Indigenous peoples and non-Indigenous allies to work toward a truly just society, and this is not something that can be achieved unilaterally. As Said (1993: 7) has argued, 'none of us is outside or beyond geography' and there is a need in colonial and postcolonial contexts to operate with an understanding of 'overlapping territories and intertwined histories' in order best to understand a sociopolitical reality and effect positive change.

In Indigenous scholarship and theorising developed and adopted by helping professionals, there have been a number of approaches put forward as a means to help remedy a host of social, economic, political and rights-based inequities stemming from colonialism. Two-eyed seeing, as articulated by Bartlett *et al.* (2012), is an important (if limited for its emphasis on just two cultural ways of seeing) approach to bridging the cultural divide and resisting the foregrounding of mainstream knowledge through an integrative, transdisciplinary, transcultural method. Recently in a social work class with one of the authors, an Indigenous student identified the limits of two-eyed seeing and articulated her preference for the idea of multiple-eyed seeing because of its greater inclusivity. Others have written of holistic Indigenous models for healing and balanced relationships and interrelationships with self, community and creation (Baskin 2011; Mawhiney and Nabigon 2008; Verniest 2006). These are invaluable contributions to both the Indigenous intellectual tradition and to social work scholarship and practice. A problem, however, not with these works but with the climate in which these works circulate, is the mainstream cultural proclivity to cast Indigenous peoples in spiritual terms: that is, many non-Indigenous people see Indigenous peoples as being spiritual but neglect the other three dimensions of personhood as described in the Indigenous holistic model (physical, emotional, psychological), and the dominant culture reinforces this understanding through discursive formations, a culture that celebrates the reified ecological/spiritual Indian but allows little room for the flesh and blood political, intellectual, athletic Indigenous person.

In response to this climate of gross stereotyping in which the other is constructed and then reinscribed through quotidian social, cultural and media practices, we have deliberately resisted any discussion of Aboriginal spirituality in its more generic sense and argued in favour of the particular. If one is to discuss Aboriginal spirituality, it is probably best done in the context of the specificities of a particular community, for it is in the minutiae of such context-specific details that the possibility of stereotyping, whether negative or positive, romanticised or deprecated, is eradicated and that true understanding of Aboriginal spirituality and the robust nature of its situatedness and interconnectivity emerge. In making this case for the particular, we are not lapsing into an uncritical postmodern relativism; rather, this is a strong moral argument for attending to specifics so as not to risk participating in those practices that constrain Indigenous persons' lives and perpetrate an ontological violence through profoundly limiting Indigenous ways of being, both in understanding and in practice. Essentialism can certainly be powerfully strategic when adopted and enacted by a group for political ends but not when imposed upon a people in an etic manner by a dominant group with a history (and contemporary practices) of colonialism.

Conclusion

Indigenous scholars and activists in Canada are making tremendous strides in the various areas outlined by Cardinal (1969) requiring redress: Aboriginal rights (Alfred 1999; Christie 2006;

McNeil 2007; Slattery 2005), education (Battiste 2000; Henderson 2000; Little Bear 2000), social issues (Baskin 2011; Blackstock 2007, 2009, 2011) and economic development (Jobin 2013; Wuttunee 2004). Indeed, Indigenous peoples are succeeding at making advances in all these areas despite the reluctance and lack of political will demonstrated by the government and mainstream society.

Indigenous spiritualities, both the understandings and practices of, are unequivocally a part of this process. However, to reduce Indigenous peoples to their spirituality and to ignore the many other dimensions of what constitutes Indigeneity is problematic. For any social worker, especially non-Indigenous social workers who want to be Indigenous allies, desiring to work in an Indigenous community or work with Indigenous service users elsewhere, it is necessary to be aware of the historical, political, cultural and social (perhaps linguistic) practices and realities of a specific community before assuming an understanding of spiritual dimensions. Without such grounding in specificities true dialogic relationship is not possible, and without dialogism, all that remains are the unproductive monologues that have characterised non-Indigenous relations with Indigenous peoples in this country since the seventeenth-century annals of the Jesuits.

Acknowledgement

The authors are grateful for the wisdom and encouragement of our colleague Val Napoleon in the development of this chapter.

References

Abbott, S. (1989) 'The origins of God in the blood of the lamb', in J. Plant (ed) *Healing the Wounds*, Philadelphia: New Society Publications.

Aldred, L. (2000) 'Plastic shamans and astroturf sun dances: new age commercialization of Native American spirituality', *The Native American Indian Quarterly*, 24(3): 329–52.

Alfred, T. (1999) *Peace, Power, Righteousness: an Indigenous manifesto*, Don Mills, ON: Oxford University Press.

Appiah, K.A. (1994) 'Identity, authenticity, survival: multicultural societies and social reproduction', in A. Gutmann (ed), *Multiculturalism*, Princeton: Princeton University Press.

Bartlett, C., Marshall, M. and Marshall, A. (2012) 'Two-eyed seeing and other lessons learned within a co-learning journey of bringing together indigenous and mainstream knowledges and ways of knowing', *Journal of Environmental Studies and Sciences*, 2(4): 331–40.

Baskin, C. (2011) *Strong Helpers Teachings: the value of Indigenous knowledges in the helping professions*, Toronto: Canadian Scholar's Press.

Battiste, M. (ed) (2000) *Reclaiming Indigenous Voice and Vision*, Vancouver: UBC Press.

Berkhofer, R.F. (1976) *The White Man's Indian: images of the American Indian from Columbus to the present*, New York: Vintage Books.

Blackstock, C. (2007) 'Residential schools: did they really close or just morph into child welfare?', *Indigenous Law Journal*, 6(1): 71–8.

Blackstock, C. (2009) 'The occasional evil of angels: learning from the experiences of Aboriginal peoples and social work', *First Peoples Child and Family Review*, 4(1): 28–47.

Blackstock, C. (2011) 'The Canadian Human Rights Tribunal on First Nations Child Welfare: why if Canada wins, equality and justice lose', *Children and Youth Services Review*, 33(1): 187–94.

Canadian Human Rights Tribunal (2016) *CHRT Ruling on First Nations Child Welfare Discrimination*, Ottawa: CHRT.

Cardinal, H. (1969) *The Unjust Society: the tragedy of Canada's Indians*, Edmonton: M.G. Hurtig.

Christ, C. (1990) 'Rethinking theology and nature', in I. Diamond and G.F. Orenstein (eds) *Reweaving the World: the emergence of ecofeminism*, San Francisco: Sierra Books.

Christie, G. (2006) *Aboriginality and Governance: a multidisciplinary perspective*, Penticton, BC: Theytus Books.

Christie, G. (in press) 'Impact Benefit Agreements, *Tsilhqot'in Nation*, and indigenous sovereignty', in A. Dylan and B. Smallboy (eds) *Impact and Benefit Agreements: their meaning for the future of the relationship between Indigenous peoples and Canada*, Toronto: University of Toronto Press.

Coulthard, G.S. (2014) *Red Skin, White Masks: rejecting the colonial politics of recognition*, Minneapolis: University of Minnesota Press.

Friedland, H. and Napoleon, V. (2015) 'Gathering the threads: developing a methodology for researching and rebuilding Indigenous legal traditions', *Lakehead Law Journal*, 1(1): 16–44.

Harding, R. (2005) 'The media, Aboriginal people and common sense', *The Canadian Journal of Native Studies*, 25(1): 311–35.

Hart, M.A. (2002) *Seeking Mino-Pimatisiwin: an Aboriginal approach to helping*, Halifax: Fernwood Publishing.

Henderson, J. (2000) 'Postcolonial ghost dancing: diagnosing European colonialism', in M. Battiste (ed) *Reclaiming Indigenous Voice and Vision*, Vancouver: UBC Press.

Heron, B. (2007) *Desire for Development: whiteness, gender and the helping imperative*, Waterloo: Wilfrid Laurier University Press.

Jennissen, T. and Lundy, C. (2006) *Keeping Sight of Social Justice: 80 years of building CASW*. Online. Available HTTP: www.casw-acts.ca/sites/default/files/attachements/CASW%20History.pdf (accessed 26 February 2016).

Jobin, S. (2013) 'Cree peoplehood, international trade, and diplomacy', *Revue générale de droit*, 43(2): 599–636.

King, T. (2012) *The Inconvenient Indian*, Toronto: Doubleday Canada.

Krech, S. (1999) *The Ecological Indian: myth and history*, New York: W.W. Norton & Company.

Little Bear, L. (2000) 'Jagged worldviews colliding', in M. Battiste (ed) *Reclaiming Indigenous Voice and Vision*, Vancouver: UBC Press.

Mawhiney, A.M. and Nabigon, H. (2011) 'Aboriginal theory: a Cree medicine wheel guide for healing First Nations', in F.J. Turner (ed) *Social Work Treatment: interlocking theoretical approaches*, 5th edn, New York: Oxford University Press.

McCabe, G. (2008) 'Mind, body, emotion, and spirit: reaching to the ancestors for healing', *Counselling Psychology Quarterly*, 21(2): 143–52.

McGregor, D. (2009) 'Honouring our relations: an Anishnaabe perspective on environmental justice', in J. Agyeman, P. Cole, R. Haluza-DeLay and P. O'Riley (eds) *Speaking for Ourselves: environmental justice in Canada*, Vancouver: UBC Press.

McNeil, K. (2007) *The Jurisdiction of Inherent Right Aboriginal Governments*, Ottawa: National Centre for First Nations Governance.

Miller, J.R. (2003) *Shingwauk's Vision: a history of Native residential schools*, Toronto: University of Toronto Press.

Mullaly, B. (2007) *The New Structural Social Work*, Toronto: Oxford University Press.

Proulx, C. (2011) 'A critical discourse analysis of John Stackhouse's "Welcome to Harlem on the Prairies"', in H.A. Howard and C. Proulx (eds) *Aboriginal People in Canadian Cities: transformations and continuities*, Waterloo: Wilfrid Laurier University Press.

Riverwind, J. (2006) *The Basic Indian Stereotypes*. Online. Available HTTP: www.corvallis.k12.mt.us/middle/staff/craigc/nas/links/documents/indian_stereotypes.pdf (accessed 26 February 2016).

Ruether, R.R. (2001) 'Deep ecology, ecofeminism, and the Bible', in D.L. Barnhill and R.S. Gottlieb (eds) *Deep Ecology and World Religion*, Albany: State University of New York Press.

Said, E.W. (1993) *Culture and Imperialism*, New York: Vintage.

Shewell, H. (2004) *Enough to Keep Them Alive: Indian welfare in Canada, 1873–1965*, Toronto: University of Toronto Press.

Sinclair, R. (2004) 'Aboriginal social work education in Canada: decolonizing pedagogy for the seventh generation', *First Peoples Child and Family Review*, 1(1): 49–61.

Slattery, B. (2005). 'Aboriginal rights and the honour of the crown', *Supreme Court Law Review*, 29: 433–45.

Strickland, R. (1997) 'Coyote goes Hollywood', *Native Peoples,* fall issue. Online. Available HTTP: www.nativepeoples.com/Native-Peoples/September-October-1997/Coyote-Goes-Hollywood/ (accessed 26 February 2016).

Tallbear, K. (2000) *Shepard Krech's "The Ecological Indian": one Indian's perspective*. Online. Available HTTP: www.iiirm.org/publications/Book%20Reviews/Reviews/Krech001.pdf (accessed 26 February 2016).

Thwaites, R.G. (ed) (1898) *The Jesuit Relations and Allied Documents*, vols. 1–71, Cleveland: The Burrows Brothers.

Verniest, L. (2006) 'Allying with the medicine wheel: social work practice with Aboriginal peoples', *Critical Social Work*, 7(1). Online. Available HTTP: www1.uwindsor.ca/criticalsocialwork/allying-with-the-medicine-wheel-social-work-practice-with-aboriginal-peoples (accessed 26 February 2016).

Wolfe, P. (2006) 'Settler colonialism and the elimination of the native', *Journal of Genocide Research*, 8(4): 387–409.

Wuttunee, W. (2004) *Living Rhythms: lessons in Aboriginal economic resilience and vision*, Montreal and Kingston: McGill and Queen's University Press.

Zemon-Davis, N. (1996) 'Polarities, hybridities: what strategies for decentring?' in C. Podruchny and G. Warkentin (eds) *Decentring the Renaissance: Canada and Europe in multidisciplinary perspective, 1500-1700*, Toronto: University of Toronto Press.

7

The sacred in traditional African spirituality

Creating synergies with social work practice

Raisuyah Bhagwan

Introduction

African spirituality embraces not only the whole and unbridled humanity of all Africans, but of humankind the world over. This notion is cradled within the ancient Akan proverb *Nnipa nyinaa ye Onyame mma, obi nye asase ba*, which means that all human beings are the children of God (Nkulu-N'Sengha 2009: 143). The African spiritual heritage stands, unequivocally salient amid the landscape of other global spiritual traditions. Despite the intrusiveness of colonisation and the imposition of capitalism, traditional African spirituality has remained unfettered (Serequeberhan 1999) and faithfully resilient, through a deep desire to maintain its tradition (Mazrui 1986). The richness of this heritage has withstood the fractures of a myriad other cultural and spiritual invasions with solemn resilience (Asante and Mazama 2009), giving Afrocentric scholars a much needed voice amid the scholarly discourse on other world religions.

It is in this context that the African contribution as a true wellspring of African identity is deserving of a scholarly space within the literature on spiritually sensitive social work practice. African transcendent expression is unitary and has evolved over the centuries through the legacies of the African heritage. Conceived through the accumulated experiences and sagacious reflections of the ancestors, it is understood as a meaningful experience, rather than a toilsome journey through life (Asante and Mazama 2009). This chapter presents a deeper understanding of the African worldview and spirituality while advancing its implications for social work practice. The emphasis on righteous living, search for the eternal, reverence for ancestors, the deep appreciation for family and communal wellbeing and the unique healing methodologies underpinning its philosophy, grounds the need to advance further intellectual inquiry in this area, particularly in relation to its implications for social work intervention. This chapter forms a starting point for a journey into this inquiry and attempts to interweave some of the core characteristics of its philosophy and relatedness to social work practice.

The traditional African worldview

African spirituality is deeply embedded in the psyche of African people. It remains aloof from Western notions of polytheism, as African people believe in a Supreme God, who created the

Universe (Lugira 2009b). Despite this monolithic view of African religion, rich variations to its characteristics, rituals and ceremonies, colour the African continent. 'God', 'The Great Spirit' and the 'Creator and Sustainer of the Universe', is referred to as the 'Originator' (*Borebore*), 'The Beginner' (*Ebangala*), 'the One who Bears the World' (*Mebee*) and 'the Very Source of Being' (*Orise*) (Nkulu-N'Sengha 2009: 290). The most salient attributes of this Supreme God or Deity has been described as one who brings rain, who gives life, who gives and destroys, who humbles the great, who you meet everywhere, who brings sunshine, who is the father of little babies and the Universal Father-Mother. Undeniable, however, is the notion of this Almighty as one who brings justice to the earth and ensures morality, social order and fertility (Asante and Mazama 2009).

The African spiritual legacy was born from the teachings of the ancestors who have provided spiritual guidance embodied in the Creator, the giver of life, harmony, balance, cosmic order, peace and healing (Solomon and Wane 2005). It continues faithfully to be handed down through the oral repository of African mythology, legends tales, songs from which its people have drawn their construction of spirituality and their healing methodologies for peace, wellbeing and balance (Thabede 2008). Religious consciousness then is transmitted in African society ubiquitously from heart to heart, rather than through the written word (Cook and Wiley 2000). In the absence of a formal sacred narrative or texts it is the forefathers, then, who have served as the generators of societies and civilisations (Asante and Mazama 2009).

In African spirituality there are no temples or shrines for the worship of the Supreme Being; instead there exists a boundless space for connecting with this Being (Asante and Mazama 2009). Mbiti (1969) reiterated that religious practices are not confined to sacred buildings or to one holy day of the week, and religious and spiritual expression and experiences can occur at any time.

Humankind is linked to the Supreme Being through an eternal divine connection, hence the belief in the enduring presence of the ancestors, collective existence and collective responsibility for uplifting each other (Ntseane 2011). Most Afrocentric scholars include spirituality in their definition of healthy psychological functioning throughout life (Ani 1997; Asante 2007; Nobles 1978; Schiele 1994; Welsing 1991). Collectively they define spirituality as a vital life force that animates humankind and propels them towards the rhythms of the universe, nature, ancestors and the community (Bujo 1992; Setiloane 1986). Spirituality in an African context is also described as participation in the metaphysical world and a duty to take care of one's ancestors, extended family and community (Ntseane 2011). These conceptualisations shed light on the pathways that need to be embraced for psycho-spiritual healing, growth and transformation.

African spirituality exemplifies an interdependent cosmological view and all elements whether animate or inanimate have a spiritual base (Schiele 1994). A typical traditional African cosmology, then, is a non-fragmented universe wherein humankind, plants, animals, ancestors, the earth, sky and the universe co-exist in varying states of balance between order and disorder, harmony and chaos. This interconnectedness and interdependency is predicated on the belief that there is a universal link that flows from the Creator (Akbar 1984; Schiele 1994). Hence, there is no fragmentation between the living and non-living, natural and supernatural, material and immaterial, conscious and unconscious. All natural phenomena such as the rivers and mountains represent powerful aspects of the Supreme and all living things have the potential to be consecrated as sacred. These unified entities remain in dynamic interrelationships, with the past, present and future harmoniously inter-weaving into one another. Reciprocity, circularity and continuity permeate this flow and at the core of this is the belief that ancestors remain active in the community of the living (Asante and Mazama 2009). Cook and Wiley (2000) have asserted that the Supreme God is approached through worship, prayers, sacrificial offerings, singing and dancing, rituals, and human and spiritual intermediaries.

African cosmology is influenced by the ontological principle of 'Human-Nature Unity', or 'Harmony with Nature' (Baldwin 1986: 243). Dixon (1976) described this humanity as inseparable from nature, which creates a communal phenomenology (Baldwin 1986). The African worldview, therefore, has a deep interconnectedness with all things and its spiritual philosophy makes no distinction between the scared and mundane. The divide then between the secular and the sacred, which afflicts the Western world, dissipates within the realm of African spirituality (Asante and Mazama 2009), grounding a deep need for its consideration of the spiritual in therapeutic work with African clients. To ignore the cultural rituals and rites and healing methodologies at its core will only further distance it from spiritually sensitive practice. The sections that follow relate to community, the ancestors, traditional healing and rituals. This is followed by a discussion on their relatedness to and forming synergies with social work intervention.

Community

The essence of being human in African religious tradition, termed 'Bumuntu', relates to the capacity to 'express compassion, reciprocity, dignity, harmony and humanity in the interests of building and maintaining community' (Nussbaum 2009: 100). Bumuntu is the African vision for a person with good character, who respects all life in the Universe and is in a tripartite relationship with the transcendent beings (God, ancestors, spirits), humankind and the natural world (Nkulu-N'Sengha 2009). It is believed that all people are born whole and are endowed with the potential for right and wrong, and good character relates to an inner orientation towards doing good for others (Bhagwan 2002).

People are seen as part of a larger community and it is this community that facilitates psychological growth and transformation (Akbar 1984; Setiloane 1986; Theron *et al.* 2012). Psychological development and change is thus not an individual journey, but occurs with a community of other people (Mkhize 2004). African people value a good moral life and its laws, customs, behaviour are held scared. Violation of the acceptable social order is thus seen punishable by both the Supreme God and ancestors (Ekeopara and Ekeke 2011).

African people call this collective way of living 'Ubuntu' (Mokwena 2007), which translates into 'I am because we exist' (De Liefde 2007: 52). The community then forms the realm for the manifestation of Ubuntu or humaneness and is imbued with a deep level of social consciousness. It inculcates respect for the inherent dignity of all humankind and a deep reverence for human interdependence (Mnyaka and Motlhabi 2005). The dissolution of the individual, through an emphasis on practical service to humanity, creates a 'family community', wherein prayer, rituals and harmonious living are valued (Mkhize 2006).

It is this humanness to care for the disadvantaged, the sick, poor and the bereaved (Mnyaka and Motlhabi 2005) that makes people and their communities a huge spiritual resource to those facing difficulty. Even child rearing and caring for the elderly are collective responsibilities of the extended family system and community (Mkhize 2004). Ross (2010) emphasised the importance of the extended kinship networks in providing moral support in times of trouble and a space for belonging and security. Apart from traditional healers, the elders in African kinship networks are considered spiritually strong and are consulted for wisdom and guidance when people experience difficulties. These then are important spiritual systems that must be considered when developing a social work intervention plan.

Ancestral spirits

The traditional African worldview thus upholds that the world is animated by a multitude of invisible spiritual entities, particularly the ancestral spirits (Bojuwoye 2005; Mbiti 1969). When someone dies it is believed that they are transformed into an ancestral spirit and death does not preclude a person from being part of his or her social unit, family, clan tribe or village.

These ancestors are then actively involved in the lives of their descendants and are seen as the custodians of the social and moral world, ensuring that group solidarity is maintained (Breidlid 2009; Mokwena 2004). All good deeds, fertility both in the abundance of the harvest, the productivity of women and joy of family are related to the ancestors. In this vein, misfortunes and other life challenges can be attributed to unhappy ancestors and affliction can be traced to a lack of ritual and sacrifice. The ancestors are seen to be able to intercede in most aspects of life, including marital and interpersonal relationship conflicts, health issues, and can avert natural disasters (Ngubane 1977) and should not be excluded when considering the context of the presenting problem and developing the therapeutic plan.

Rituals

The African propensity to seek and maintain balance and reciprocity is grounded within rituals that strengthen individual family and community life. In fact, African spirituality marks through ceremony and ritual, salient moments related to birth, death, marriage, initiation and it is the traditional rituals that facilitate this process (Wheeler *et al.* 2002). African rites of passage are practices, customs and ceremonies that help African people move smoothly through the stages of life from birth, childhood, puberty, initiation, marriage, aging and death, last funeral rites and finally, the processes of reincarnation (Lugira 2009a).

Often, African people assimilate rituals held by families and carry these down through time and space. Traditional healers may also prescribe rituals to help with personal and family difficulties and restore harmony in families and communities (Bojuwoye 2005).

A ritual ceremony brings people and all elements (living and non-living) of the universe together. It serves as a means by which people are united together and creates opportunities for mediating relationship behaviours, so as to influence the way individuals and families treat each other (Bojuwoye 2005). Traditional African religion is underpinned by a belief that harmony in nature is not self-generated but is gained through personal community with other people. Most African spiritual rituals involve rhythmic drumming, dancing and use of trance as catharsis and call-response that encourages active participation in worship (Wheeler *et al.* 2002). It is believed that personal growth and development occurs through ritual ceremonies, where people are helped to break their isolation and find support through their experiences as they eat, dance and rejoice together. In this way people share their burdens, communalise their problems and find a way to de-stress and get support (Bojuwoye 2005).

Traditional healing in the African world

African healing and its relatedness with social work practice

Despite Western influence, African people continue to honour their ancient traditions as a source of healing (Bojuwoye 2005; Moodley and West 2005; Solomon and Wane 2005). These ancient traditions continue to permeate contemporary sacred teachings, ceremonies and healing methodologies. In times of crisis, African spirituality is paramount (Mbiti 1969).

Africans conceive of psycho-social problems and illness in a holistic manner and of having a deep spiritual and metaphysical nature and causation (Ogungbile 2009). In most African cosmologies, illness and personal and family difficulties are related to super sensible origins, such as the wrath of divinities and neglected ancestral spirits. Traditional healing is holistic and encompasses biopsycho social and spiritual aspects, which results in wellbeing and wholeness. Healing is a sustained ritual process of correcting the disequilibrium generated by spiritual, natural, psychological and social factors that manifest through illness and other psychological difficulties (Adogame 2009).

This mirrors the biopsycho social and spiritual paradigm in social work that posits that these facets are interweaved, thereby necessitating a holistic approach to intervention (Bhagwan 2002). Similarly, African psychotherapy is conceptualised as holistic and views the individual as a total system with biopsychosocial and spiritual facets (Awanbor 1982).

Traditional healers and their methodologies

African people who are experiencing individual or family-related difficulties will consult first with a healer who diagnoses the problem and sets in place a treatment plan. This mirrors the social work process of assessment followed by therapeutic intervention. Each healing ritual is unique to the person requiring healing and to the healer (Solomon and Wane 2005). Traditional or spiritual healers are those who intercede on behalf of those needing help, to bring healing, peace and harmony (Solomon and Wane 2005). Even in contemporary times these healers are called herbalists (iyanga); diviners (commonly known by their Zulu name as Sangomas) and faith healers (umthandazis) (Gurung 2013; King 2012; Washington 2010), who are consulted first in times of crisis. Herbalists use various herbs to treat physical and psychological problems, by preparing a mixture of roots, leaves, barks, fruits and animal parts. The healer invokes the appropriate deity to give power to the mixture, before it is given to clients, by using certain expressions and invocations that embody spiritual references (Ogungbile 2009). Sangomas, on the other hand, are reputed for their clairvoyance, their abilities to read a person's mind and to use cosmic energy to ensure health and wellbeing (Sodi *et al.* 2011). They also have a closer relationship with the ancestral spirits, and can act as a conduit between the ancestral spirits and a person in the healing process.

The process of assessment within the African milieu begins with the healer going into an altered state of consciousness, by entering into a trance and meditating. The healer then communicates with the ancestral spirits through divination. Pieces of stones, shells, bones and tree barks are the divination instruments that are cast and the position of the falling objects provides clues related to the difficulty being experienced. These are seen as messages from the ancestors with regards to a person's problems. The diviner then communicates with the ancestors by dancing and singing their praise, so as to appease them for any wrong doing and by securing help with the problem (Bojuwoye 2005). In some instances rituals and sacrifices are undertaken for the spirit to sustain the immutability of this power (Adogame 2009).

Healing itself follows a comprehensive approach, which includes psychotherapy, soma-therapy, metaphysicotherapy and hydrotherapy in an African context (Ogungbile 2009). *Soma-therapy* focuses on the application of a physical measure such as tying a consecrated thread or chain on a person's wrists, neck or waist, which symbolically counters bad energies and brings harmony. *Hydrotherapy* in contrast uses water for healing due to the belief in its power and efficacy within African ethno-cosmology (Ogungbile 2009). *Metaphysicotherapy* utilises the traditional leader, as discussed, to actively engage with the Spiritual Being, to effect healing.

African healing in a social work context

African people and those of the African diaspora 'harbour a tenacious distrust of scientific theory,' as colonialism is perceived to be synonymous with the West (Wheeler *et al.* 2002: 74). Western social work theories advocate autonomy and independence, which is antithetical to the type of interdependency that African-centred psychology is predicated upon. The latter embraces the extended network system, family and community that must be considered as a source of strength during crises (Wheeler *et al.* 2002).

African spirituality ultimately is 'what healing is all about' (Idowu 1992: 193). This allows for a natural conception with spiritually-based social work interventions. African spirituality influences African people's thinking, sense of security, life challenges, identity development, behaviour, decision making and problem solving (Idowu 1992). Spiritual interventions may therefore only be conceived within the context of African families and communities, and when practitioners engage their clients with sensitivity, awareness and ethical wisdom. Clients from the African spiritual tradition may view history taking as intrusive and hence it is important to demonstrate genuine caring from the onset (Cook and Wiley 2000). In fact, their deep personal spirituality may prevent them from engaging with social workers in the first instance, as even in contemporary times they will first seek the help of traditional healers, spiritual leaders and family elders for problems related to interpersonal conflict, emotional trauma or family disputes (Ross 2010). Even those who seek social work services for material help or who seek counselling will engage African spiritual healing methodologies first.

Psychotherapy within an African context refers to the use of symbolic elements, actions and words that could enable equanimity and provide wellbeing. From birth Africans are socialised into rituals, songs, proverbs, fables and religious ceremonies as part of daily life. These may easily be infused into spiritually-based social work intervention.

A spiritual assessment is crucial to illuminating their personal spiritual world view, the African spiritual resources, rituals and practices, and the healing methodologies that they use, to support ethical spiritual interventions. Spiritual systems that can be included in assessment and intervention include transpersonal encounters with the Supreme Being as well as elders, community leaders and traditional healers. It is always helpful to explore what the clients' conception of their Supreme Being is, as meditative imagery can be used as part of therapeutic intervention. There are also ancient stories or narratives passed down through the generations from the elders that can also offer wisdom, guidance, strength and support, and point to enabling ways of coping with adversity (Bhagwan 2002).

Narratives and stories are important ways that social workers can get clients to share about their lives, family and community. This is salient to the African community where history and meaning is passed down through an oral tradition (Bhagwan 2002). While storytelling provides a way to learn about their spiritual history, their spiritual rituals and ceremonies, it is also through the telling of the story that therapeutic benefits can be achieved. Other African forms of expression include poetry, dance, music and song (Shorter 1996), which can be synchronised with contemporary social work intervention.

Collaboration with traditional healers, and referrals to spiritual support systems – be it healers or elders groups – are important sources of strength for clients and valuable resources for practitioners. Awanbor (1982) referred to the community as a therapeutic milieu, because African spirituality is communal (Nobles 1972). Both emotional and material resources can be provided through informal family and community-based networks, where sharing is dictated by the concept of Ubuntu.

Often interpersonal difficulties and other forms of distress are attributed to the inscrutable acts of the spirits, violations of taboos or rituals, or disrespect towards the ancestors (Bojuwoye 2005). It is therefore important to consider this as significant in therapeutic work and support referrals to traditional healers to venerate the ancestors and perform worship and prayers that may ease their difficulties.

Ancestors are believed to bestow protection and guidance and are seen as the guardians of the family and community's traditions, ethics and affairs (Bhagwan 2002). It is thus crucial that they be invoked or venerated through ritual and prayer. Rituals are 'codified spiritual practices' (Hodge and Williams 2002: 588) and form an important part of enabling the therapeutic plan. Through libation and the offering of food, those in distress seek their help and blessings through diverse rituals and rites. These rituals are believed to bring strength, equanimity, blessings, and good health and fortune (Asante and Mazama 2009).

Rituals and prayers are often undertaken with music, which is viewed as a sacred pathway for African people to connect with the supernatural world, where God or the spirits live (Ross 2010). Most African musicians understand and play certain rhythms for God and the spirits, as it is believed that this extends an invitation to them and also directs the flow of the supernatural. Drumming is used extensively, as it is believed to serve as the conduit for communication between humans and ancestral spirits and has significant healing qualities (Harrison 2009). In fact, there is a wealth of empirical evidence that attests to the wide benefits of engaging in community rituals with the intent of relieving loneliness and isolation, easing anxiety, enabling feelings of belonging and feeling loved, and providing comfort, reassurance and security (Pargament 1997; Worthington *et al.* 1996).

Conclusion

This chapter has drawn attention to the rich opportunities presented by the African worldview, for a natural integration of its wisdom with social work interventions. Despite the historical reluctance of social work to engage with traditional therapies, it is crucial that practitioners give consideration to the full integration of traditional healing practices where appropriate. The synergies created with modern social work interventions will inevitably lead to a more holistic approach that harmonises the biopsychosocial and spiritual paradigm to enable healing and transformation with clients from the African community. Therapeutic success, however, lies with a welcoming and respectful approach to acknowledging African spiritual histories and to utilising its knowledge, beliefs and rituals as a powerful resource within the milieu of social work practice.

References

Adogame, A. (2009) 'Zulu' in M.K. Asante and A. Mazama (eds) *Encyclopaedia of African Religion*, Thousand Oaks: Sage.

Akbar, N. (1984) 'Africentric social sciences for human liberation', *Journal of Black Studies,* 14(14): 359–414.

Ani, M. (1997) *Let the Circle Be Unbroken: the implications of African spirituality in the diaspora*, New York: Nkonimfo.

Asante, M. (2007) *An Afrocentric Manifesto*, Cambridge: Polity Press.

Asante, M. and Mazama A. (eds) (2009) *Encyclopedia of African Religion*, Thousand Oaks: Sage.

Awanbor, D. (1982) 'The healing process in African psychotherapy', *American Journal of Psychotherapy,* 36(2): 206–13.

Baldwin, J.A. (1986) 'African (black) psychology: issues and synthesis', *Journal of Black Studies,* 16(3): 235–49.

Bhagwan, R. (2002) 'The Role of Religion and Spirituality in Social Work Practice: Guidelines for curricula development at South Africa schools of school work'. Unpublished PhD thesis, University of Natal.

Bojuwoye, O. (2005) 'Traditional healing practices in Southern Africa', in R. Moodley and W. West (eds) *Integrating Traditional Healing Practices into Counseling and Psychotherapy*, Thousand Oaks: Sage Publications.

Breidlid, A. (2009) 'Culture, indigenous knowledge systems and sustainable development: a critical view of education in an African context', *International Journal of Educational Development*, 29(2): 140–8.

Bujo, B. (1992) *African Theology in Its Social Context*, Nairobi: St Paul Publications.

Cook, D.A. and Wiley, C.Y. (2000) 'Psychotherapy with members of African American churches and spiritual tradtions', in P.S. Richards and A.E. Bergin (eds) *Handbook of Psychotherapy and Religious Diversity*, Washington, DC: American Psychological Association.

De Liefde, W.H.J. (2007) *Lekgotla: the art of leadership through dialogue*, 2nd edn, Pretoria: Jacana Media.

Dixon, V.J. (1976) 'World views and research methodology', in L.M. King, V.J. Dixon and W.W. Nobles (eds) *African Philosophy: assumptions and paradigms for research on black persons*, Los Angeles: Fanon R & D Center.

Ekeopara, C.A. and Ekeke, E.C. (2011) 'The relevance of African traditional religion in an HIV/AIDS environment', *Research Journal of International Studies*, 19: 43–52.

Gurung, R.A.R. (2013) 'A multicultural approach to health psychology', *American Journal of Lifestyle Medicine*, 7(1): 4–12.

Harrison, R.K. (2009) *Enslaved Women and the Art of Resistance in Antebellum America*, New York: Palgrave Macmillan.

Hodge, D.R. and Williams, T.R. (2002) 'Assessing African American spirituality with spiritual ecomaps', *Families in Society*, 83(5–6): 585–95.

Idowu, A.I. (1992) 'The Oshun festival: an African traditional religious healing process', *Counseling and Values*, 36(3): 192–200.

King, B. (2012) 'We pray at the church in the day and visit the sangomas at night: health discourses and traditional medicine in rural South Africa', *Annals of the Association of American Geographers*, 102(5): 1173–81.

Lugira, A. (2009a) 'Africism', in M. Asante and A. Mazama (eds), *Encyclopedia of African Religion*, Thousand Oaks: Sage.

Lugira, A.M. (2009b) *African Traditional Religion*, 3rd edn, New York: Infobase Publishing.

Mazrui, A. (1986) *The Africans: a reader*, New York: Greenwood Press.

Mbiti J.S. (1969) *African Religions and Philosophy*, Nairobi: Heinemann.

Mkhize, N. (2004) 'Sociocultural approaches to psychology: dialogism and African conceptions of the self', *Self, Community and Psychology*, 5(1): 5–31.

Mkhize, N. (2006) 'African traditions and the social, economic and moral dimensions of fatherhood', in L.M. Richter and R. Morrel (eds) *Baba: men and fatherhood in South Africa*, Cape Town: HSRC Press.

Mnyaka, M. and Motlhabi, M. (2005) 'The African concept of Ubuntu/Botho and its socio-moral significance', *Black Theology*, 3(2): 215–37.

Mokwena, M. (2004) 'Integrating traditional African spirituality through a gendered lens', *Agenda*, 18(61): 86–91.

Moodley, R. and West, W. (2005) *Integrating Traditional Healing Practices into Counselling and Psychotherapy*, London: Sage.

Ngubane, H. (1977) *Body and Mind in Zulu Medicine*, London: Academic Press.

Nkulu-N'Sengha (2009) 'African traditional religions', in M. De la Torre (ed) *The Hope of Liberation in World Religions*, Waco, TX: Baylor University Press.

Nobles, W.W. (1972) 'African philosophy: foundations for black psychology', in R.L. Jones (ed) *Black Psychology*, New York: Harper & Row.

Nobles, W. (1978) 'African consciousness and liberation struggles: implications for the development and construction of scientific paradigms', unpublished manuscript, San Francisco: Westside Community Health Center, Inc.

Ntseane, P.G. (2011) 'Culturally sensitive transformational learning: incorporating the Afrocentric paradigm and African feminism', *African Education Quarterly*, 61(4): 307–23.

Nussbaum, B. (2009) 'Ubuntu: reflections of a South African on our common humantiy', in M.F. Murove (ed) *African Ethics: an anthology of comparative and applied ethics*, Scottsville: University of Kwa-Zulu Natal Press.

Ogungbile, D. (2009) 'Serpent', in M. Asante and A. Mazama (eds) *Encyclopedia of African Religion*, Thousand Oaks: Sage.

Pargament, K. (1997) *The Psychology of Religion and Coping*, New York: Guilford Press.

Ross, E. (2010) 'Inaugural lecture: African spirituality, ethics and traditional healing – implications for indigenous South African social work education and practice', *South African Journal of Bioethics and Law,* 3(1): 44–52.

Schiele, J. (1994) 'Afrocentricity as an alternative world view for equality', *Journal of Progressive Human Services,* 5(1): 5–25.

Serequeberhan, T. (1991) *African Philosophy: the essential readings,* New York: Paragon House.

Setiloane, G. (1986) *African Theology: an introduction,* Johannesburg: Skotaville.

Shorter, A. (1996) *Christianity and the African Imagination,* Nairobi: Paulines Publications Africa.

Sodi, T., Mudhovozi, P., Mashamba, T., Radzilani-Makatu, M., Takalani, J. and Mabunda, J. (2011) 'Indigenous healing practices in Limpopo Province of South Africa: a qualitative study', *International Journal of Health Promotion and Education,* 49(3): 101–10.

Solomon, A. and Wane, N. (2005) 'Indigenous healers and healing in a modern world', in R. Moodley and W. West (eds) *Integrating Traditional Healing Practices into Counselling and Psychotherapy,* London: Sage.

Thabede, D. (2008) 'The African worldview as the basis of practice in the helping professions', *Social Work/Maatskaplike Werk,* 44(3): 233–45.

Theron, L.C., Theron, A.M.C. and Malindi, M.J. (2012) 'Toward an African definition of resilience: a rural South African community's view of resilient Basotho youth', *Journal of Black Psychology,* 39(1): 63–87.

Washington, K. (2010) 'Zulu traditional healing, Afrikan worldview and the practice of Ubuntu: deep thought for Afrikan black psychology', *The Journal of Pan African studies,* 3(8): 24–39.

Welsing, F.C. (1991) *The Isis Papers: the keys to the colors,* Chicago: Third World Press.

Wheeler, E.A., Ampadu, L.M. and Wangari, E. (2002) 'Lifespan development revisited: African-centred spirituality throughout the life cycle', *Journal of Adult Development,* 9(1): 71–8.

Worthington, E.J., Kurusu, T., McCullough, M. and Sandage, S. (1996) 'Empirical research on religion and psychotherapeutic processes and outcomes: a 10 year review and research prospectus', *Psychological Bulletin,* 119(3): 448–87.

8

Studying social work

Dilemmas and difficulties of Ultra-Orthodox women

Nehami Baum

Introduction

Ultra-Orthodox Jews, termed Haredim in Hebrew, are fundamentalist Jews committed to particularly strict interpretation of Jewish religious law. Concentrated in large cities in the United States and Europe, they comprise a small but unknown percentage of the Jewish people worldwide. However, in Israel, where they are found in several locations, it is estimated they comprise approximately 15–17 per cent of the Jewish population (Central Bureau of Statistics 2006).

Wherever they live, they are a self-secluding group, who separate themselves from the larger society, Jewish and non-Jewish alike, through their choice of distinctive dress, widespread use of Yiddish in daily conversation (among those of European descent) and, most substantively, by a lifestyle centred on precise observance of the many Jewish religious laws that govern all areas of life, from prayer, ritual observances and diet, through family relationships and relations with others (Friedman 1991; Shalhav 2005). Even though Haredi society consists of often fractious and vying factions, all Haredim view the spiritual, cultural, social and political phenomena of the surrounding society as corrupting and as a threat to their values and lifestyle (Caplan 2007; Friedman 1991). Blocking out the surrounding society, they live in Haredi neighbourhoods and send their children to gender-separated Haredi schools, which focus on religious education and do not prepare their pupils for matriculation. To block out information and ideas that are unacceptable to the community's highly conservative worldview, most secular literature is deemed out of bounds, television is forbidden, and internet use is restricted to a few closely supervised Haredi sites. Special cell phones block Sabbath calls.

For the most part, too, higher (non-religious) education has been out of bounds. Haredi men, encouraged to engage in lifelong religious study, have had a very low participation in the workforce (Hakak 2004), whereas Haredi women are expected to support their families economically, despite marrying young and bearing many children. However, the strong emphasis placed on female modesty in the Haredi lifestyle restricts higher education for women. In addition to requiring full body coverage (except for the hands and face), the preservation of modesty means that women must avoid unnecessary contact with men and refrain from activities in the public domain (Caplan 2007; El-Or 1997; Shalhav 2005) as the mingling of the sexes violates the strict gender separation practiced by Haredi society. Contact with non-Haredi students and faculty raises fears of 'assimilation' into the wider society. Furthermore, much of secular learning is viewed with a combination of disdain and apprehension, both as unimportant and as a source of ideas that may undermine the Haredi lifestyle and values.

In recent years, several developments have led to growing recognition in Haredi society of the need for post-high school academic education (Caplan 2003). One is the increasing economic pressure on the average Haredi family. These are large families, where the parents married in their late teens and early twenties and who, in their strict adherence to the commandment to 'be fruitful and multiply', typically have many children. The resulting poverty has been exacerbated by the reduction of special government economic benefits to members of the Haredi community, at much the same time that growing numbers in the community have become less willing to accept poverty as a way of life (Jerby and Levy 2000). Moreover, the community and its leaders, the rabbis, have become increasingly aware of the need for well-qualified professionals from within the community who understand its ways (Aviram and Dahan 2002). Finally, in the wake of the numerical growth of the community, there are an increasing number of individuals within it who want higher education (Sheleg 2000).

Social work is one of the areas where the need for professionals from the community has been strongly felt. After many years of denial, the Haredi community now admits the existence of social problems such as family violence and children's behavioural difficulties, in its midst. Haredi rabbis have come to recognise that social work intervention can be useful in helping community members cope with such difficulties as personal and family problems, normative life transitions and crises such as illness and unexpected death.

The need for Haredi professionals could not be met, however, by any of the institutions of higher education in Israel. Haredi society is characterised by strict gender separation anchored in the Haredi interpretation of Jewish law. Since all of Israel's colleges and universities are co-educational, the required gender separation obviously makes it impossible for Haredim, whether women or men, to attend them. Moreover, the self-imposed cultural segregation of the Haredi community and its fear of contamination through contact with non-Haredim and/or through exposure to information and ideas that are not accepted in the Haredi worldview constitute barriers to their attending any non-Haredi educational institutions, whether co-ed or not.

The outcome has been the beginning of a slow and as yet still limited entrance of Haredi men into the workforce and some acceptance, albeit grudging, from among the rabbis that women have to receive higher education that will better enable them to support their families. Until quite recently, the main profession for which Haredi women were trained was teaching. However, for many years now the number of young Haredi women who wanted to earn their living by means of professional employment has far outnumbered the positions available in teaching.

In the 1990s, these developments in the Haredi community converged with the policy adopted by the Israeli government to bring the increasingly numerous Haredim into the workforce, for which academic education was understood to be necessary. Thus, at about the same time as higher education in general was being expanded in Israel (Shavit *et al.* 2007), the country's Council for Higher Education set out to create culturally-appropriate academic frameworks that would meet the special needs of the Haredi community (Kalaagi 2007).

Establishing a social work programme for Haredi women

The first step in the process was the establishment of a number of colleges for Haredi women, which avoid challenging the values of the Haredi community. A prime example is the Haredi College for Women in Jerusalem. Like other Haredi colleges, it trains the students in practical occupations in which they can obtain gainful employment. In addition to social work, it offers degree programmes in education, medical technology, communication disorders, management, economics and computers. An in-house rabbi is employed to vet the study materials and to advise the students, and day-care is provided on the premises for newborns through toddlers. Where male students are admitted, as is now the case, strict gender separation is maintained. Males and females attend different classes, use the library at different hours, and even walk along different routes in the corridors and on campus so that they do not see members of the opposite sex.

Social work was included among the colleges' programmes of study only after considerable hesitation by the Haredi leadership. The psychological contents of social work education were viewed as alien to Haredi concepts of human behaviour. There was also concern that fieldwork encounters with drug users, persons with psychiatric illnesses, and other social work populations would spoil the Haredi students' innocence. It was only the recognised need for social work intervention in the Haredi community that finally overcame these deterrents. Moreover, since only a BSW is required in Israel for licensing as a social worker, social work studies were regarded as an efficient and practical way to employment.

To be included in the college, social work was defined as a 'sensitive program' (Aviram and Dahan 2002). Although the programme was designed to resemble as closely as possible social work programmes in other academic institutions in Israel, adjustments were made so that culturally sensitive contents were treated with care. For example, contents involving sex were introduced slowly, in careful gradations and avoiding graphic language. Films showing unclothed arms and legs were not shown. Books with long descriptions of behaviours were not used.

The students' experiences

The remainder of this chapter will describe and discuss the findings of research into the motivations and experiences of Haredi social work students in Israel.

Method

Data on 66 current students and 76 graduates of the social work programme were obtained from the files of the Haredi College administration office. The students were between 18 and 51 years (M=22.8, SD=6.53) old when they were accepted to the programme. At the time of acceptance, 70 per cent had never been married, 29 per cent were married, and 1 per cent were divorced; 15 per cent had children (M=4 children); 48 per cent reported that had been Haredi all their lives, 4 per cent that were 'newly Haredi', and 48 per cent that they were 'national-religious', that is modern Orthodox and not Haredi. The participants who had graduated from the social work programme were employed. Most were employed in the Haredi community, though some worked in settings catering to the entire population, such as hospitals.

Thirty-two Haredi students and graduates were recruited to participate in one of four hour-and-a-half long focus groups. Each focus group was led by two social workers with experience with group facilitation and qualitative research. All the interviews were tape recorded and transcribed. Each group opened with a statement informing the participants that we were interested in learning about their decision to study social work at the college and about the processes involved. The participants introduced themselves by first name without providing any other information. They were invited to talk freely. We did not ask specific questions so as not to lead them in a preconceived direction. As they spoke, however, we at times asked them whether they could expand on what they were saying or provide details or examples.

As befitting a subject about which little is known, cross-case thematic content analysis using a phenomenological approach was separately conducted by two coders (Berg 2001; Giorgi 1997). Two main issues were identified. One was the opposition to and support for higher education for women that the study participants encountered before they began their social work education. The other was their dilemmas and ways of coping during their education.

Findings

All in all, the findings tell the story of a relatively small vanguard of women who went on to pursue an academic education, which until very recently no Haredi woman and very few Haredi men in Israel had done. As the interviewees present it, they are exposed to two messages from their communities. One, the traditional message, sounded by their teachers and the older and more conservative members of the community, is that they should not go on to study at all, lest their exposure to the secular education in particular and the outside world in general undermine their religious observance and the cohesion of the community. As they explained it, the opposition was grounded on fear that exposure to the outside world, whether through contact with non-Haredi persons or the secular contents of their studies, would corrupt their innocence, draw her away from Haredi religious practices, and thus undermine the entire Haredi society and way of life. Some interviewees put it succinctly: 'What's the chance you'll stay Haredi if you go on to study?' Others elaborated on the perceived dangers:

> It's scary to someone who raises Haredi children. Exposure to the world outside is very tempting. But not everything that glitters is gold. ... Exposure to certain contents before the right time is problematic. It can cause loss of innocence, which is one of the advantages of Haredi society. Wherever boundaries are broken, one can very quickly fall into the abyss. My Haredi sister-in-law went to study in a non-Haredi religious college. She tells that very quickly she stopped wearing her wig, then started to go about without stockings. If you're not strong enough ...

A related concern that the interviewees reported was that higher education for girls stood in opposition to the value that Haredi society places on family. The concern was that such education would conflict with her designated role as wife and mother and would dim her chances of finding a desirable husband:

> There's tremendous opposition to girls going to college – because it means they'll go on to a career. ... It's something that's not wanted ... as there are higher values: family.

> They [the high school teachers] brainwashed me: "No one will want to marry you", and all kinds of things like that ...

The women were exposed to a tremendous amount of pressure. They were pressured not to matriculate, so as not to be able to meet the prerequisite for higher education, and not to go to college. They were made to feel that they were violating basic religious tenets. 'They believed that matriculation is blasphemous', one interviewee told of her high school teachers. They were made to feel that they were acting in an untoward, totally unacceptable way: 'I was the only one [who went to college] out of all the girls in my cohort. They were really against it... They kept saying to me... "How can you do it?"' In a society where marriage and family are the most important things in life, the prospect of not being able to marry constituted a real threat.

The opposition was not across the board, however. Most of the interviewees told that women in their immediate environment encouraged them and that some even expressed envy:

> When I went to study [social work] I thought all the girls in my class would say "no", "don't do it". Actually, all of them congratulated me, and a lot of them were really supportive. Even now, women who are just my neighbors say, "How great that you had the courage to do that, and that your parents supported you". Wow, you're going to have a career and me ... what am I going to do in another year or two?

Most of the women also received encouragement from their rabbi. In all cases, this encouragement was restricted to study of a clearly defined occupation at the college for Haredi girls. As the following quotation indicates, the rabbis' support was predicated on the notion that having an occupation would increase the girls' earning power and thereby improve their ability to fulfill their role as family provider:

> The rabbi knew about it and encouraged me... Actually, this rabbi encourages any woman who wants to learn an occupation. He told me, "you're going to build a home, you need to have food on the table".

The rabbis' support was not unqualified. Thus, one student told that her rabbi personally approved of her going on to study, but also brought to her attention that not marrying might be the price she would have to pay: 'Who will you marry? ... I'd say you can go to college ... but if you want to find a match, just bear in mind that most men won't want to marry you.' In short, what emerges is a contradiction between the notion that by pursuing an academic education, these women will be doing a vital service for their families and community and the high personal price that the community will exact for their doing it.

Like the rest of the Haredi community, the women interviewed were concerned with how they could pursue their studies while preserving the religious purity of the society and their traditional role as wives and mothers. Their concerns reflect their internalisation of the values of their community and of its perception of higher education as potentially dangerous to the Haredi lifestyle.

Virtually all the interviewees found or crafted ways of overcoming the external opposition to their studying and of mitigating their own inner conflicts. The most common coping tactic, employed by almost all the interviewees, was framing their studying so that it accorded with Haredi values. The women all insisted that they were not pursuing higher education for its own sake or for a career, that they viewed their role in life as wives and mothers, and that their studies were aimed at enabling them to fulfill their obligations as Haredi women to provide economic support for their families.

Another common form of coping was to compromise in their field of study. Most of the interviewees reported that they chose to study social work because social work studies were available at the Haredi college for women. This was the only place where they could go to study, given that their primary consideration was that their place of study be a gender separated Haredi institution. It is quite conceivable that had a wider selection of courses been available, at least some of the women might have chosen a different field. Since, for most of the interviewees, the field of study was apparently secondary to the place of study, however, few of them actually felt that they were making a compromise and few mentioned another field of study that they might have preferred.

The exception was a small number of interviewees who told that they would have preferred studying psychology. Some of them gave up on this preference on their own, stating as their reasons that psychology was not taught at the Haredi college, that it required too many years of study and that it was incompatible with their role as Haredi wife and mother. A few interviewees reported having been strongly pressured not to study psychology. The pressure that was reported came from respected authority figures: a career counsellor chosen by the community or from a rabbi, an esteemed religious leader, who dismissed the possibility and laughed at the woman who raised it. There was no way that these women, brought up in the community and sharing its values, could possibly have acted against the rabbis' directives. In contrast to those who opted for social work without considering other alternatives, these women strongly felt that they had given up something that they wanted, and anger and resentment could be heard in their voices.

Once the students started to study, they encountered two main difficulties: that the contents of their courses were inconsistent with the perspectives of the Haredi community and that the fieldwork expectations and requirements violated the Haredi rules of gender separation. With respect to the course contents, many of the women indicated that they were exposed for the first time to topics whose open discussion is practically taboo in the Haredi community. The topics most frequently mentioned were men, premarital sex and rape. As one put it: 'Thinking about the values I was taught in high school, men were never mentioned in our classes. It's much more open here.'

Also upsetting to the students was their exposure to Freudian theory, which they variously termed 'bizarre', 'funny' and 'totally unacceptable' without further elaboration. The single student who in any way indicated what her objections were referred to Freud's contention 'that a person acts only on the basis of impulses and drives'. This she considered an offensive and 'shameful' claim that denied a person's responsibility for their choices.

With respect to their fieldwork, students told of feeling awkward when a male extended his hand for them to shake and described the thought of having to sit alone in a room with a man as 'scary'. Home visits with single men, even elderly or disabled, were entirely out of bounds. As one student put it: 'Being alone with a man is a violation of religious law, and I don't have to commit that violation just because I'm studying here. I'm not studying in order to stop being Ultra-Orthodox.'

Most of the Haredi students made determined efforts to cope with their distress, to learn the course material, to carry out their fieldwork assignments and to reconcile the discrepancies between their deeply-held Haredi values and ways and the incompatible course contents and expected behaviours. The married students among them, who constituted about half the student body, made the effort even as they fulfilled their responsibilities as mothers and wives in a society where the burden of housework and childcare still falls almost entirely on the woman.

Three types of coping were employed to deal with offensive course contents. The least functional professionally consisted of minimisation and blocking of the course contents, by referring to them as 'bizarre' and 'funny'. This approach was adopted to avoid having to really know and engage with the material. Adopted at an early stage of professional training, this approach makes it impossible for students to properly judge the theory and make an informed choice.

More functional was compartmentalisation, both of course contents and clients' disclosures, adopted to enable the student to deal with the offensive contents in her work while keeping them out of her personal life. This strategy has the advantage of enabling the students to maintain a sense of personal integrity while acknowledging the 'other'.

The most functional strategy, adopted by most of the students, was searching for correspondences with Judaism. This was a way of trying to bridge the discrepancies between the two worlds so as to be able to engage with and integrate unfamiliar, unsettling social work concepts and contents into their worldview with Torah at the centre. In essence this strategy compelled those who adopted it to engage with the contents, enabled them to absorb the material and would later enable them to incorporate what they learned into their professional practice.

Most of the study participants reported seeking rabbinic advice on how to meet the professional demands placed on them without violating the prohibitions. They described their rabbinic consultations as a means of enabling them to carry out problematic fieldwork assignments:

> If you know what to do in advance, and if you ask the right questions, you can overcome the difficulties … There can be a lot of obstacles, but Jewish Law has solutions for every situation.

The interviewees reported different solutions to the prohibitions against handshaking and against being alone with a man in a closed space. They avoided handshaking by politely explaining that it was forbidden them. So as not to be alone with a man in a closed space, they refused to make home visits to male clients and kept their office doors open when they met with their male clients there. On the whole, the students felt that their clients understood and respected their position, However, one student felt that keeping the door of her office open might impair her intervention:

> We sit together, and don't completely shut the door. The door is left open a crack. You can't leave the door wide open. It disrupts the therapeutic process if the door is wide open. If I'm meeting with a woman, I lock the door.

None of the students even mentioned the inconvenience that their refusal to visit single male clients at home might cause.

Where the discrepancies could neither be smoothed over nor compartmentalised within the professional realm, the students used two other means of coping to reduce the dissonance and conflict the discrepancies caused. One was to go through the motions of learning the unacceptable material without internalising it and, in fact, blocking its meaning and implications: 'I have to study it – so I study it. I don't recall finding anything that's contrary to Judaism …' The other was to prioritise the Torah over the thinking and values of the profession: 'I'm not at all sure that we have to "buy" everything they try to sell us. The values of the Torah are much more important, and what we're learning carries no weight in comparison.'

Issues for social work education in fundamentalist religious communities

The findings of the study show how very difficult it is to create a culturally sensitive social work programme for members of a fundamentalist enclave community, which meets both the requirements of the profession and the needs of the students. For virtually all the students, the discrepancies were a source of considerable distress. The students were shocked, discomforted and outraged by the sexual contents and the notion of the unconscious they encountered in their classes and fieldwork. They felt awkward and scared in the face of the potential breaches of the rules of gender separation that confronted them in their fieldwork. In both areas, at least some students felt that their most basic values were being overlooked, ignored and even challenged.

The contents that were problematic for the students were references to sexual matters and instruction in Freudian theory. In theory, it might be argued that these contents are not essential to social work training. Social work training and practice in Israel, however, still retain a strong clinical underpinning. The programme at the Haredi College was designed so that its graduates would be qualified to work in any social work agency in Israel, not only in the Haredi community. Even though a key motive in establishing the programme was to provide Haredi social workers for the Haredi community, the programme's founders were adamant not to restrict the employability of the students or to provide them with a different, potentially second rate, degree. Since a BSW in Israel, whether at the Haredi College or elsewhere, entitles those who possess it to be employed as licensed social workers, it would be counter-productive to eliminate course contents that students find unacceptable or distressing, especially since they will probably encounter some of those contents in their fieldwork and professional lives. With this, it would be advisable to consider whether and how shocking or objectionable contents can be presented in a more palatable, less jarring way and, following the students' lead, to try to draw connections between the contents and the Torah.

With respect to the gender contact prohibitions, it is clear that concessions must be made by the training institution. Given their prioritisation of religious teachings and the rabbis' views, the students will not bend on this matter. Despite the inconvenience that their adherence to the prohibitions may entail for their clients and agency, it may be argued that the same sensitivity be shown in training programmes for distinct populations as is today the accepted norm in social work with persons of different cultures. At the same time, so as to minimise any detrimental impact on the clients, the students should be made aware of the impact that their observances may have on their clients and, to a lesser extent, on their co-workers.

References

Aviram, U. and Dahan, N. (2002) *Mifgash Ben Tarbuti: tachnit nisyonit shel hauniversita haivrit beyerushalayim lehachsharat nashim haradiot leavodah sotzialit* [*Intercultural Meeting: an experimental program of the Hebrew University of Jerusalem for qualifying ultra religious women in the field of social work*], Jerusalem: Ministry of Science, Education and Sport.

Berg, B.L. (2001) *Qualitative Research Methods for the Social Sciences*, 4th edn, Boston: Allyn and Bacon.

Caplan, K. (2003) 'The Haredi society in Israel', in E. Sivan and K. Caplan (eds) *Israeli Haredis: integration without assimilation?* Jerusalem: The Jerusalem Institute for Israeli Studies.

Caplan, K. (2007) *Besod Hasiach Haharedi* [*In the Internal Popular Discourse in Israeli Haredi Society*], Jerusalem: Zalman Shazar Center.

Central Bureau of Statistics (2006) *Yearbook 2006*, Jerusalem: Central Bureau of Statistics.

El-Or, T. (1997) 'Visibility and possibilities: ultraorthodox Jewish women between the domestic and public spheres', *Women Studies International Forum*, 20(5–6): 665–73.

Friedman, M. (1991) *Hahevrah Haharedit – mekorot, megamot vetahalichim* [*Haredi Society: origins, trends and processes*], Jerusalem: Jerusalem Institute of Israel Studies.

Giorgi, A. (1997) 'The theory, practice, and evaluation of the phenomenological method as a qualitative research procedure', *Journal of Phenomenological Psychology*, 28(2): 235–60.

Hakak, Y. (2004) *Vocational Training for Ultra-Orthodox Men*, Jerusalem: The Floersheimer Institute for Policy Studies.

Jerby, I. and Levy, G. (2000) *The Socio-economic Gap in Israel*, Jerusalem: The Israeli Democracy Institute.

Kalaagi, T. (2007) *Conservatism and Openness in a Segregative Fundamentalist Society – The Struggles Revolving Around the Academization Process in the Haredi Sector in Israel in the Beginning of the 21st Century: establishment of the Haredi College in Jerusalem*, Ramat Gan: Bar Ilan University.

Shalhav, Y. (2005) 'Nashim Haradiot ben shnai olamot [Ultra-Orthodox women between two worlds]', *Mifne*, 46–47: 53–5.

Shavit, Y., Ayalon, H., Chachashvili-Bolotin, S. and Menahem, G. (2007) 'Israel diversification, expansion, and inequality in higher education', in Y. Shavit, R. Arum and A. Gamoran (eds) *Stratification in Higher Education: a comparative study*, Stanford, CA: Stanford University Press.

Sheleg, Y. (2000) *The New Religious*, Jerusalem: Keter Publishing.

9

Western Buddhism and social work

Caroline Humphrey

Introduction

Buddhism was transported from the Asian continent to Europe, North America and Australia from the nineteenth century onwards when representatives of colonial powers analysed Buddhist scriptures, art and architecture. At the same time, Asian émigrés were forming Buddhist enclaves in the West (Chappell 2004a). In the twentieth century, Western converts who had been immersed in a Buddhist culture or ordained by a Buddhist preceptor instituted Buddhist orders and meditation centres for Westerners (Chappell 2004b). For example, Roshi Glassman founded the Zen Peacemaker Order in North America (now the Zen Peacemakers) and Sangharakshita established the Friends of the Western Buddhist Order in Britain (now Triratna or The Three Jewels). This coincided with the persecution of Buddhism in swathes of Asia, and Buddhist leaders-in-exile such as the Dalai Lama and Thich Nhat Hanh started to convey Buddhism to a worldwide audience. By the turn of the millennium, information and communication technologies enabled spiritual seekers in the West to access Buddhist writings and participate in online Buddhist conferences (Chappell 2004b). Such an exponential growth of a religion transplanted outside of its cultural milieux entrains the twin dangers of a superficial familiarity alongside profound misunderstandings (Sangharakshita 1996; Wilber 2006). When aspects of this ancient Eastern religion are conjoined with modern Western social work, further confusion could be on the horizon.

The aim of this chapter is to dispel the confusion by distinguishing three levels from which Westerners may approach Buddhist principles and practices. First, the secular level is available to people of any faith or no faith as it invites us to inspect these principles and practices for ourselves, relying upon our human faculties for sensory experiencing, cognitive processing, moral evaluation and scientific investigation. Second, the spiritual level revolves around a transpersonal experiencing of these principles and practices 'from the inside', so it can surface within atheists or Christians who venture into Buddhist territories, although it does not propel them towards abjuring their (non-) religious standpoint. Third, the religious level is chosen by converts who place their faith in the Buddha and who interpret their everyday and esoteric experiences within a Buddhist framework. By deploying this multi-levelled approach to the Buddha's Enlightenment, his teachings on suffering and Buddhist practices to transform our mind and our world, we will be able to pinpoint where Buddhism and Western social work make easy bedfellows, and where they may part company.

The Buddha's Enlightenment

The man who was to become the Buddha was born as Prince Siddhartha Gautama in Northern India (now Nepal) in the fifth century BCE. His excursions beyond the palace unveiled the reality of human suffering (he witnessed old age, sickness and death) and the possibility of a release from suffering (he saw a holy man, a wandering mendicant, at peace with himself). So Siddhartha escaped incognito from the palace in order to pursue a spiritual quest to make sense of and surmount the suffering of the world. He perfected the art of sitting in silence and still-ness under a tree, an introspective practice that became known as meditation, and that yielded Enlightenment (Trainor 2004). It enabled him to comprehend and control the workings of his own mind, as representative of all human minds. It also revealed a trans-human reality, com-prising the evolutionary recycling of species that unfolded in accordance with their condition-ing in the realm known as Samsara, and the distinctively human potential for liberation in an unconditioned realm dubbed Nirvana. When Siddhartha arose from his meditation, he was no longer recognisable. He was asked whether he was a god, a ghost or a man? His reply was that he had destroyed all the conditionings that give rise to such forms and so he was a Buddha – this transliterates as 'one who is awake' in the sense of having awakened to transcendental reality (Sangharakshita 1996: 30–1). He devoted the rest of his long life to expounding his realisations to disciples, lay publics and political rulers in teachings on psychology, morality, meditation and wisdom (the Dharma) and developing communities for monks and nuns (Sanghas).

The Buddha imparted the Dharma in different ways to different audiences in order that the maximum number of people would be able to absorb its messages at a level congruent with their conditioning, their stage of spiritual development and their aspirations (Blum 2004a). Therefore, it is fitting to adopt a multi-levelled approach to the story of the Buddha's Enlightenment. Secular Westerners tend to treat him as an ordinary human being whose insights into humanity and reality can be verified by anyone who deploys his method of meditative introspection and who reflects upon his teachings in relation to world history. As such, they will be adhering to the Buddha's exhortation that everyone should test out his teachings for themselves and follow their own inner light (Ellsberg 2001), but are likely to discard many of the subsequent scriptures as myths. Spiritual seekers and secularists who sustain a meditation practice are likely to experi-ence some transpersonal aspects of the Dharma for themselves, at which point they may hail the Buddha as an extra-ordinary human being, more akin to the mystics of all religions. Given the close association between spirituality and the perennial philosophy, those who reach the Buddha on a spiritual level are likely to believe that once we abstract from the specifics of a given cultural-historical era, the kernel of the Dharma can be found in all moral and religious tradi-tions (cf. Ellsberg 2001; Kabat-Zinn 2005). Western converts partake in a Going for Refuge ceremony, taking refuge in the Three Jewels of the Buddha, the Dharma and the Sangha. They believe that Siddhartha-the-man died under the Bodhi tree and that the Buddha was born as an Enlightened Mind inhabiting Nirvana, and they seek to follow in his footsteps. Enlightenment is bound to be an enigma for non-enlightened minds, so conversion to Buddhism entails a quantum leap of faith (Sangharakshita 1996).

After the demise of the historical Buddha, this new religion evolved into diverse traditions, and the Mahayana tradition predominates in Western Buddhism. Mahayana signifies 'the great vehicle' as it allows for laypeople as well as monks and nuns to attain Enlightenment, but it harbours contradictory strands. On the one hand, there are schools of meditation (Chan in

Chinese, Zen in Japanese), which cultivate the simplicity of mindfulness in everyday life (Blum 2004b). This can appeal to any secularist or spiritual seeker, and Western Buddhists in the caring professions tend to be trained in Zen meditation (e.g. Brazier 2001; Brenner and Homonoff 2004). On the other hand, Mahayana scholars solved the death of the historical Buddha by elaborating cosmologies with an array of archetypal Buddhas and Bodhisattvas (Blum 2004a). Given that this Buddhist pantheon does not feature in the cultural heritage of most Westerners, it requires a vivid spiritual imagination to entertain it, and relevant transpersonal encounters or religious faith to endorse it. The Mahayana ideal is the Bodhisattva – a being who seeks Enlightenment for the sake of all sentient beings and who vows to return to Earth again-and-again until all are free from suffering. The Dalai Lama is regarded as the reincarnation of the Bodhisattva of Compassion, and this Bodhisattva is also the ideal for Buddhist social workers (Canda and Furman 1999). A reconciliation between these Mahayana strands is possible insofar as the Buddha recalled previous lifetimes as a Bodhisattva (see Conze 1959). But Westerners may prefer to interpret Buddhist symbolism through the lens of depth psychology, conceiving of a Bodhisattva as an aspect of our higher self, whether as a conscious ideal or as a hidden potential (cf. Sangharakshita 1996). Such a reading is compatible with the Mahayana belief that an embryonic 'Buddha nature' undergirds all beings since it is co-terminous with cosmic reality itself (Brazier 2001).

The non-duality between Samsara and Nirvana is a core tenet of Mahayana Buddhism. The Buddha referred to himself as the Tathagata, which is translated as 'going the way of suchness or thusness' and applied to one who sees and responds to reality 'as it is' in every moment (Brazier 2001: 37–38). More mysteriously, all Buddhas are Tathagatas insofar as they are 'thus come' and 'thus gone' i.e. they are no-one, 'coming from nowhere and going nowhere', as they inhabit Nirvana, which transcends time, place and personhood (Conze 1959: 166–7). Although all of us are embryonic Buddhas (Tathagata-garbhas), it is only those who have extinguished the sources of delusion who are awake in Samsara, and Nirvana refers to this extirpation of Samsaric conditioning, or the radical purification of consciousness, rather than the exiting of Samsara itself (Ellsberg 2001). A living Bodhisattva embodies Enlightenment on Earth, and Nirvana is only sustainable within Samsara if they represent two different ways of being-on-the-earth, perceiving-the-world and engaging-with-reality, rather than two literal realms. This is why the non-dual has become the philosopher's stone of Western Buddhism (Wilber 2006).

However, the Buddha extemporised his insights into reality with reference to two orders of reality, as they only become one for the Enlightened Mind, and the non-dual can only remain silent when confronted with the artificial divisions of human language (Sangharakshita 1996). This engenders the great chasm in Mahayana scriptures between 'conditioned' and 'uncondi-tioned' reality – so there are psychological and historical truths about the empirical and condi-tioned reality of life-on-Earth now ratified by Western sciences, and cosmic and metaphysical truths about an ultimate, underlying and unconditioned reality disclosed by and to the Buddha (Blum 2004a; Ellsberg 2001; Sangharakshita 1996). To bypass this distinction courts the risk of misunderstanding some doctrines in Western Buddhism and misapplying them to Western social work. This will be exemplified later with reference to the doctrine of emptiness and the associated notions of no-self and non-attachment.

Suffering and its overcoming

The Buddha taught that the conditioned reality of life-on-Earth is characterised by the imper-manence of all things and the inevitability of suffering for sentient beings as their bodies undergo birthing, ageing, decaying and dying. In the case of the human species, the mind amplifies suffering in myriad ways. We develop attachments to our bodies, identities, homes, careers, families, nations and religions. In tandem with this, we are burdened with aversions to disability and mortality, the loss of cherished people and places, and criticisms of our worldviews. The mind also ruminates on wounds from the past and hopes for the future, further compounding our suffering in the present. But the core neurosis is our attachment to the 'self' – in the absence of a belief that 'I' and 'you' exist as separate entities, there can be no other attachments or aversions, as there is no-one to cling to anything, and no-one to love, mourn or despise (Brazier 2001).

The toxic ingredients of attachments and aversions are stirred together in the cauldron of delusion, which refers to our ignorance of the law of conditionality and of our true (Buddha) nature, which lies hidden beneath the debris of conditioning. The law of conditionality is technically rendered as the law of conditioned co-production or the law of dependent origination. In its most general form, it states that whatever arises, arises in dependence upon the preceding conditions, and that whatever changes or ceases, changes or ceases by virtue of a transformation or cessation of the preceding conditions (Conze 1959). In the human world, it also manifests as the law of karma since intentional actions generate consequences; whenever we set out to heal or hurt someone, we are sowing positive or poisonous karmic seeds that will bear fruit in the future; and karma operates within and between lifetimes (Sangharakshita 1996). The Great Physician is another appellation of the Buddha, since he revealed how the mind sows the seeds of suffering, and how we can dig up poisonous roots and plant nutritious seeds in their stead (Brazier 2001).

Abiding by ethical precepts and principles is the first step on the journey towards Nirvana. There are five prohibitions to prevent us from causing suffering to ourselves and others, which are correlated with five injunctions designed to cultivate peaceful and present-focused states of mind, as illustrated in Table 9.1 and adapted from Sangharakshita (1996).

If we practise the virtues we cannot succumb to the prohibitions, but if the virtues are not perfected we will lapse into the vicious cycle of conditioned reactivity – for example, by seeking vengeance upon those who injure us rather than showing them loving-kindness.

It is only when we are steadfast in our morality and the positive psychology associated with it that we are ready to embark upon the next stage of the journey towards Nirvana, i.e. insight-based meditation and the transcendental wisdom it eventually yields (Conze 1959). Transcendental wisdom is the gateway to the unconditioned reality of Nirvana, but this can only be traversed when we have undone the entirety of our conditioning, including our division of the world into self and other, and our assumption that these cultural signifiers point to actual substances. The Buddha saw the universe as a web of interconnections stretching across the infinity of space-time, wherein all elements and entities are in a perpetual process of becoming, transforming from within, transacting with each other and transmuting into each other. At

Table 9.1 Buddhist morality

	Negative prohibitions (Shilas or ethical precepts)	Positive injunctions (Dharmas or ethical principles)
1	Harming sentient beings	Loving-kindness to all sentient beings
2	Taking the not-given	Generosity of giving
3	Sexual misconduct	Contentment of mind and body
4	Untruthful and unkind communications	Truthful and helpful communications
5	Imbibing intoxicating substances	Awareness or mindfulness

this metaphysical level there is only interbeing – a term coined by Thich Nhat Hanh (Ellsberg 2001), but perhaps more accurately rendered as interbecoming. The Buddhist doctrines of 'emptiness' (shunyata) and 'no-self' (anatman) flow from this, since everything and everyone is devoid of an inherent or immutable essence. By extension, this metaphysics overturns conventional morality since nothing and no-one can be intrinsically 'good' or 'bad' (Blum 2004a).

Most secularists raise no objections to the Buddha's teachings on suffering and morality. Beyond a minimal level of maturity, we are cognisant of transitoriness and unsatisfactoriness from our own life-experience, and those who enter the caring professions witness the causes and consequences of suffering in the lives of others. The conduct prohibited by the Buddha is reflected in civil and criminal law, and the positive injunctions are aligned with virtue ethics in the caring professions (Øvrelid 2008). If we peel back the metaphysical layers of the law of conditionality, it is the most ancient rendering of the scientific law of cause-and-effect and systemic theory. A spiritual appropriation of these teachings is accessible to most of us too. The Dalai Lama has pointed out that spiritual seekers and scientists alike are waking up to the reality of interconnectedness (2006), and he acclaims the universal validity of Buddhist virtues at a secular-spiritual level beyond religious disputes (2011). But only a minority of Westerners subscribe to metaphysical beliefs in karmic re-becoming. Their quest is for a radical de-conditioning that destroys all karmic traces, both 'good' and 'bad', in order to become a Bodhisattva or a Buddha in this or a subsequent lifetime (Sangharakshita 1996).

The Buddhist view of suffering and its overcoming may be more contentious among Western social workers. Classic Buddhist scriptures trace all suffering to the root poisons in the human mind, resulting in an introspective and individualistic approach to its overcoming (Mascaró 1973). Although engaged Buddhists acknowledge the societal structures and cultures underpinning inequality and violence, these are also ultimately traceable to destructive mind-states such as greed and hatred. This is reversed in the social work ethos of anti-oppressive practice, where prejudices and predispositions at a personal level are grounded in cultures and structures, so that the diminution of suffering presupposes the dismantling of social systems (Thompson 2012). While destructive mind-states and destructive social systems are two sides of the same coin, which one we prioritise has major implications for practice. Øvrelid (2008) contends that social workers aggravate their suffering by wanting to change the world, and that if they could see societal reality as it is, as a network of causes and conditions beyond their control as individuals, it would release more energies for casework. This resolves the dilemma only if we assume that social work and casework are synonymous, an assumption that can also be challenged from a Buddhist standpoint, as we shall see later.

Social workers may be more perplexed by the idea that nothing is inherently 'good' or 'bad'. Let us recall the great chasm of Mahayana Buddhism. The moral truth that slavery is 'bad' can be juxtaposed to the metaphysical truth of interbecoming, which implies that there is no such thing as 'slavery'. The law of conditionality at a cosmic level means that all phenomena are equally indispensable to the evolution of the universe, so without people-becoming-slaves there would be no people-freeing-slaves either. Definitive moral judgements at an ultimate level are then only possible from the standpoint of infinity and eternity. This yields a supra-mundane morality rather than non-morality, as the Great Compassion arises precisely when we no longer discriminate between self and other, friend and foe, good and bad (Ellsberg 2001). To eschew this transcendental wisdom is to misunderstand Buddhism and to turn away from the Great Compassion; but to interpret it as a licence for doing nothing in the face of societal injustices such as slavery is to misapply transcendental truths to concrete facticities in the socio-historical world. Buddhists are exhorted to live and labour at the interface of two realities, which demands a dialectical movement between engaging with the world as it is in order to alleviate suffering, and retreating from the world in order to touch the transcendental reality that is the ultimate source of healing and understanding. Only Buddhas resolve the tensions of this dialectic by fully realising Nirvana within Samsara (Sangharakshita 1996).

Meditation practices

Westerners who take up meditation in an educational or health care setting are exposed to a secular version of this practice. Pacification meditations are designed to calm the body and clarify the mind so they function as stress management strategies for agitated and anxious people. In strict Buddhist terms, they are methods of purifying our psychology and morality, thus preparing us for the insight-based meditations which engender transcendental wisdom.

While the simplicity of the Zen method of just sitting (zazen) is attractive, it is also arduous, and alternatives such as walking or lying meditations can be more accessible for beginners (Kabat-Zinn 2005). Sitting meditations are facilitated by concentrating on a mantra (phrase) or mandala (image), since when we concentrate on something it allows the debris in our minds to disperse, providing a respite from our internal chattering. The mindfulness of breathing is the most popular concentrative practice, but the modern term 'mindfulness' can be misunderstood (Kabat-Zinn 2005). It is wise to recall the older translations of 'watchfulness' or 'wakefulness' (Mascaró 1973) since the meditator is aware of but not attached to the machinations of the mind, or emptying rather than filling the mind. When we tune into the breath the mind is returned to its rightful place in the body here-and-now; lapses of concentration are also vital to the process, since they tell us about the toxins we carry, and furnish us with opportunities to return to the breath; this in turn demonstrates that we can transcend our mind and its toxins. There is evidence of the benefits of meditation for clinical and non-clinical populations, and an understanding of its operations that is faithful to both Buddhist and Western psychology (cf. Groves 2014; Kabat-Zinn 2005), so it is not surprising that it has been included as an optional module in some social work programmes (Birnbaum 2008).

Meditation acts as a stimulant to spiritual development for many erstwhile secularists, including social work students who have only been exposed to an eight-week course (Birnbaum 2008). In Buddhist terms, when pacification meditations generate an experience of bliss, we have arrived at the first dhyana, a transpersonal state of consciousness that propels us beyond discursive, discriminatory and dualistic thought, unveiling the first glimpses of our Buddha nature (Sangharakshita 1996). The hallmark of transpersonal experiences is a dissolution of boundaries between self and others, and there are loving kindness meditations to enhance our receptivity to this. Here, loving kindness is initially directed towards one's self, then re-directed to loved ones, strangers and enemy figures, and eventually radiated out to all sentient beings (Kabat-Zinn 2005).

Buddhists who meditate on a religious level undergo a journey of spiritual death and rebirth. Sangharakshita (1996) sketches out two insight-based meditations reserved for people ordained into his Western Buddhist Order. The six-element practice confronts us with our mortality as we meditate upon the demise of the body and mind, relinquishing each of the elements constitutive of our being (earth, water, fire, air, space and consciousness) to the universe from which they emerged, and realising that none of them ever belonged to us, that we are not identical with elements, body or mind, that 'I' am no-thing and no-one at all. This is an experiential realisation of the doctrines of emptiness and no-self (cf. Kabat-Zinn 2005). It is also the void from which we can be reborn within this lifetime, or the great opportunity for breaking the chains of our conditioning. Ordination involves being given a new name and a seed mantra related to a Buddha or Bodhisattva, and ordained members undertake a daily visualisation meditation to nurture this seed. So a committed Buddhist becomes a midwife charged with the birth and growth of a transcendental self, which recognises that the division between self and others is illusory.

Meditation at the secular-spiritual interface would be beneficial to most social workers, particularly if cultivated in a consistent manner so that it becomes a preventative rather than remedial approach to stress management. Birnbaum (2008) makes a convincing argument that the admixture of awareness-with-acceptance in mindfulness meditations is an antidote to the endless rounds of theoretical analysis and critical reflection in social work education, promoting a more healthy balance between the senses and the mind, emotions and cognition, striving for achievements and letting-be or letting-go. The most scholarly students, as well as their academic educators, can encounter more pitfalls in meditation. Intellectuals are more likely to be weighted down by a discursive mode of consciousness; if they manage to jettison this, they are more likely to soar into space, detaching their mind from their body and the world; and this is tantamount to an alienated rather than integrated awareness (Sangharakshita 1996). The message is that *all* of our experiencing has to be cooked in the pot of mindfulness. The paradox is that the cooking takes place all by itself, and our only contribution is to sit down in the non-doing of a non-discursive and non-discriminatory attentiveness (Kabat-Zinn 2005).

The erasure of self, others and attachments at the spiritual-religious interface is troubling for social workers. Once again we need to distinguish between metaphysical and psychological layers of truth and reality. It is impossible to relinquish one's self or to countenance spiritual death-and-rebirth if one has not yet attained authentic selfhood on a psychological level, so a Buddhist monk or nun retains their individuality and integrity in everyday life (Wilber 2006). Similarly, non-attachment is more pertinent for adults facing significant losses around divorce, disability and death (Masel *et al.* 2012), and may be harmful if applied to young children who need secure attachments as the incubator for psychological maturity. In concrete terms, this means that a social worker who encouraged a vulnerable adult to free themselves of ego or a child to weaken their attachments to care-givers in the name of Buddhist principles, would be guilty of misunderstanding and misapplying them.

Worldly engagements

The phrase 'engaged Buddhism' was coined by Thich Nhat Hanh in the 1960s. He developed a School of Youth for Social Services in Vietnam as an offshoot of his Order of Interbeing, and trained social work students in mindfulness before sending them out into rural areas, initially to educate children, and later to rebuild villages after their bombardment (Ellsberg 2001). In the Western world, it is best exemplified by Roshi Glassman's Zen Peacemaker Order. He initiated street retreats where his students lived on the streets of New York among homeless people, an experiential exercise in seeing 'reality as it is' from the perspective of disprivileged others. Informed by this grassroots perspective, the students set up affordable housing managed by the residents, a bakery providing apprenticeships for those deemed unemployable and a health care centre for people with HIV/AIDS (King 2009).

Viewed from the outside, such endeavours are scarcely distinguishable from the work of community-oriented social workers who often subscribe to a secular ideology. But we do not have to delve far into the inside to bear witness to the spiritual underpinnings of socially engaged Buddhism. It is predicated upon interbeing, so when Western Buddhists mobilise for environmental protection, they invent rituals to cultivate empathy for the suffering of all sentient beings and planet Earth (Macy 2007). By contrast, its specifically religious core is often concealed from the Western gaze. The Dalai Lama's peaceful negotiations with the Chinese government that desecrated his country are rooted in a belief in karma. Karmic logic intimates that the Tibetans may have perpetrated injustices against their Chinese neighbours in the distant past, in which case they must bear the consequences. Furthermore, the Tibetans can be grateful towards the Chinese for an opportunity to perfect the virtues that will expunge their karma, so the oppressors who have not yet harvested the fruits of their violence are in greater need of compassion than their victims (King 2009).

Western social workers are likely to repudiate the doctrine of karma. A retrospective reading of karma is oppressive if it showers praise or blame upon people for what in secular terms is an accident of birth, while legitimating status hierarchies around caste, disability and gender. A prospective reading of karma is more empowering as it imparts the message that our fate is in our own hands, given that our future is already being incubated in our present, which is always malleable to some extent (King 2009). Social work would be more enriched by locating itself within the community of interbeing. This presupposes a reformulation of our conception of the person-in-their-environment so that it encompasses our earthly habitat, along with the abandonment of socialist economics that also exploits scarce natural resources to cater to spiralling human greed (Coates 2007). Contra Øvrelid (2008), this is an entreaty to social work as a profession to reorient itself towards communities and take on the suffering of the world.

In the meantime, Western social workers will continue to undertake casework. A small-scale study of Zen-trained social workers in North America showed that the main contribution of Zen was to enable them to empty themselves of ego on the one hand, and professional theories and techniques on the other, in order to be fully present with clients in the here-and-now (Brenner and Homonoff 2004). But this is only one side of the equation, and the danger is that the client's self-absorption can increase in tandem with the professional's self-emptying, with ruminations on the past and the future being reinforced by our discursive methods (Brazier 2001). The other conundrum is that Zen masters are renowned iconoclasts, prepared to jettison venerable teachings and to improvise as they see fit at any given time. So in Brandon's (1976) candid account of his Zen-inspired social work in Britain, we find departures from standard practices and even professional ethics. In a youth offending context, he threw the ignition keys of a teenager's motorcycle down a drain; and when dealing with domestic violence, he threatened to assault the husband if the latter assaulted his wife again, and then carried out this threat.

From a Buddhist perspective, the question is whether such spontaneous acts reflect a conditioned human nature or the Buddha nature? From a social work perspective, the problem is that however we answer this question, our codes and curricula seem irrelevant. My advice is that social workers should treat their theories, techniques and codes in the way that Buddhists treat the Dharma. The Buddha's analogy was that the Dharma is a raft ferrying us across the ocean of Samsara, a raft which can be abandoned when we reach the shore of Nirvana insofar as it may become an obstacle to the rest of our journey (Ellsberg 2001). The corollary is that a premature dismantling of the raft could drown us.

Conclusion

Globalisation facilitates and necessitates a multi-levelled approach to Buddhism, which has been depicted here as a continuum between the secular, the spiritual and the religious, a continuum that allows for both intersections and quantum leaps between levels. Most social workers and clients in Western countries will be operating at the interface of the secular and the spiritual when applying Buddhist principles and practices, and they have latitude in whether to adopt a more secular or spiritual orientation. It is only when social workers are committed Buddhists or when they are dealing with clients from Buddhist communities that the religious level comes to the foreground (Wisner 2011). While a religious orientation to Buddhism has spawned sublime ideals, ranging from the Bodhisattva of Compassion to the community of interbeing, it is inseparable from a metaphysics that can be misappropriated by Westerners, particularly if it is not recognised as such.

References

Birnbaum, L. (2008) 'The use of mindfulness training to create an "accompanying place" for social work students', *Social Work Education*, 27(8): 837–52.

Blum, M.L. (2004a) 'Mahayana Buddhism', in K. Trainor (ed) *Buddhism: the illustrated guide*, 2nd edn, London: Duncan Baird.

Blum, M.L. (2004b) 'Chan and Zen: the way of meditation', in K. Trainor (ed) *Buddhism: the illustrated guide*, 2nd edn, London: Duncan Baird.

Brandon, D. (1976) *Zen in the Art of Helping*, London: Routledge and Kegan Paul.

Brazier, D. (2001) *Zen Therapy: a Buddhist approach to psychotherapy*, London: Constable and Robinson.

Brenner, M.J. and Homonoff, E. (2004) 'Zen and clinical social work: a spiritual approach to practice', *Families in Society*, 85(2): 261–9.

Canda, E.R. and Furman, L.D. (1999) *Spiritual Diversity in Social Work Practice: the heart of helping*, New York: The Free Press.

Chappell, D. (2004a) 'The expanding community', in K. Trainor (ed) *Buddhism: the illustrated guide*, 2nd edn, London: Duncan Baird.

Chappell, D. (2004b) 'Society and the Sangha', in K. Trainor (ed) *Buddhism: the illustrated guide*, 2nd edn, London: Duncan Baird.

Coates, J. (2007) 'From ecology to spirituality and social justice', in J. Coates, J.R. Graham, B. Swartzentruber and B. Ouellette (eds) *Spirituality and Social Work: selected Canadian readings*, Toronto: Canadian Scholars' Press.

Conze, E. (1959) *Buddhist Scriptures*, London: Penguin.

Dalai Lama (2006) *The Universe in a Single Atom: how science and spirituality can serve our world*, London: Little, Brown.

Dalai Lama (2011) *Beyond Religion: ethics for a whole world*, London: Rider.

Ellsberg, R. (2001) (ed) *Thich Nhat Hanh: essential writings*, New York: Orbis.

Groves, P. (2014) 'Buddhist approaches to addiction recovery', *Religions*, 5(4): 985–1000.

Kabat-Zinn, J. (2005) *Coming to Our Senses: healing ourselves and the world through mindfulness*, London: Piatkus.

King, S.B. (2009) *Socially Engaged Buddhism*, Honolulu: University of Hawai'i Press.

Macy, J. (2007) 'Eco-spirituality', in F. Gales, N. Bolzan and D. McRae-McMohan (eds) *Spirited Practices: spirituality and the helping professions*, Crows Nest, New South Wales: Allen and Unwin.

Mascaró, J. (1973) *The Dhammapada*, London: Penguin.

Masel, E. K., Schur, S. and Watzke, H. H. (2012) 'Life is uncertain. Death is certain. Buddhism and palliative care', *Journal of Pain and Symptom Management*, 44(2): 307–12.

Øvrelid, B. (2008) 'The cultivation of moral character: a Buddhist challenge to social workers', *Ethics and Social Welfare*, 2(3): 243–61.

Sangharakshita (1996) *A Guide to the Buddhist Path*, Birmingham: Windhorse.

Thompson, N. (2012) *Anti-Discriminatory Practice: equality, diversity and social justice,* 5th edn, Basingstoke: Palgrave Macmillan.

Trainor, K. (2004) 'The career of Siddhartha', in K. Trainor (ed) *Buddhism: the illustrated guide*, 2nd edn, London: Duncan Baird.

Wilber, K. (2006) *Integral Spirituality: a startling new role for religion in the modern world*, Boston: Shambhala.

Wisner, B.L. (2011) 'Exploring the lived religion of Buddhists: integrating concepts from social work and religious studies', *Journal of Religion and Spirituality in Social Work*, 30(4): 385–404.

10

Achieving dynamic balancing

Application of Daoist principles into social work practice

Celia Hoi Yan Chan, Xiao-Wen Ji and Cecilia Lai Wan Chan

Introduction

Daoism (also known as 'Taoism') is one of the great indigenous philosophical traditions in Chinese communities, which encompasses philosophical and/or religious teachings and practices. The primary tenets were described in *Dao De Jing*, the most influential classic text. This chapter will briefly discuss the essential principles of Daoist teachings, based on the basic tenets of Daoist philosophy including 'Dao' (the way), 'De' (virtue) and 'Yin-Yang perspectives'. On the basis of a comprehension of these three concepts, 'Wuwei' (non-coercive action), 'Ziran' (naturalness), 'Su' and 'Pu' (simplicity) will be introduced, which can also serve as the theoretical underpinnings in developing contemporary social work practice.

Daoist teachings acknowledge that human beings are living in a world with constant changes, which may bring pain and suffering in life. People are asked to go with the flow of nature and the universe so as to achieve personal growth and self-transformation. Informed by Daoist teachings, we proposed a new concept in psychosocial intervention termed 'dynamic balancing', explained as a constant self-transforming process interacting with the ever-changing external environment. By adopting a moving symbolic representation of Yin-Yang symbols, dynamic balancing can be comprehended as a state of mind or a way of living addressing the co-existence of strengths and weaknesses, resilience and vulnerabilities, positivity and negativity. This is in keeping with the person-centred and strength-based orientation of social work practices.

In this chapter, we aim to:

1   demonstrate how the Daoist concepts can be applied into social work practice, such as by enhancing clients' internal capacity in facing life transitions and changes;
2   discuss the emotional competences of human service professionals with reference to elements in Daoist teachings;
3   review empirical studies that demonstrated the application of Daoist teachings into social work practice and research; and
4   introduce the body-mind-spirit techniques that have developed based on Daoist philosophy, which aims to help people achieve the internal state of dynamic balancing, accept changes in life and be aware of afflictive attachment to any desire.

Basic tenets of Daoist teachings

Daoism is an ancient Chinese tradition. Its primary tenets were recorded in *Dao De Jing* and were considered as the most influential classic texts in Daoist teaching and philosophy. Derived from Daoist teaching, a series of regime practices has been developed by followers over the centuries.

Dao and De

Dao, as interpreted and embedded with rich connotations, represents the way of nature and the universal laws (Lee 2003). The Chinese character 'Dao' consists of two pictorial parts: 1) 'to go' and 2) 'head', which also means the origin. The combined characters signify the meaning of going with the natural and right way by following the origin. The spiritual aspect of Dao is considered as a metaphysical path referring to 'a vast oneness … generate the endlessly diverse forms of the world', that has no form and cannot be described but can be perceived in its process of dynamic transformation between opposites (Lee *et al.* 2009: 70), such as Yin-Yang, moon–sun and female–male that describe the dynamic flux of the universe. As summarised by Chang (1977: 27), the meaning of Dao is 'the substance of the cyclic and dynamic universe. It (Dao) seems empty but full, static but dynamic; it contains spiritual and materialistic attributes, time and space; and it produces and regulates activities of all beings'.

As elucidated in the classic texts of *Dao De Jing*, De is another pivotal concept, which was denoted as harmony with fellow human beings in terms of humanistic behaviours, virtues, characters, influences or moral forces. The Chinese character 'De' consists of three pictorial parts: 1) 'to go' or behaviours, 2) values or standards and 3) the heart or attitude. The word 'De' implies motivation by inward rectitude (Lee 2003). Watson (1993) defined De as moral virtue or power that one acquires through being in accordance with Dao; that is what one gets from Dao.

Actionless/non-coercive action

According to *Dao De Jing*, 'Wuwei' means non-action or non-doing. Human beings are supposed to be in harmony with the 'Dao' if they behave in a natural or uncontrived way (Yeates 2015). Therefore, the goal of Daoist practice is the attainment of the natural way of behaving, whereas purposeful manipulation or control will result in a counterproductive effect because it usually runs against natural rules or the Dao. Wuwei, as a non-acting status of an individual, can be applied into social work practice by facilitating people to be and become part of the universe. As elaborated by Chen and Holt (2002), Wuwei does not mean doing nothing; instead, it emphasises the importance of following the way of nature by doing nothing purposefully but accomplishing things as they unfold. It is the 'good order' illustrated by Laozi, the author of *Dao De Jing*, when he wrote, 'When there is this abstinence from action, good order is universal' (Chapter 3) and 'The Dao in its regular course does nothing (for the sake of doing it), and so there is nothing which it does not do' (Chapter 37).

Metaphor of water-representation of Dao and De

Water is an effective metaphor Laozi used to describe Dao because water resembles Dao's attributes of softness/weakness, subordination and non-completion (Chen and Holt 2002). For example, in the *Dao De Jing* it is written:

> The highest excellence is like (that of) water. The excellence of water appears in its benefiting all things, and in its occupying, without striving (to the contrary), the low place which all men dislike. Hence (its way) is near to (that of) the Dao ... And when (one with the highest excellence) does not wrangle (about his low position), no one finds fault with him.
>
> (Chapter 8)

Moreover, the cyclical movement of water also features functions of dynamic and vigorous Dao. As Yu (2012) further argued, Dao flows as a river, continuously gaining strength by gathering streams together and exerting its impact by downward flowing without contentiousness. Thus, such features of water also denote essentials of the De (virtue) that is the operation of Dao in social and moral senses that can be perceived and performed by human beings. Lee (2008) further posited personality aspects of 'wateristic' features with five essential components: 1) altruism, 2) modesty, 3) flexibility, 4) transparency and honesty and 5) gentleness with perseverance. By nourishing everything in a non-coercive way and assembling strengths through weakness and from lower places, water-like characteristics give a reified image of De.

Ziran (naturalness) and Su and Pu (simplicity)

Along with the notion of Wuwei and the water metaphor, Daoist teachings take much notice of the concepts of naturalness and simplicity. Naturalness is the supreme principle (Dao is modeled on naturalness) that reflects ultimate concerns toward the world and human beings (Liu 2004). Meanwhile, Su and Pu (simplicity) are aligned with naturalness that describes a natural state of humanity. 'Su' refers to raw silk that is unstained and 'Pu' refers to an unprocessed log; both of which are in their natural state, and therefore praised by Laozi. In order to stay Su and Pu, one also needs to limit one's own selfish desire. In this sense, simplicity does not mean an uncultivated state but a state that preserves the original beauty of human nature and avoids contamination by lusting on it. Thus, followers of Daosim over the centuries have spoken of the need to 'return to Pu (simplicity) and back to Zhen (authenticity)', which is now a well-known phrase in the Chinese community. This idea is crucial when living in an ever-changing world along with the flow of universal forces that denote impermanence and transition from one state to another (Yeates 2015). Therefore, Daoism advocates that human beings should live harmoniously with nature in a state of simplicity, following the universal laws and principles of nature that are beyond the will of human beings.

Theoretical underpinnings of Daoist teachings in social work practice

Maintaining harmony with nature and the universe

An ideal relationship between human beings and nature is 'Tian Ren He Yi', which means humans are absorbed into nature and the universe, and all are unified into oneness (Lee *et al.* 2008). To reach this state of oneness, an individual needs to cultivate 'Qi' and have a healthy lifestyle, harmonic life attitude and perform energy-generating physical exercise. One of the most distinctive practices is Qigong (Ai *et al.* 2001). Qi is a dynamic energy that flows constantly. The balanced Qi-flow through and around the body can lead to an intuitive connection to Dao (Kohn 2011). Qigong involves training in Qi-regulation that is vital to an individual's life, and can facilitate communication between human beings and nature. Another traditional healthcare practice in cultivating Qi is acupuncture, which has long been utilised in Traditional Chinese Medicine. Qi, combined with Jing (life essence) and Shen (spirit), are three important life energies in Daoism (Chan *et al.* 2014a). External energy is inhaled and progressively converted into higher forms (from Qi to Jing to Shen), and refined energy returns to the outside environment (Yeates 2015). Hence, by practicing Qigong, Taiji (one kind of dynamic Qigong, relative to static Qigong), the body and mind will be closely connected to the greater universe with the state of no-self (body-self), no-desire and authentic spirit as body-form merges with cosmic forces (Kohn 2011).

Dynamic balancing through Yin-Yang completion

Dynamic balancing in life is considered as the unification of two opposite but complementary forces, namely Yin and Yang. The existence of both Yin and Yang keeps a balanced equilibrium in the universe. When the two types of force join together and complement each other, balance will be achieved and Qi will also be generated. As written in Chapter 42 of the *Dao De Jing*:

> All things leave behind them the Obscurity (Yin, out of which they have come), and go forward to embrace the Brightness (Yang, into which they have emerged), while they are harmonised by the Breath of Vacancy.

Yin-Yang concepts are another fundamental and primitive metaphor rooted in Daoism. Everything in the world comprises Yin and Yang. Yin and Yang are considered as related to Qi in Daoism. There is a waxing and waning relationship between Yin and Yang and they can transformed into each other. As Yang expands, Yin reduces and vice versa. They are interdependent with and cannot exist without each other, with Yang giving birth to Yin and Yin giving birth to Yang. Hence, Yin-Yang is not static but dynamic; their nature flows and changes with time and context. The key attributes of Yin and Yang are described in Table 10.1.

Dynamic balancing highlights the transformational nature of Yin and Yang rather than being a comparison between polar opposites (Grønning *et al.* 2011). All entities are correlated with each other in this universe, and there is no cut-off or absolute essence of events. As noted in the *Dao De Jing*, the movement of Dao is in a manner of 'to return'; hence, nature acts in a cyclical instead of linear pattern connoted in dynamic balancing. It also resembles the on-going process of life with co-existing opposite forces complementing and mutually transforming each other in a non-coercive manner, which has informed the existential concern of life and death, ups and downs in life, strengths and weaknesses. Basically, an on-going process of life is dynamic that is driven by various forces and keeps moving in physiological and mind–spiritual senses.

Table 10.1 The attributes and symbols of Yin and Yang

Yang	Yin
Masculinity	Femininity
Positivity	Negativity
Sun	Moon
Light	Dark
Active	Passive
Fire	Water
Hot	Cold
Strengths	Weaknesses
Expressive	Calm
Birth	Death

Thus, there is always a chance to change and to keep one's balance alongside/inside dynamics of 'the way' by gradual strength-gaining processes, especially when an individual is struck with numerous life predicaments that can include physical illness, psychological distress and spiritual disorientation.

Self-cultivation: observing and respecting the cycles of life

In conventional social work practice, one of the objectives is to empower people to survive and thrive when confronting adverse life events. In order to facilitate better worker–client connections, which support people facing difficulties, practitioners have to learn to observe and respect the flow of developmental life cycles. It is the dynamic of action and non-action in the course of helping, especially when people are dealing with life unpredictability. The personhood of the practitioner can be understood as the emotional capacity to provide support to negative and vulnerable clients and not be prevented in the helping process. Therapeutic alliances built on a safe and nurturing environment could facilitate the therapeutic relationship between practitioner and client.

As informed by the *Dao De Jing*, the characteristics of softness and modesty are essential strengths needed in order for people to confront negative predicaments. Famous analogies of grass and tree, and tongue and teeth depict Laozi's philosophy of 'softness overcoming hardness', denoting that when storms come, strong wood is more easily broken than soft grass. Similarly, it has been proposed that the soft tongue survives longer than hard teeth when aging. From this perspective, life difficulties can be understood as necessary developmental processes. Staying strong or hard is not necessarily an effective strategy in coping with stressful life events. Non-action in terms of acknowledging limitations and vulnerabilities and respecting simplicity is a way to maintain dynamic balancing in life. An individual needs to be aware of the calamity brought by being preoccupied with the physical self; as well as the need to reduce selfish and excessive desires (Chen and Holt 2002).

Applications of Daoism into contemporary social work practice

A growing body of literature has examined and discussed the applicability of Daoist philosophy to healthcare practices. Specifically, Traditional Chinese Medicine practices, such as Qigong, Taiji and acupuncture, which are derived from Daoism, have received attention from practitioners and researchers.

To capture the ideal state of Daoist practice, Yeates (2015: 22) proposed the term 'flow state experiences' (FSEs) in Taiji practices for patients with neurological conditions, which is defined as 'experiential continuity, deep absorption, and a merging of self-awareness and activity'. Research has revealed unique benefits of long-term practice of Taiji (Wei *et al.* 2014). Given that neurological patients experience incoherent and fragmented cognitive states, Taiji is considered an effective intervention to facilitate consistency in FSEs. Various studies have also evaluated the efficacy of Taiji in other clinical groups. It has been reported that Taiji can improve physical functioning (flexibility, balance, muscular strengths, etc.) as well as some aspects of physiological wellbeing, such as cardiovascular function and immune system (Klein and Adams 2004; Lee *et al.* 2007). When compared with sitting meditation in dealing with uncontrollable rumination, Taiji practice can minimise the teaching and instruction of verbal knowledge and focus on embodied movement. A more recent review addressed psychological benefits that can be gained from Taiji, especially among those suffering from depression (Wang *et al.* 2014).

Table 10.2 Body–mind techniques developed from Traditional Chinese Medicine

Body–mind techniques	Descriptions	Objectives
One-second techniques	'Easy to learn' physical exercises that involve moving or massaging various parts of body, which can be practiced in various settings (such as taking bus, watching TV or strolling)	Nourish one's bodily well-being Use the movement of body to connect emotion
Ten-minute longevity acupressure	Bodily massage of meridian in ten points of whole body within ten minutes	Stimulate blood circulation and relax body
Clapping-hand Qigong	Classic exercise of Daoism regime. Splay ten fingers and clap two hands strenuously	Stimulate acupoints at hands, circulate blood through whole body, and nourish Qi and blood
Six healing breaths techniques	Inhale deeply through nose and exhale slowly through mouth with six different exhalations, each one involving one of six Chinese characters (Xi, He, Wu, Xu, Chui, Si)	Regulate Qi to balance associated with five organs

Likewise, different forms of Qigong were also found effective in improving holistic wellbeing. Recently, Chan and her associates have conducted a series of clinical trials examining the effectiveness of Baduanjin (also translated as Eight Section Brocade) on a wide range of physical and psychosocial areas including sleep quality, depression, anxiety, fatigue, physical functioning and telomerase activity for people with chronic fatigue syndrome, insomnia, depression and anxiety (Chan *et al*. 2014c; Ho *et al*. 2012).

Based on Daoist teachings and health philosophies in Traditional Chinese Medicine, Chan and associates (2002) developed the Integrative body-mind-spirit (I-BMS) social work practice. It embraces a holistic orientation, and the interconnectedness of body, mind and spirit as well as the environment. Further, I-BMS provides a unique framework in understanding changes, transition and illness, which emphasises mutuality, complementarity and balance. If a system is out of balance, it tends to polarise forces and the individual becomes disconnected and stagnant, manifested by bodily and emotional symptoms. A selection of body–mind techniques are described in Table 10.2.

In addition to body–mind exercise, Daoist philosophical themes comprise a far richer comprehensive implication in social work practice. A study found that rumination can predict chronicity of depressive disorder and anxiety symptoms, and it may be a particular feature of mixed anxiety/depression symptoms (Nolen-Hoeksema 2000). Setting off personal maladaptive attachments and excessive rumination results in states of imbalance and the need to depolarise these negative forces so as to return to a state of dynamic balancing.

Empirical studies of I-BMS approach

Informed by Daoist teaching, the affliction and equanimity framework is a valued effort to redefine the concept of wellbeing by emphasising the interconnectedness of body, mind and spirit (Chan *et al*. 2014a). Affliction is conceptualised as a consequence of maladaptive attachment. Affliction manifests as emotional vulnerability, including displays of resentment, jealousy and bitterness. Somatically, the affliction is in the form of irritability and nervousness. In the spiritual domain, an existential threat underlies affliction when the individual loses their direction and meaning of life. On the contrary, equanimity is perceived as an ideal state of wellbeing, which is achieved by internal cultivation of mindfulness and compassion, while also abolishing the illusion of self. Specifically, equanimity encompasses a mindful awareness toward internal and external stimulus, a bodily vitality and expanded self in relatedness to others and the whole world. This framework has been operationalised by Chan and her colleagues (2014b) into a Holistic Wellbeing Scale (HWS).

I-BMS intervention has been found effective in various clinical trials since 2000. Recent research showed that people with anxiety and depression benefitted after participating in the I-BMS group intervention (Chan *et al.* 2012; Ho 2014; Sreevani *et al.* 2014). Beside psychosocial parameters, spiritual wellbeing was also enhanced as measured by the subscales of spiritual disorientation and spiritual self-care in HWS (Chan *et al.* 2014b). Similar results have been found in other effectiveness studies on sleeping disturbances and mood distress (Chan *et al.* 2015), and in our recent research on people living with psoriasis.

Spiritual growth through dynamic balancing: ways of living with psoriasis

From a perspective of dynamic balancing, clients coming to I-BMS groups are usually those feeling that their life is out of balance, and are finding it difficult to harness the energy and strengths needed to attain tranquility. That is to say, their life energy is mostly blocked in one pole. Accordingly, the I-BMS approach aims at facilitating participants to regain a new distinct form of dynamic balancing from their previous state via self-cultivation and self-transformation in the face of their personal difficulties. In the specific case of psoriasis patients, the main goal is to help them to find inner resources that can aid them to accept and appreciate themselves while living with this incurable chronic disease. Some participants realised a process of self-transformation from an ill patient to a helper, and were then able to benefit others with what they had learnt from I-BMS. Although they still face symptom fluctuations and difficulties in life, the participants became more aware of their relations to uncontrollable things and learnt to preserve their equanimity.

From resolution to non-coercive action

It is not uncommon that patients tend to treat disease as their opposite, the rival, enemy, and thus intend to defeat it for good as soon as possible. Yet, this may not be possible for patients with chronic physical conditions where the disease is incurable and the aetiology is also not clearly explained. Psoriasis is one such disease. In addition to a patient's appearance being impacted, invisible joint pain is also common among sufferers. Mr T. is one of these patients. At the completion of the course, he had transformed his intention of curing his disease into an overcoming process with non-coercive action. He tells his story:

> I have this chronic illness for more than 30 years. I always want to "overcome" or "solve" the psoriasis. But it was quite often that consequence did not meet my expectation, then I would become more depressed, unhappier resulting in generating negative energy. This conditions would definitely affect my illness negatively in return. Worker remind me of that indeed, the process of "overcoming" the problem is also important … working on something to solve the problem is already a very good attitude. Although things often do not come out in particular way we wished, you still can have some gains during the whole process. After I become aware of this point. I relax myself a little bit. I know there is no need to perceive solution of problem as a must … Body scan is also beneficial … when I

am scanning some painful joints before sleep, I will also smile to accept this fact gently that it is pain ... today I feel painful, but I may have another kind of feeling tomorrow.

Flow with the 'naturalness'

In the I–BMS framework, participants learn to experience a sense of simplicity and naturalness, by using simple body–mind exercises adopted to circulate Qi and blood inside participants and to facilitate interaction with the wider world. Through body–mind practices and spiritual reflection on Yin-Yang balancing, learning of acceptance and non-coercive action, Ms L. was able to respect and follow the flow of life, foster her physical and emotional capacities as well as transform her difficulties into life wisdom:

> Psoriasis is really very dreadful ... it can be very severe ... I plan to insist practicing things I learnt here and try to contribute my limited time to share with others and spread the benefits to other patients ... When we do the reflection this week, I realised that for many things, I can let them go, do not need to bear them all.

In addition to Qigong movement, Mr Y. found that activities focusing on self-reflection and self-connection also helped to move him from psychological senses:

> Despite the body exercises, the most impressive moment is the lesson focusing on who I am. Previously, I never tried to inner talk before. I feel that this skill (talk to myself) I learnt from this course is very beneficial. I will do it regularly ... Although I am quite nerdy and seldom went out before. Yet, after attending this courses every Saturday, I plan to commit myself to all these physical exercises, mindfulness and self-connections to keep it (the balancing) running.

Likewise, Mr S. felt he had overcome some of the negative impacts of his illness, and kept a healthy lifestyle by doing aerobic exercises. However, there were still some things he could learn to do in order to enhance the dynamic balancing he had already attained:

> Here I found that there are a variety of ways to express emotions. This is really a holistic course. Before this, my solution was quite unilateral. I found that there are many other means to keep myself healthy in mind-spiritual aspects ... also, during sharing sessions, I witnessed various kinds of energy were released.

Challenges and future directions

Despite the promising results in empirical studies, the application of Daoist teachings into contemporary social work practices is still experiencing great challenges. The more salient predicament is the modern translation of Daoist concepts. Daoism has been developed and evolved through centuries, and the foundational tenets have been interpreted by scholars in various ways. Our work primarily focuses on the teachings generated by Laozi so as to avoid excessive complexity. Other Daoist Masters' works (i.e. *Nan Hua Zhen Jing* of Zhuangzi) are still worthwhile to investigate.

In terms of the practices developed under Traditional Chinese Medicine, Qigong, Taiji and acupuncture feature as the most well-known, while the spiritual practices and reflections of Daoist teachings are largely neglected. I–BMS is almost the first attempt to address the core concepts of Daoism and to integrate them into social work practices. Incorporating Daoist philosophy into healthcare or social work practice is still under an initial stage of construction.

Future research should be conducted to connect the theoretical underpinnings of Daoist teaching with the experiential practices of Qigong and TCM, as well as to investigate how effective it is in holistic patient care services. Given that Daoism bears strong features of Chinese culture, exploration into how it can be translated into other cultures with sensitivity would need effortful commitment. In terms of research, rigorous RCT studies and innovative study designs, such as Whole System Research (WSR), are warranted (Verhoef *et al.* 2005).

Conclusion

Daoist teachings and regime practices place great value on whole-person wellbeing in terms of dynamic balancing, which has been gradually recognised in the field of clinical social work. Concepts of 'non-action', 'simplicity' and 'naturalness' communicate ways of Dao achievement. In the context of social work practice, it can be understood and experienced through teaching and physical exercises so as to activate the flow of Qi. On the basis of Yin-Yang theory, the framework of dynamic balancing depicts a self-adjusted process in an ever-changing world. For the personal and professional development of the practitioner, water-like qualities can always be sources for self-reflection. Increasing evidence shows that practices rooted in Daoism can improve the total wellbeing of various groups of clientele.

References

Ai, A.L., Peterson, C., Gillespie, B., Bolling, S.F., Jessup, M.G., Behling, B.A. and Pierce, F. (2001) 'Designing clinical trials on energy healing: ancient art encounters medical science', *Alternative Therapies in Health and Medicine*, 7(4): 83–90.

Chan, C., Ying Ho, P.S. and Chow, E. (2002) 'A body-mind-spirit model in health: an eastern approach', *Social Work in Health Care*, 34(3–4): 261–82.

Chan, C.H.Y., Chan, T.H.Y. and Chan, C.L.W. (2014a) 'Translating Daoist concepts into integrative social work practice: an empowerment program for persons with depressive symptoms', *Journal of Religion and Spirituality in Social Work*, 33(1): 61–72.

Chan, C.H.Y, Chan, C. L.W., Ng, E.H., Ho, P.C., Chan, T.H., Lee, G.L. and Hui, W.H.C. (2012) 'Incorporating spirituality in psychosocial group intervention for women undergoing in vitro fertilization: a prospective randomized controlled study', *Psychology and Psychotherapy: Theory, Research and Practice*, 85(4): 356–73.

Chan, C.H.Y., Chan, T.H.Y., Leung, P.P.Y., Brenner, M.J., Wong, V.P.Y., Leung, E.K.T., Wong, X., Lee, M.L., Chan, J.S.M. and Chan, C.L.W. (2014b) 'Rethinking wellbeing in terms of affliction and equanimity: development of a Holistic Wellbeing Scale, *Journal of Ethnic and Cultural Diversity in Social Work*, 23(3–4): 289–308.

Chan, J.S., Ho, R.T., Chung, K.F., Wang, C.W., Yao, T.J., Ng, S.M. and Chan, C.L. (2014c) 'Qigong exercise alleviates fatigue, anxiety, and depressive symptoms, improves sleep quality, and shortens sleep latency in persons with chronic fatigue syndrome-like illness', *Evidence-Based Complementary and Alternative Medicine*. 2014(2014):1–10.

Chan, J.S.M., Chan, C.L.W. and Yuen, L.P. (2015) 'Qigong improves depressive symptoms, hope and mental functioning in persons with insomnia and depressive disorders: a RCT', *Annals of Behavioral Medicine*, 49(Suppl 1): S247.

Chang, Y.M. (1977) *The Thoughts of Lao Tzu*, Taipei: Li Ming.

Chen, G.M. and Holt, G.R. (2002) 'Persuasion through the water metaphor in Dao De Jing', *Intercultural Communication Studies*, 11(1): 153–71.

Grønning, K., Lomundal, B., Koksvik, H.S. and Steinsbekk, A. (2011) 'Coping with arthritis is experienced as a dynamic balancing process: a qualitative study', *Clinical Rheumatology*, 30(11): 1425–32.

Ho, R.T.H., Chan, J.S.M., Wang, C.W., Lau, B.W.M., So, K.F., Yuen, L.P., Sham, J.S.T. and Chan, C.L. (2012) 'A randomized controlled trial of qigong exercise on fatigue symptoms, functioning, and telomerase activity in persons with chronic fatigue or chronic fatigue syndrome', *Annals of Behavioral Medicine*, 44(2): 160–70.

Klein, P.J. and Adams, W.D. (2004) 'Comprehensive therapeutic benefits of Taiji: a critical review', *American Journal of Physical Medicine and Rehabilitation*, 83(9): 735–45.

Kohn, L. (2011) *Living Authentically: Daoist contributions to modern psychology*, Dunedin, FL: Three Pines Press.

Lee, M.S., Pittler, M.H. and Ernst, E. (2007) 'Is Tai Chi an effective adjunct in cancer care? A systematic review of controlled clinical trials', *Supportive Care in Cancer*, 15(6): 597–601.

Lee, M.Y., Ng, S.M., Leung, P.P.Y. and Chan, C.L.W. (2009) *Integrative Body-Mind-Spirit Social Work: an empirically based approach to assessment and treatment*, Oxford: Oxford University Press.

Lee, Y.T. (2003) 'Daoistic humanism in ancient China: broadening personality and counseling theories in the 21st century', *Journal of Humanistic Psychology*, 43(1): 64–85.

Lee, Y.T., Yang, H. and Wang, M. (2009) 'Daoist harmony as a Chinese philosophy and psychology', *Peace and Conflict Studies*, 16(1): 68–71.

Lee, Y.T., Han, A., Byron, T. and Fan, H. (2008) 'Daoist leadership: theory and application', in C.C. Chen and Y.T. Lee (eds) *Leadership and Management in China: philosophies, theories and practices*, New York: Cambridge University Press.

Liu, X.G. (2004) 'An outline of Laozi's humanistic naturalness' *Philosophical Researches*, 12(12): 24–32 (in simplified Chinese).

Lu, Y. (2012) 'Water metaphors in Dao de jing: a conceptual analysis', *Open Journal of Modern Linguistics*, 2(4): 151–8.

McLaughlin, K.A. and Nolen-Hoeksema, S. (2011) 'Rumination as a transdiagnostic factor in depression and anxiety', *Behaviour Research and Therapy*, 49(3): 186–93.

Nolen-Hoeksema, S. (2000) 'The role of rumination in depressive disorders and mixed anxiety/depressive symptoms', *Journal of Abnormal Psychology*, 109(3): 504–11.

Sreevani, R., Reddemma, K., Chan, C.L., Leung, P.P.Y., Wong, V. and Chan, C.H.Y. (2013) 'Effectiveness of integrated body–mind–spirit group intervention on the wellbeing of Indian patients with depression: a pilot study, *Journal of Nursing Research*, 21(3): 179–86.

Verhoef, MJ., Lewith, G., Ritenbaugh, C., Boon, H., Fleishman, S. and Leis, A. (2005) 'Complementary and alternative medicine whole systems research: beyond identification of inadequacies of the RCT', *Complementary Therapies in Medicine*, 13(3): 206–12.

Wang, F., Lee, E.K.O., Wu, T., Benson, H., Fricchione, G., Wang, W. and Yeung, A.S. (2014) 'The effects of Tai Chi on depression, anxiety, and psychological wellbeing: a systematic review and meta-analysis', *International Journal of Behavioral Medicine*, 21(4): 605–17.

Watson, B. (1993) 'Introduction', in S. Addiss and S. Lombardo (translators) *To Te Ching*, Indianapolis: Hackett Publishing Company.

Wei, G.X., Dong, H.M., Yang, Z., Luo, J. and Zuo, X.N. (2014) 'Tai Chi Chuan optimizes the functional organization of the intrinsic human brain architecture in older adults', *Frontiers in Aging Neuroscience*, 6:74.

Yeates, G. (2015) 'Flow state experiences as a biopsychosocial guide for Tai Ji intervention and research in neuro-rehabilitation', *Neuro-Disability and Psychotherapy*, 3(1): 22–41.

11

Celtic spirituality

Exploring the fascination across time and place

Laura Béres

The study of Celtic spirituality and changing priorities over time

Although the current interest in Celtic spirituality is 'perhaps most evident in the form of attractively packaged commodities which can be purchased at the postmodern spiritual supermarket' (Bradley 2010: vii), despite this more commercial manifestation, interest is also demonstrated in the popularity of pilgrimages to Celtic holy sites and workshops. Modern-day pilgrims to these Celtic sites include 'New Agers, feminists and deep ecologists, as well as liberal, evangelical, and charismatic Christians, [who] identify with its ethos and message and call for a recovery of its key principles' (Bradley 2010: viii). In his 2009 book *Pilgrimage: a spiritual and cultural journey*, Bradley points out that over 250,000 people visit the tiny isle of Iona each year, with as many as 1,600 each day in the summer months. This is significant on a small island that has only just over 100 year-round residents, and as it takes such a long time to travel there.

If, as Bradley says, people are drawn to the ethos and key principles of Celtic spirituality, what *are* the ethos and key principles, and why are people today drawn to them? What might the answers to those questions imply for social work academics and practitioners?

Celtic spirituality is a term that is often used with little acknowledgment of how imprecise a description it actually is. Since the texts that inspire an understanding of Celtic spirituality are early Celtic Christian texts, I will use both terms: Celtic spirituality and Celtic Christianity. Some scholars (Davies and O'Loughlin 1999; O'Loughlin 2000; Sheldrake 2013) suggest, however, that both these terms are a little misleading since they point out there was never any unified Celtic identity, or unified Celtic Church separate and distinct from the Roman Church during the historical period that gives rise to most of what is now referred to as Celtic spirituality. Although some say the origins of the term 'Celts' was in Greek and Roman geographical and ethnographical writing 'from the sixth to fourth century B.C.[E] ... the term had no precise ethnic signification and [the] Celts merely designated those people who lived in the west' (Davies and O'Loughlin 1999: 4). Alternatively, Chadwick suggests the Celts were a recognisable people in Central Europe by 500 BCE and it was only with Roman conquest in Europe that the Celts were pushed west to those areas we think of as Celtic today: Ireland, Scotland, Wales and parts of England (Chadwick 1970).

The history of the Celts is important because, as Sheldrake points out:

Spiritual traditions do not exist on some ideal plane above and beyond history. The origins and development of spiritual traditions reflect the circumstances of time and place as well as the psychological state of the people involved. They consequently embody values that are socially conditioned. … This does not imply that spiritual traditions and texts have no value beyond their original contexts. However, it does mean that to appreciate their riches we must take context seriously.

(Sheldrake 2013:12.)

In the early medieval period (the period in which we find the first descriptions of what is called Celtic spirituality), religious and spiritual practices were far more likely to be fundamentally local, without any over-arching religious unity, as would have been supported and valued after the 'neo-imperialism of Charlemagne in the ninth century' (Sheldrake 2013: 68). This is one argument why, despite the recent interest in Celtic spirituality as a separate and distinct form of spirituality, it is not possible to support an argument that there was one form of Celtic spiritual-ity totally distinct from other local forms of spirituality practiced in Britain at the time. None the less, the spread of Celtic spirituality and Celtic Christianity has been described as having sprung from Ireland, moved to Iona with Columba setting up a monastery there, and then spread through Scotland and northern England. Of particular note, monks travelled from Iona to Lindisfarne in Northumbria where another Celtic monastery was set up by Aidan. These early churches and monasteries were not separate from the political, cultural and royal concerns of the time; when the Northumbrian King Oswald, who had been influenced by Celtic spirituality in Iona, married a Queen who had been raised in the south of England and influenced by the Roman Church, the royal couple began to experience challenges in their differing faith prac-tices particularly in relation to the date for celebrating Easter, and so a gathering was organised at Whitby in 664. Bradley (2010) reports that many suggest this meeting marks the ousting of Celtic spirituality in Britain, but he states,

It may be true that the Synod of Whitby did mark the end of a distinctive native Celtic Christianity in Britain. But that end took a long time coming – if, indeed, it has ever come … [It] continued as a fairly distinct and recognizable entity in several parts of the British Isles for another 500 years after Whitby.

(Bradley 2010: 25)

Celtic spirituality/Christianity continued to be practiced in Iona, and was ultimately only pushed back into Ireland from there due to Viking raids. So, despite arguments that a separate Celtic spirituality or Celtic Church did not exist, there is also some evidence that the Roman Church recognised there were Celtic practices occurring and they attempted to bring them more in line with their own.

Focus on the natural geographical and social context of the development of Celtic spirituality requires consideration of early medieval Ireland (Bradley 2010; Sheldrake 2013). Since Ireland was never part of the Roman Empire and so no Roman city or road system was developed at that time, the Irish landscape remained largely wilderness, and since it was a relatively small island, the sea remained a dominant feature, particularly as a means of transport, rather than traveling through an inhospitable interior; 'it does not take a vast leap of imagination to make connections between these realities and a particular spiritual "temperament"' (Sheldrake 2013: 68). What was characteristic of the early Irish Church, or 'Celtic spirituality', were the follow-ing: asceticism; solitude; a profound sense of a Trinitarian God, saints and angels all around in the day-to-day lives of people; natural imagery in prayers and poetry; a wandering form of pilgrimage seeking a 'place of resurrection'; a focus on the spiritual needs of individuals; spiritual guidance and the importance of 'soul friends' (anam cara); private confession and penance (Sheldrake 2013).

Any world religion attempting to make an impact in a new indigenous culture will inevitably experience 'some degree of fusion or coalescence ... between the new religion and the religious forms it is seeking to replace' (Davies and O'Loughlin 1999: 12). In relation to Celtic spirituality, or Celtic Christianity, pre-Christian and pagan paradigms were influential. They were often centred on particular sacred places in the natural world, especially those where water was a key feature. Birds, animals and nature generally are important in Celtic spirituality and are represented often in the art and poetry associated with it (Davies and O'Loughlin 1999).

Pelagius is a significant representative of early Celtic Christianity. Having been born somewhere in Britain or Ireland (Bradley 2010) around 350, he studied in Rome and travelled through North Africa and Palestine, being influenced by the Dessert fathers and other Eastern traditions. He was excommunicated by the Roman Catholic Church as a heretic due to his disagreement with St. Augustine of Hippo's statements on original sin and the need for grace, which had become the teaching of the Roman Church while Pelagius remained committed to the earlier Christian (and Celtic) position 'that babies were born innocent and that baptism was a sign and seal of God's gracious love for them rather than an operation which had to be performed to avoid their dispatch to Hell' (Bradley 2010: 63). Pelagius also stressed the essential goodness of nature, with a divine spark existing within all of creation (Bradley 2010; Newell 2008). 'The Celts felt the presence of Christ almost physically woven around their lives ... and a conviction that the presence of God was to be found throughout creation' (Bradley 2010: 33) as depicted by the intertwining ribbons of the Celtic knot. This leads to the suggestion that the Celts have a great deal to teach us today about our relationship to the rest of the Earth, and it is this aspect that makes Celtic spirituality of interest to those committed to deep ecology and a renewed sense of stewardship of the world's resources.

The Celts' awareness of the divine presence in all things has been described as being similar to an experience with Buddhist mindfulness, moving beyond the physical to an embrace of the spiritual world. In particular, the Celts 'felt the narrowness of the line that divides this world from then next' (Bradley 2010: 37). More recently, George MacLeod, who accomplished the rebuilding of the abbey on Iona in the middle of the twentieth century, also stressed the manner in which the physical world is 'shot through with the spiritual' (Bradley 2010: 107). MacLeod has been described as 'unselfconsciously' speaking of angels and feeling the nearness of heavenly hosts: 'Pilgrim and poet, he tirelessly preached the oneness of creation and the thinness of the line that divides this world and the next' (Bradley 2010: 108). As 'angels' are a further popular area of fascination, it is possible that for many people their interest in Celtic spirituality, and pilgrimages to Celtic sacred places, are motivated by an interest in the possibility of a direct experience with something mystical and unmediated by organised religion and religious leaders.

Exploring people's engagement with Celtic spirituality and place

On my first visit to Iona in June of 2010, when I began a series of research interviews with people regarding their engagement with this setting, which has been described as a thin place, I met a couple of regular visitors from Ireland. They suggested that it would be impossible to understand Celtic spirituality without visiting Ireland, so in October of 2010 I made my way there. I visited with both of them and conducted research interviews with two interesting contacts they provided: the first was a self-labeled Celtic monk, who chose to leave the Roman Catholic priesthood in order to commit to the practice of Celtic spirituality; the second was a Roman Catholic priest, who described himself as having been able to integrate Celtic spirituality into his Roman Catholic faith. These two opposing methods of engaging with Celtic spirituality provide examples from the two extremes of the continuum we may experience as we meet people in professional practice: those who combine alternate spiritual practices within organised religion, and those who take up alternate practices instead of being affiliated with organised religion. Social work practitioners need to recognise and support whatever practices are providing people with a sense of meaning and purpose in their lives, and not assume that one way is more legitimate than another.

On Inis Mor, the largest of the Aran Islands off the west coast of Ireland, which attracts as many as 400,000 tourists/pilgrims each year, I interviewed Dara Molloy (Molloy 2009), whose biography can be found on his website (Molloy 2012). He was ordained a Roman Catholic priest in 1979, and while working with youth in his community he was provided with contacts on Inis Mor and arranged for a short camping trip there with a youth group. At that time, he had already been unsure if it was right for him to continue on in the priesthood and he said he would describe himself as having been on a search, although he would not have been able to say what he had been searching for. He had been offered opportunities to travel overseas to become a missionary, but was sure he should stay in Ireland. While visiting Inis Mor that first time, he knew at once that this was where he should return to live: It was his 'place of resurrection', as the Celtic monks of the early medieval ages would have described a place that called to them and suggested that they should stop there to live out the rest of their days. Dara explained that for the first time in his life he felt immersed in his Gaelic heritage, which he said he had lost. He felt drawn to reconnect not only to the language, but to the spirituality, beliefs and values of those early Celtic monks who had lived on Inis Mor.

Dara knew that I was interested in learning about people's engagement with thin places so he said he would start by talking with me about that topic, although he also said this wasn't his 'favourite word'. He went on to suggest he preferred the terms 'threshold places and threshold times'. He suggested that there are times in life and during the day that are like thresholds and he thought these were consistent with threshold places, leading to moments of insight in people's journeys and in their stories. He also added that he believes that the fact someone is searching for something does not mean what they find is inauthentic.

Dara went on to say that for him Inis Mor is a threshold place, feeling as though it is on the edge of the world. He remarked that certainly in medieval times, people in Europe truly believed it was on the edge of the world, since they knew of nothing further west. Inis Mor, as an island off the west coast of Ireland, and Iona, off the west coast of Scotland, would have both been considered on the edge of the known world and, therefore, on the threshold of other possible worlds. Due to the length of time it continues to take to access these places today it still feels as though you are on the edge of the world when there, despite our current understanding of geography.

Dara explained that he was drawn to the simplicity and imagery of Celtic spirituality and felt it needed to resist any attempt made from outside to impose a structure. He did not want merely to take up a superficial use of certain Celtic prayers and hymns and integrate them into organised religion, but rather wanted to live differently. Since giving up his role in the Church and relocating to Inis Mor, he has married and now has two children, making an income providing various ceremonies as a priest, monk, druid or lay person, dressing however the people requesting the ceremony would like him to. However, he says he chooses to call himself a Celtic monk in order to 'liberate the term from its institutional framework'. For him a Celtic monk chooses to follow a spiritual path at every level of life. For him, Pelagius' notion was not new and heretical at the time he was excommunicated but rather represented original Irish commitments, resisting the imposition of the Roman Catholic Church's teaching. Dara also said he speaks about aspects of God being in the sea, or aspects of the Goddess being in the river, because he likes this imagery but he is speaking metaphorically. He said that 'the Divine is so vastly beyond us' and the notion of us having been made in God's image 'is a bit arrogant' but he believes that there is a spark of the divine in everything and so everything can begin to move us towards the Divine.

At the other end of the continuum, I then met Fr. Frank, who had been the priest at Ballintubber Abbey in County Mayo for 25 years at that time. Ballintubber Abbey, which was built in 1216 and celebrates its eight-hundredth anniversary in 2016, marks the beginning of Tóchar Phádraig (St. Patrick's Causeway), a 35 km pilgrimage to Croagh Patrick (a 764 metre mount), which Frank explained has been, according to archaeological excavation, a site of worship since 3000 BCE. Frank also took me to Church Island, near Ballintubber Abbey, which is a small island on which people lived more than 3,000 years ago, and on which also stood an ancient monastery in the past, according to carbon dating. Currently it has a tiny chapel and a few other buildings used for retreats. The chapel is the fifth built on that site, having been completed in the fourteenth century, but containing a small window area above the altar from the sixth century. Frank led me on a pilgrimage around the island, recounting the history of people through Biblical stories from creation through the gospels by reflecting on images present in the natural environment. Time and again Frank came back to the need to learn from Celtic traditions and their respect for nature in such a way as to stay connected to the love of Christ (or the Divine), but he suggested that this would also need to be 'demonstrated through our treatment of people, especially those who have been marginalised from the love of God somehow'. He focused on the interconnectedness of all of the created universe (similar to Buddhist principles again) and the need to look after creation rather than using and abusing it. Frank believed the majority of people had become much more concerned with a search for power and prestige, rather than on fostering community and a love of the environment.

During my interview of Frank and his reactions to my questions about 'thin places', he related his thoughts to the story of the fall of Adam and Eve in Eden. He said he thinks of us as still living in Eden but being unaware of it. Frank believes the other world, both good and evil, is all around us. He conceded that some places may be 'thinner' and so it might be easier to connect to the other world in those places, such as Ballintubber Abbey where there is always someone present praying and the act of ongoing prayer keeps the space special. He also spoke about pilgrimage and the need to engage in pilgrimage with an openness to the whole process rather than a focus on just the end goal. Frank does not think many people have experiences like Paul's on the Road to Damascus (no big 'aha' moments in a 'thin place'), but rather most people have a more gradual experience over a longer journey. When preparing young people for the Tóchar Phádraig, Frank tells them that one of the 'rules' for the walk is that there must be no complaining. He said that he tells them just to say 'Thanks be to God' at any moment when they might otherwise want to complain. This has much in common with Buddhist approaches to acceptance and non-attachment, which I believe offer people a much more peaceful engagement with life in contrast with mainstream approaches of struggling to try to fix and control circumstances. Of course, there has been a parallel growing interest in Mindfulness and Eastern religions in the West at the same time as the interest in Celtic spirituality has been growing. Again, the focus on simplicity and an alternative to the fast-paced world where we each must be independent and in control may be part of what is appealing. I also suspect that as more people in the West become interested in Aboriginal spiritualities and they struggle with not appropriating Indigenous knowledges, they may turn to their own roots, many of which are in Celtic Indigenous traditions.

Conclusions: informing social work practice now[1]

Despite declining rates of affiliation with organised religions in the West, and a continuing mainstream preoccupation with the accumulation of money and prestige, along with the power to purchase and consume, many people are searching for alternatives to this fast-paced, individually-focused lifestyle. There is a growing interest in down-sizing and simplicity (Elgin 1981; Henning 2002), and as people grapple with the insecurity of employment, they may also begin to consider committing to nurturing place and community before following multinational companies' precarious jobs, which are all consistent with Celtic spirituality-inspired lifestyle choices.

People's interest in Celtic spirituality also appears to be partly due to their search for something meaningful (spiritual) in their lives at a time when they may have become dissatisfied with organised religion. For some, they will be able to meet those needs separate from any formal church, while for others, they will be able to integrate these aspects into attendance at church, recognising that these forms of practice were historically present in the Early Christian Church. Keating, for instance, describes centring or contemplative prayer as a form of mindfulness that developed from a commitment to practicing interior silence leading to compassion and service to others (Keating 1992: 14–5). He describes how in the sixth century Pope Gregory (also known as Gregory the Great, who came from a monastic tradition) would have encouraged a form of personal reflection and contemplative prayer that would have allowed the common person to experience the Divine without the interference of the Church. By the sixteenth century, contemplative prayer was being described by the Church as extraordinary and only possible for the few. He suggests the 'rush to the East is a symptom of what is lacking in the West. There is a deep spiritual hunger that is not being satisfied in the West' (Keating 1992: 31). Celtic spirituality offers something similar to that offered by the Eastern religious practices and so is meeting some of those same needs people are experiencing that motivate them to search for different practices: a wish to connect with the Divine without needing priests to mediate on their behalf. Celtic spirituality, however, offers those people with roots in Britain or Europe an opportunity to reconnect to their own cultural heritage and to re-integrate these practices into local Western Church practices should they wish.

Another significant aspect of Celtic spirituality is the idea of there being a spark of the Divine in all of nature and in all people (similar to the underlying principle of saying 'Namaste' in yoga practice: the divine in me bows before the divine in you). This reminds social workers to look for the good in people despite outer layers of behaviours, and to be more concerned for the natural world in which we all live. Zapf (2007, 2010) has much to say about the need for social workers to take much more seriously the concept of person in environment, where the environment is not considered merely a backdrop but also as something of importance. Berry (1988, 2009) provides reflections on the sacredness of the universe and eco-spirituality, which also share something in common with Celtic spirituality.

In conclusion, I wish to highlight the manner in which my study of Celtic spirituality has recently assisted me in ethically engaging with a remote fly-in First Nations community in the far north of Canada. I have had the opportunity over the last two summers to travel with a colleague (a Roman Catholic priest and Religious Studies faculty member) and a small number of Religious Studies and Social Work students to a northern First Nations community, which is primarily Catholic. A number of First Nations communities and reserves come together for the first week of July each year on a small island for a Roman Catholic retreat, but also as a way of reconnecting to the land and some of their traditional cultural practices. July 2015 saw them celebrating their twenty-fifth anniversary on the island.

As a social work academic trained to take into account the effects of colonisation and the oppression of marginalised communities, I was initially concerned about the fact these communities appeared so disconnected from their traditional Aboriginal spiritual practices. As a white woman visiting the communities with primarily white colleagues and students, I was worried about inadvertently continuing to support what could have been considered proselytising and colonising practices. Speaking with Elders in the community, I asked how I might be able to engage ethically and if there was anything they could imagine I could do that might be of use. They asked me to start sharing stories of what their lives are like. It is their belief that most people in the rest of Canada, let alone the rest of the world, have no idea of what life is really like for them there.

I asked about traditional Aboriginal spiritual and healing practices and was told that, because as Dene communities they had lost most of those practices, they would need to invite outsider Aboriginal people, like the Cree, to come and teach them their practices, but they do not want that. They have taken up Catholic spiritual practices and they say they are happy with those. Many of the Elders have taken up lay person roles in the Church and provide Catholic services to the community when the priest who rotates between communities is not available.

As my relationships continue to develop with other Dene community members, I am beginning to see more of how some of their traditional Aboriginal stories and cultural practices are continuing and are being interwoven into their Catholic spiritual practices. Reflecting on the manner in which Christian practices were influenced as they integrated with pre-Christian Celtic traditions and seeing how a respect for nature and imagery can be honoured within Christian practices has assisted me in realising that these Canadian Christian Aboriginal communities may have also influenced their practice of Catholicism (Blondin 1997; Goulet 1998; Riddington and Riddington 2013). This insight further supports my respect for the choices my Aboriginal community friends have made and continue to make when they choose to be so involved in the Catholic Church. It has also influenced the next step of my research process as we engage Elders in the community in sharing the stories of this ongoing process of celebrating cultural traditions at the same time as they participate in Catholic practices.

As Sheldrake (2013) points out, spiritual practices are not static and will continue to adjust to the cultural and psychological needs of various communities. Social workers need to become more informed about the spiritual and religious practices of the people and communities with whom they work, realising that practices change over time and can be unique in various local contexts. This is not about imposing one truth or one way of being on all people. This is about social work practitioners showing respect to aspects of people's lives that give them a sense of meaning, purpose and hope, even if those practices and beliefs are different from the social workers' own.

Note

1 I have previously presented clinical social work case examples of how I have integrated my interest in Celtic spirituality and spirituality more generally. Please see Béres (2012, 2013, 2014).

References

Béres, L. (2012) 'A thin place: narratives of space and place, Celtic spirituality and meaning', *Journal of Religion and Spirituality in Social Work*, 31(4): 394–413.
Béres, L. (2013) 'Celtic spirituality and postmodern geography: narratives of engagement with place', *Journal for the Study of Spirituality*, 2(2): 170–85.
Béres, L. (2014) *The Narrative Practitioner*, Basingstoke: Palgrave MacMillan.
Berry, T. (1988) *The Dream of the Earth*, San Francisco: Sierra Club Books.

Berry, T. (2009) *The Sacred Universe: earth, spirituality, and religion in the twenty-first century*, New York: Columbia University Press.

Blondin, G. (1997) *Yamoria, the Lawmaker: stories of the Dene*, Edmonton: NeWest Press.

Bradley, I. (2009) *Pilgrimage: a spiritual and cultural journey*, Oxford: Lion Hudson.

Bradley, I. (2010) *The Celtic Way*, new edn, London: Darton, Longman and Todd.

Chadwick, N. (1970) *The Celts*, New York: Penguin Books.

Davies, O. and O'Loughlin, T. (1999) *Celtic Spirituality*, New York: Paulist Press.

Elgin, D. (1981) *Voluntary Simplicity: toward a way of life that is outwardly simple, inwardly rich,* 2nd revised edn, New York: Harper.

Goulet, J.A. (1998) *Ways of Knowing: experience, knowledge, and power among the Dene Tha*, Lincoln: University of Nebraska Press.

Henning, D.H. (2002) *Buddhism and Deep Ecology*, Bloomington: 1st Books.

Keating, T. (1992) *Open Mind, Open Heart: the contemplative dimension of the gospel*, New York: Continuum International Publishing.

Molloy, D. (2009) *The Globalization of God: Celtic Christianity's nemesis*, Inis Mor: Aisling Publications.

Molloy, D. (2012) *A Biography*. Online. Available HTTP: www.daramolloy.com/biography.html (accessed 8 August 2016).

Newell, J.P. (2008) *Christ of the Celts: the healing of creation*, Glasgow: Wild Goose Publications.

O'Loughlin, T. (2000) *Celtic Theology: humanity, world, and God in early Irish writings*, London: Continuum.

Riddington, R. and Riddington, J. in collaboration with Elders of the Dane–Zaa First Nations (2013) *Where Happiness Dwells: a history of the Dane-Zaa First Nations*, Vancouver: UBC Press.

Sheldrake, P. (2013) *Spirituality: a brief history*, 2nd edn, Oxford: Wiley-Blackwell.

Zapf, M.K. (2007) 'Profound connections between person and place: exploring location, spirituality, and social work', in J. Coates, J.R. Graham and B. Swartzentruber with B. Ouellette (eds) *Spirituality and Social Work: selected Canadian readings*, Toronto: Canadian Scholars Press.

Zapf, M.K. (2010) 'Social work and the environment: understanding people and place', *Critical Social Work*, 11(3): 30–46. Online. Available HTTP: www1.uwindsor.ca/criticalsocialwork/social-work-and-the-environment-understanding-people-and-place (accessed 8 August 2016).

12

Material spirituality

Challenging Gnostic tendencies in contemporary understandings of religion and spirituality in social work

Russell Whiting

Introduction

The basic premise underlying this chapter is that the material is spiritual. What is resisted is the pre-supposition, labelled as Gnostic here, that the spiritual realm and the material world are somehow separate and distinct from each other. This latter notion, it will be argued, is an often accepted although possibly not thought through assumption in much contemporary discussion of religion and spirituality in social work, and it leads to workers treating issues of religion and spirituality as somehow different and separate from their day-to-day practical work. This presupposition will be challenged by a focus on the meaning of 'the body' in spiritual terms in social work practice.

As an example of how the discussion might be framed, I recall an occasion when working as an admissions tutor at a UK university, which was offering qualifying social work education. At a recruitment event, a prospective student asked me, 'Do you need to be a vegetarian to be a social work student?' At the time I laughed off this question and thought it said something superficial about the image of social workers in the UK. But actually it can potentially be seen as a starting point for a deeper discussion on the social worker's engagement with and attitudes towards the wider world and spirituality. How an individual should view the world and the place of their own body within it and hence what they should consume are actually the central topics of Gnostic thinking. This question can therefore be used to contextualise a discussion on Gnosticism and religion and spirituality in social work and it will be returned to later in the chapter.

The first section of this chapter will consider briefly how Gnosticism has been defined, its history and development; it will outline my own personal faith position in relation to these beliefs and draw on the work of Wendell Berry (1997) to consider the implications of Gnosticism in contemporary society. The chapter does not hold a position favouring religion or spirituality, and Gnosticism is shown as potentially damaging, in different ways, to both. The next section, which will look briefly at the recent good work that has been done on the body and embodiment in social work (Cameron and McDermott 2007; Ferguson 2011; Price and Walker 2015), notes that Walsh (2009) has begun the work of connecting up these ideas to the thinking on spirituality but that this has not yet been taken further. The implications for social work practice of an unthinking Gnostic or dualistic view of the body and the spirit are considered via a discussion of *anorexia nervosa*, sometimes called The Gnostic Syndrome. Looking for positive interpretations of the body in social work, this chapter examines the potential of mindfulness (Lee *et al.* 2009) in this regard. Finally, the ideas of phenomenological writers such as Heidegger (1962) and Levin (1985) will also be offered as a helpful way forward.

Definitions, doctrines and a brief history of Gnosticism

Gray (2015) has claimed that Gnosticism is the predominant set of beliefs of most educated people in modern society, particularly in the West. By Gnosticism he means the primacy of knowledge (science) and faith in the human capacity for advancement through such science. Gray has little time for such an exalted view of the human and the self. Voegelin (1975) describes the entire renaissance and humanist/enlightenment project through to the Marxist totalitarian state as the Gnostic Age because he argues it is a period that sees elevation of the human to the divine. It may be helpful, however, before engaging with contemporary speculations about the usefulness and relevance of the term Gnostic, to begin with a more detailed account of the origins and doctrines of historical Gnosticism.

Gnosticism emerged contemporaneously with Early Christianity. There is much debate among scholars (George 1995) about whether it should be seen as a separate religion or as an off-shoot of or heresy within Christianity. Certainly there were Gnostic movements that were wholly separate from Christianity; the religion founded by Mani in Iran, which went on to be known as Zoroastrianism, is the most notable. However, it is not necessary to get into a technical discussion on precedence and primacy. The essential doctrines of Gnosticism, whether it operated within or without Christian groupings, are broadly similar. The Christian theologian Leech (1981) describes Gnosticism as having three main traits; first, a stress on secret knowledge or *gnosis*; second, 'the division of the world into … the *illuminati*, those who are "in the know" and the rest of mankind, the common herd; thirdly, the location of evil in *matter*' (Leech 1981: 32). This chapter will focus predominantly on the last trait but the other two will also be briefly discussed. The secret knowledge of historical Gnosticism was not science in general but can be summed up in the phrase 'I am God' or 'the divine within'. Houtman and Aupers, in their account of contemporary New Age spirituality in social work, write:

> This, then, is the principal doctrine of New Age spirituality: the belief that in the deepest layers of the self "the divine spark"—to borrow a term from ancient Gnosticism—is still smouldering, waiting to be stirred up and supersede the socialised self.
>
> (Houtman and Aupers 2010: 211)

The key point is that the Gnostic looks inward, to the inner life, for their explanations and meaning. They do not look outward to the world because they believe that the world, all matter in fact, to be bad or evil. This is what is meant by the description of Gnosticism as a dualistic religion (Runciman 1947). It keeps the spirit pure by separating it entirely from the material world. Any concept of the divine cannot be of a creator god because creation is clearly impure. Therefore, Gnostics often have complex explanations for the creation of the world as made by a demigod, angels, demons or the devil. The divine must be wholly separate from impure creation although through such secret knowledge initiates could in themselves become divine. This is how they at least begin to address the perennial problem of the existence of evil.

Official church histories portray a narrative of Gnosticism being one of the principal Christian heresies, which was overcome by the Early Fathers at the councils of the Church. Gnosticism was known to have persisted, dwindling in popularity although continuing in pockets in heretical churches such as the Paulicans, the Bogomils in Bosnia and the Cathars in southern France

(Runciman 1947), who were finally defeated and massacred in the 1200s. In actual fact, a strong argument can be made that the ideas of Gnosticism survived and were incorporated within Christianity itself:

> Although the orthodox teaching held that the material world is good, mainstream Christian history offers many examples of teaching and practices that seem rather "world hating", the charge the orthodox levelled against the Gnostics.
>
> (George 1995: 25)

One of the central doctrines of the Church, original sin, has strong Gnostic overtones. St. Augustine, the first and principal propagator of the doctrine, had originally been a Manichean. Chittester, a Christian feminist theologian, has argued that theological dualism, the fear of the body and the patriarchal power structures of the Church are closely inter-related:

> Bodies, with their drives and needs, their impulses and urges, warranted basic distrust by virtue of their threat or right reasoning, if nothing else. And women, most of all, the blatantly natural, and totally carnal, the most bodily of bodies, epitomised the hazard and jeopardised the rationality, of the male soul.
>
> (Chittester 1998: 23)

Certainly dualist, anti-materialist, patriarchal tendencies have remained a significant feature of the Christian religion to up the present day but there is a risk that such dualism is so deep-rooted that alternative spiritualities, such as New Age thinking and the 'spiritual but not religious' discourses, are likewise at risk of polarising the body and the spirit. Leech adds:

> The rejection of art and beauty, of human passion and amusement derives from a more fundamental rejection of, and mistrust of, the body. It is this which is fundamental to Gnosticism in every age, including our own.
>
> (Leech 1981:36)

It is necessary at this stage to be clear about my own faith position, which is one that believes as Psalm 24.1 says 'The Earth is the Lord's and the fullness thereof'. Such a belief does not accept the separating out of 'the world' from 'the holy' and I believe, with Macintyre, that 'the purpose of religion is the hallowing of the world' (MacIntyre 1985: 1). This is an outward-looking faith that seeks to find the finger of God in the created world and the face of God in other people rather than in the depths of one's own soul. My own working out of these beliefs is Christian (Whiting 2015) and aligns with Christian humanism but there are also clearly many other inter-pretations of the rejection of the division of the material and the spiritual in other faiths such as Judaism (Koltun-Fromm 2010), Shamanism (Jordan 2001) and Shintoism (Whiting and Gurbai 2015) but not, and this will be quite important in the discussion that follows, in Buddhism (Lee at al. 2009), which maintains a very clear division between the two.

The implications of Gnostic thinking for contemporary society

Gray (2015) and Voegelin (1975) were mentioned briefly as arguing that Gnosticism is perva-sive in modern society. I do not wish, however, to engage more extensively with these texts. Instead, I will focus on Wendell Berry's (1997) *The Unsettling of America*. It may appear surpris-ing to take as a starting point for an analysis of the contemporary significance and resonance of

Gnosticism a book written originally in 1982 and predominantly about the consequences of the industrialisation of agriculture in the USA.[1] In addition, Berry never even uses the word Gnostic in his text. But in facing his problems as a farmer in the late twentieth century, he sums up eloquently the human condition and in particular the impact of the separation of body and spirit or 'the world' and 'the holy' on human society. Much of the rest of this section is therefore given over to Berry and uses his words directly and extensively to comment on the prevalence of Gnostic ideas in contemporary society. Only brief comments are made on Berry's text, usually to make explicit the links to social work.

Berry notes first that:

> The word health belongs to a family of words, a listing of which will suggest how far the consideration of health must carry us: *heal, whole, wholesome, hale, hallow, holy* … If the body is healthy, then it is whole … Blake said that "Man has no Body distinct from his Soul" and thus acknowledges the convergence of health and holiness. In that, all the convergences and dependences of creation are surely implied.
>
> (Berry 1997: 103)

The key word here is creation. Berry is a creationist but this does not mean creationist as opposed to evolutionist. It means holding particular views about the world as a good gift to humanity. He adds:

> Our bodies are also not distinct from the bodies of other people, on which they depend in a complexity of ways from biological to spiritual. They are not distinct from the bodies of plants and animals, with which we are involved in the cycles of feeding and the intricate companionships of ecological systems and of the spirit.
>
> (Berry 1997: 103)

The point about personhood resting in the body but only in relation to other people and their bodies is one that will be picked up and discussed further in relation to social work and phenomenology. Berry further notes:

> A medical doctor [or social worker] uninterested in nutrition, in agriculture, in the wholesomeness of the mind and spirit is as absurd as a farmer who is uninterested in health. Our fragmentation of this subject cannot be our cure, because it is our disease. The body cannot be whole alone. Persons cannot be whole alone … To try to heal the body alone is to collaborate in the destruction of the body.
>
> (Berry 1997:103)

This is why, to make matters explicit, the prospective student's question on vegetarianism discussed in the introduction should not be taken as superficial. A good social worker will see the link between their own nutrition, that of others and the wider impact of such small-scale decisions as what a person eats. Berry further adds:

> It is clear to anyone who looks at any crowd that we are wasting our bodies exactly as we are wasting our land. Our bodies are fat, weak, joyless, sickly, ugly, the virtual prey of the manufacturer of medicine and cosmetics … As for our spirits, they seem more and more to comfort themselves in buying things.
>
> (Berry 1997: 108)

111

This text was written originally by Berry in the 1980s, but the realities and consequences of a lack of care of the body and the distracting trivialities of the consumer society are all the more apparent today.

As noted previously, Gnosticism can be seen to be as prevalent within the Christian Church as outside it. Berry comments eloquently:

> For the churchly, the life of the spirit is reduced to a dull preoccupation with getting to Heaven. At best the world is no more than an embarrassment and a trial of the spirit, which is otherwise radically separated from it.
>
> (Berry 1997: 108)

If the engagement of the churches with the world is superficial or fake in the way that Berry describes, that has serious consequences in a situation (such as currently in the UK) where churches are increasingly being seen to be stepping back into social work. If such work in 'the world' is only about rescuing 'the lost' for Heaven, then church social work will be, as an existentialist might say, inauthentic. Berry sees this problem as a chronic one for the churches:

> The ... separation of the soul from the body and from the world is no disease of the fringe, no aberration, but a fracture that runs through the mentality of institutional religion like a geologic fault. And this rift in the mentality of religion continues to characterize the modern mind, no matter how secular or worldly it becomes.
>
> (Berry 1997: 108)

This last is also an important point. Secularism or worldliness does not diminish the likelihood of a Gnostic response to 'the world'. It might be argued, for example, that since Berry wrote his comments, Western society has become even more worldly. Sex and sexuality, for example, are much more prevalent and present in public life and the sexualised body is no longer hidden. But the key point stands because the flesh and the spirit are, and remain, kept apart.

Social work and the body

In recent years there has been an increased focus on the body in social work. Cameron and McDermott (2007) write eloquently about the dangers of social workers working only in their heads and being unaware of the physical world. They encourage the concept of 'body cognizant' social workers. Price and Walker (2015) have similarly written about the body in social work but with more of a focus on the body of the person with whom the social worker is engaging. They write particularly about the danger that the reality of the 'ill body' will be marginalised and ignored by society and even by social work. What neither of these texts do, however, is consider the topic of religion and spirituality in relation to either the body of the social worker or the body of the person with whom they are working. The one writer to have done so in detail to date has been Walsh (2009) and her suggestions are returned to as follows.

The Gnostic Syndrome

The previous sections have suggested that social work has not yet fully engaged with the body in relation to spirituality and has speculated that this is because of an implicit acceptance of dualistic understandings of body and spirit. But what are the consequences of this lack of engagement? This question can be helpfully considered with a discussion on work with those who have gone through more extreme interpretations of the meanings of their own bodies. The link between Gnostic thinking and eating disorders has been made previously; Barrett and Fine (1990) described *anorexia nervosa* as *The Gnostic Syndrome*. They see the behaviour of people with anorexic symptoms as resorting more and more to 'secretiveness and rituals associated with strivings for purity and control' (Barratt and Fine 1990: 268), and add:

> The therapist hopes to help his patients at least to the extent that these patients can view themselves on a certain level as material beings, not just fighting against their own bodies.
>
> (Barrett and Fine 1990: 269)

Similarly, Bell (1985), in his account of the lives and thinking of medieval saints and mystics such as St. Catherine of Siena, makes a direct and pointed link with the experience of individuals diagnosed as anorexic in the twentieth century. For Bell these women are not necessarily passive or powerless and he sees their actions as, in part, responses to the patriarchal power structures of their day. But in both accounts, of the recent and distant past, individuals are described who see the material world as to be avoided or ignored, both in terms of their own bodies and even of food itself. A third example of the possible connection between Gnostic thinking and self-starvation can be seen in the life and death of the twentieth-century philosopher Simone Weil. Weil travelled widely across the intellectual landscape of the 1930s, moving from socialist to anarchist and eventually to conservative and Catholic-influenced positions. But also in the late 1930s, Weil studied and came to sympathise with the medieval Cathars. She was very sympathetic towards the idea of a spiritual elite. She did not join the Catholic Church and kept herself apart from the masses (and the Mass). She ended her life as a sick woman refusing to take nourishment just as the spiritual elite among the Cathars had done (Hanratty 1997).

These suggestions that Gnostic beliefs are being lived out in the lives and deaths of modern people are of course speculative, but they cannot be dismissed. They should concentrate the mind of the social work practitioner on the importance of coming to a view on the meaning and significance of the body. Many people with whom they will be working, and certainly not just those who may be have eating disorders, will be carrying deeply held beliefs that their own bodies are somehow impure and that their own physicality, their own pain even (Price and Walker 2015), is to be suppressed or ignored. In recent times, one of the ways in which individuals have been encouraged to become more in touch with their own bodies has been through mindfulness. This idea will now be explored in some detail.

Mindfulness and the body

One of the most interesting texts on spirituality in social work published in recent years is by Lee *et al.* (2009). They present a model that proposes to integrate body, mind and spirit in practice. It includes two important chapters on the body in social work. They present their model based on the ideas of Yin and Yang, Taoism and Buddhism, while making it clear that:

> Our discussion focuses on these beliefs as philosophies and not as religions. Religious conversion does not have a place in the learning and practice of integrative social work.
>
> (Lee *et al.* 2009: 91)

Lee *et al.* focus on the practice of mindfulness. Since their original work on the topic, the idea and practice of mindfulness has flourished in social work circles and it is important to consider it in relation to Gnosticism. Lee *et al.* note that mindfulness originates in Buddhist teaching: 'In the Satipathanna Sutta, the Buddha described four foundations of objects of mindfulness; the body, consciousness, feelings and the Dharma' (Lee *et al.* 2009: 587).

Ostensibly, from the position taken in this chapter, the focus on the body in mindfulness appears to be an extremely positive one. The emphasis is on being present in the body in the moment. The mindful practitioner is encouraged to focus on their breathing in order to generate a calm state in which to observe bodily sensations, thoughts and feelings (MacDonagh 2014). It is clear how this could be a potentially useful skill in social work. For example, Ferguson (2011) discusses how a bodily reaction can influence a social work decision. A home may be so dirty that the social worker's skin creeps but that may not necessarily mean that a child or adult is being poorly treated in that home. So if a social worker is mindful and aware of what is happening to their own body and how that might be impacting on their thinking, this can only be advantageous in their decision making.

By way of contrast, Lee *et al.* in their explanation of the focus on the body in mindfulness, go on to add, 'The suggested focus is on the person, because we are accustomed to focus our attention on the outside, illusory world rather than the inner, real world' (Lee *et al.* 2009: 587). The Buddhist belief that the outer world is illusory is clearly a challenge to a material spirituality. Runciman, in his summary of Manichean Gnosticism, summarises the different positions well:

> To the orthodox Christian, Matter is bad, as a result of the Fall, but can be made good through Christ's Sacraments. To the Christian Dualist, Matter is irretrievably bad. To the Brahmin and, still more, to the Buddhist, Matter is an irrelevant thing.
>
> (Runciman 1947: 186)

The Buddhist focuses on the body in order to transcend it and all material reality. Although Gnosticism and Buddhism are clearly very different faith positions (and Runciman is categorical that there is no historical link between the two) in effect there is little practical difference between believing the material world is bad or that it is irrelevant. The result is the same, i.e. a turn inwards. George notes:

> Although the idea that self-knowledge alone can lead to spiritual liberation is heretical to mainstream Christianity, it is central to Buddhism. The root of suffering, according to Buddhists, is ignorance concerning the true nature of the self.
>
> (George 1995: 122)

Self-examination is clearly important but there is possibly a fine line between self-examination and self-obsession. MacDonagh (2014) wrote an excoriating piece on mindfulness after attending a series of training sessions. She comments:

> This brings me to what really annoys me about being mindful, which is that as far as I can gather, it's Mostly About Me. Sitting concentrating on your breathing is a good way to chill out and de-stress, but it's not a particularly good end in itself.
>
> (MacDonagh 2014)

She goes on to criticise mindfulness as an activity for the self-indulgent and self-obsessed with no practical outlet.

Moss (2005), in his preliminary discussion of spirituality in social work, provided a very open and inclusive definition of what spirituality might be but he also added a test for effectiveness. He argued that spirituality in social work should be affirming and outward-looking. It is worth questioning whether the particular focus on the body in some interpretations mindfulness is leading to an inwardness that may not always be conducive to good social work. Clearly social workers in their use of mindfulness might well be outward-looking and purposeful and there are certainly advocates of Buddhist practice who emphasise the importance of an active compassion (Kittisaro and Thanissara 2014). This chapter in no way wishes to denigrate or question Buddhist social work practice, simply to point out that a materially grounded spirituality is something very different. One possible way of thinking about the body in a way that might complement mindfulness is through a consideration of the academic discipline of phenomenology in relation to social work.

Phenomenology

Walsh (2009) points to the importance of the work of Levin (1985) and other prominent writers in the field of phenomenology for social work. What is phenomenology? Heidegger, one of its early proponents, writes that it is 'a special method for gaining access to our experience and making it conceptually explicit' (Heidegger 1962: 59). The works of Merlieu-Ponty (2002) and Levin (1985) have taken the discipline further with their explicit and extended focus on the body. In particular, Levin is focused on the significance of the body in relation to other bodies, so not as a turning inwards. He writes:

> It is becoming increasingly clear that … the deepening of experience must eventually be understood as an elemental groundedness as bodily beings. As bodily beings, we are graced with the sense of the body as a whole.
>
> (Levin 1985:291)

There is clearly scope for more work on the connections between a grounded spirituality and phenomenology in social work.

Conclusion

This chapter has discussed the prevalence of Gnostic tendencies in different interpretations of religion and spirituality. It has encouraged those involved in social work to consider how they might view 'the body' in relation to 'the spirit' and in particular to beware of the tendency to hive off the spiritual and to think of it as something wholly separate from the material world. The possibility that taking such thinking to its limits can result in problems such as eating disorders has been discussed from an historical perspective.

Mindfulness, as a practice that foregrounds an awareness of the body in the moment, has been noted as potentially very useful in this regard, although concerns have been raised in relation to Buddhist doctrines about 'the immaterial', which can inform some contemporary interpretations of mindfulness. Phenomenology, as an approach that does not discredit or minimise the significance of the knowledge gained through the body, has been suggested as a potentially valuable approach for practitioners although clearly more work can and should be done on developing the use of this way of thinking in relation to religion and spirituality in social work.

This *Handbook* is a physical artefact that by its very existence demonstrates how far the topic of religion and spirituality in social work has come in the last generation from a time when the topic was not given sufficient credence (Whiting 2008) to where we are today. It is a testament to the hard work and devotion of scholars in the field. But it also represents a threat or a risk. That risk is the Gnostic one, that religion and spirituality might be hived off from normal practice and treated as a specialism for those who are interested. There is then a short step from there to the secret knowledge of *the illuminate*. This is to be avoided at all costs, and if discussion of religion and spirituality in social work is to serve any purpose it must be inclusive and be for, and by, in Leech's term 'the common herd' (1981: 32). So I write, in conflict with myself, as a specialist scholar in religion and spirituality in social work rejecting the premise of specialist or elite knowledge on this subject. Every social worker should be able to know themselves in their own skin, who they are in that physical sense, and be able to use their sense of their own body in their work with other people. What this chapter has argued is for the possibility of physical awareness also linking to spiritual awareness or, more simply, a spirituality of the body.

Note

1 The writings of Wendell Berry are also discussed by Mishka Lysack in Chapter 36.

References

Barrett, D. and Fine, H.J. (1990) 'The Gnostic syndrome: anorexia nervosa', *Psychoanalytic Psychotherapy*, 4(3): 263–70.

Bell, R.M. (1985) *Holy Anorexia*, Chicago: Chicago University Press.

Berry, W. (1997) *The Unsettling of America: agriculture and culture*, 3rd edn, San Francisco. Sierra Club Books.

Cameron, N. and McDermott, F. (2007) *Social Work and the Body*, Basingstoke: Palgrave Macmillan.

Chittester, J.D. (1998) *Heart of Flesh: a feminist spirituality for women and men*, Cambridge: Eerdmans Publishing.

Ferguson, H. (2011) *Child Protection Practice*, Basingstoke: Palgrave Macmillan.

George, L. (1995) *The Encyclopaedia of Heresies and Heretics*, London: Robson Books.

Gray, J. (2015) *The Soul of the Marionette: a short inquiry into human freedom*, London: Farrar, Straus and Giroux.

Hanratty, G. (1997) *Studies in Gnosticism and the Philosophy of Religion*, Dublin. Four Courts Press.

Heidegger, M. (1962) *Being and Time*, New York. Harper and Row.

Houtman, D. and Aupers, S. (2010) 'New age ethics', in M. Gray and S.A. Webb (eds) *Ethics and Value Perspectives in Social Work*, Basingstoke: Palgrave Macmillan.

Jordan, P. (2001) 'The materiality of Shamanism as a world-view: praxis, artefacts and landscape', in N. Price (ed) *The Archaeology of Shamanism*, London: Routledge.

Kittisaro and Thanissara (2014) *Listening to the Heart: a contemplative journey to engaged Buddhism*, London: Penguin Random House.

Koltun-Fromm, K. (2010) *Material Culture and Jewish Thought in America*, Bloomington: Indiana University Press.

Lee, M.Y., Ng, S-M., Leung, P.P.Y. and Chan, C. L.W. (2009) *Integrative Body-Mind-Spirit Social Work*, London: Oxford University Press.

Leech, K. (1981) *The Social God*, London: SPCK.

Levin, D.M. (1985) *The Body's Recollection of Being*, Illinois: North Western University.

MacDonagh, M. (2014) 'Mindfulness is something worse than just a smug middle-class trend', The Spectator. Online. Available HTTP: http://new.spectator.co.uk/2014/11/whats-wrong-with-mindfulness-more-than-you-might-think/ (accessed 11 November 2015).

MacIntyre, A. (1985) *After Virtue: a study of moral theory*, 2nd edn, London: Bloomsbury.

Merlieu-Ponty, M. (2002) *Phenomenology of Perception*, London: Routledge.

Moss, B. (2005) *Religion and Spirituality*, Lyme Regis: Russell House Publishing.

Price, L. and Walker, L. (2015) *Chronic Illness, Vulnerability and Social Work: autoimmunity and the contemporary disease experience*, London: Routledge.

Runciman, S. (1947) *The Medieval Manichee: a study of the Christian dualist heresy*, Cambridge: Cambridge University Press.

Voegelin, E. (1975) *From Enlightenment to Revolution*, Durham: Duke University Press.

Walsh, A.M. (2009) 'The resonant body: preliminary considerations for social work practice', *Critical*

Social Work, 10(1): 48–58. Online. Available HTTP: www1.uwindsor.ca/criticalsocialwork/system/files/walsh.pdf (accessed 2 December 2015).

Whiting, R. (2008) 'No room for religion or spirituality or cooking tips: exploring practical atheism as an unspoken consensus in the development of social work', *Ethics and Social Welfare,* 2(1): 67–83.

Whiting, R. (2015) 'Gestures of mutuality: bridging social work values and skills through Erasmian humanism', *Ethics and Social Welfare*, 9(4): 328–42.

Whiting, R. and Gurbai, S. (2015) 'Moving from the implicit to the explicit: "Spiritual Rights" and the United Nations Convention on the Rights of Persons with Disabilities', *Canadian Journal of Disability Studies*, 4(3): 103–26. Online. Available HTTP: cjds.uwaterloo.ca/index.php/cjds/article/download/233/407 (accessed 30 November 2015).

13

Social work with Muslim communities

Treading a critical path over the crescent moon

Sara Ashencaen Crabtree

Contextualising social work with Muslim communities

Islam is part of the triumvirate of Abrahamic religions and the youngest of this group, which includes Judaism and Christianity. Accordingly there are many points of comparison across the three faiths, whose communities of believers are known as 'the people of the Book': those guided by the sacred texts of these religions; although with highly distinctive elements to each of the Abrahamic religions. The Holy Qur'an is the textual foundation of Islam, being the sacralised writings venerated by Muslims who believe that it holds the sacred word of Allah as revealed to the Prophet Mohammed (570–632 BCE), peace be upon him.[1] Death overtaking all mortal beings, upon his demise his followers sought to capture Mohammed's teachings in form of the *sunna* (the prophetic tradition), in which can be found the *hadiths* – the sayings of the Prophet guide followers in terms of religious belief, practice and conduct. A feature of Islam, which means 'to submit', is its holism in combining these three elements and encompassing the five fundamental duties for Muslims:

1   *Shahadah* – bearing witness that there is only one God and Mohammed is his Prophet
2   *Salat* – prayer, practised five times a day and fixed according to the movement of the sun
3   *Zakat* – an alms tax to support the needy in society as distributive wealth
4   *Saum* – fasting from sunrise to sunset during the holy month of Ramadan
5   *Hajj* – the pilgrimage that should be undertaken at least once in the life of the believer to the Ka'aba in Mecca, Saudi Arabia.

(Ashencaen Crabtree *et al.* 2008)

Denominational differences are found in Islam in terms of Sunni and Shi'a sects, where sectarian oppression of the latter can be observed. Sufism forms another devotional tradition, which also extends across several Muslim societies, although this is also under sectarian pressures (Ashencaen Crabtree *et al.* 2017).

Contemporary demographic data indicate that Islam is the fastest growing religion in the Global North (Al-Krenawi 2012). Gündüz (2010) comments on the rapid expansion of Muslim minority ethnic (ME) groups across Europe, which at 23 million now represents 5 per cent of the overall population (Gündüz 2010). Nevertheless, Muslim groups tend to be concentrated, with the majority (65 per cent) of Muslims in Europe residing in the UK, France and Germany (Ashencaen Crabtree 2014; Jikeli 2013). Diversity is wide in terms of ethno-cultural heritage, custom and practice (Ashencaen Crabtree *et al.* 2008) and where Muslim communities are subject to very different social policy drivers across national boundaries (Ashencaen Crabtree 2014).

Regarding professional services and Muslim communities, the secularisation of social work as enacted in Britain and other countries has been challenged as insufficiently responsive. Over the past decade, there has been a notable increase in a social work canon focusing on religion and spirituality (Furness and Gilligan 2010). However, attempts to address spiritual need have been piecemeal owing to continuing and uniformed professional assumptions. The needs of many service user and client groups have been overlooked across a range of religious and spiritual beliefs, including those of Christians, where stereotypically a self-identification of Anglicanism is too often interpreted as effectively that of 'non-believer'.

Consequently the landscape of religious piety in Britain is frequently assumed to be primarily confined to minority ethnic (ME) groups, of which Muslims form a sizeable, if somewhat unfamiliar, group, around which have coalesced many contested positions and debates. Whether or not it forms part of the new awareness of religion and spirituality as being important but often professionally neglected domains of the human experience, there is a welcome rise in the research literature on Islamic perspectives. There is a growth of research literature interrogating social work values, practice and education in terms of religio-cultural differences, in addition to a burgeoning exploration of health and social welfare services as affecting Muslim service users (Ashencaen Crabtree *et al.* 2008). These have added much to our emergent understandings of the holism of Islam in terms of belief, daily practice and how personal needs and professional responses are accordingly influenced.

Islamic perspectives have to an extent now begun to populate a vacuum of professional knowledge regarding what might be construed as appropriate and/or sensitive intervention with multifaith groups in keeping with a cultural competence agenda. While holding clear merits in raising social work awareness of the need to work effectively with diverse communities, the cultural competence approach has been critiqued on the grounds of homogeneity – the essentialising of generalised groups of people who may be quite distinctive in most characteristics, apart from a common identity as Muslims (Ashencaen Crabtree 2014).

Casting illumination over pathways to improved social work intervention with Muslim individuals, families and communities does not disguise the divergent forks in the road that are apparent. Along with greater social work awareness of these important aspects of diversity in multicultural and multifaith societies are found representations of Muslim minority groups as socially problematic in Westernised, democratic spaces; particularly when these are associated with civil subversion and terrorism.

The conception of Muslims as legitimate would-be recipients of sensitive social work intervention or the construction of Muslims as socially subversive security risks controversially carries an unavoidable common element. The latter form a symbolically ostracised group representing contested areas of belief, practice and lifestyle, feeding into contemporary mythologies of the feared and alien 'other' in our midst. However, equally the validated and thus normalised Muslim service user/client is a conceptually nebulous entity. The crucial point of similarity between the two stereotypes is that through being unlinked from familiar, 'known' identifiers such as ethnicity or nationality, Muslims are therefore recast as a unique but isolated category, as opposed to a diverse group of people of multiple heritage and customs, like any other population.

Admittedly the Islamic concept of *Ummah*, the community of the Muslim faithful, acts to form a sense of common principles of belief and common identity. This serves as a conceptual glue aiding the proselyting mission of Islam in its rapid move from a locally confined belief system to a global religion (in common with comparable elements to Christianity, unlike that of Judaism). However, whether the notion of *Ummah* was conceived as displacing ethnic and regional identifiers is, from this historical perspective, a question for further theological debate.

Here both a paradox and a hazard are together found, in that in contemporary society among nearly all other minority ethnic groups, it is the religious identifier rather than that of the ethnic identifier that demarcates Muslims from other peoples. It is also this imposed marker that can create both a specifically defined, seemingly static identity as well as a risk of separation or alienation from the wider multicultural community.

Let us pause momentarily in considering the specifics in order to better contemplate the ambiguous and ambivalent. The constructed space that is viewed as 'known' includes well established but mutable ethnic classifications, but is juxtaposed by that which is 'unknown' represented by unfamiliar, misunderstood or misrepresented belief systems. This latter space creates an area of supposed emptiness that may be filled by opinion, assumptions, misunderstandings, negative associations and prejudice. However, such spaces also hold an unbounded liminal vacuum working between the spaces of perception and realities. It is here, therefore, in this fertile void of ignorance that an exploration of how social work addresses the needs of Muslim service users, families and communities begins to establish a definite point in a complex and often poorly illuminated terrain.

In this brief chapter, areas of ambiguity and tension can merely be outlined as a backdrop to a rich tapestry made up of diverse peoples self-identifying as Muslims who, over the course of centuries, have been subject to a range of recognised citizen (and resident) entitlements. This pattern of migration and settlement (as well as conversion) is today threaded through by a current discourse of alienation with society and the threatened fragmentation of multicultural democratic ideals (Grossfoguel and Mielants 2006; Gündüz 2010: 45). It is within this uncertain and tense milieu that social work as an institution must operate; and where to compound problems in Britain, English social work is fighting a politicised rear-guard action to maintain its professional autonomy and to halt the erosion of its erstwhile splendidly expansive social work education from collapsing into a narrow training protocol to serve neo-political ends (Parker and Doel 2013).

Muslim families in Britain

The areas for intervention from micro practice to macro engagement appear legion. What is often referred to as 'effective social work practice' seeks to address micro-level need at the individual level, which in turn is embedded in meso-level community dynamics and circumstances. However, social work must also engage in problematising overlapping and competing discourses that shape macro policy and social attitudes, and in so doing articulate clear responses to events taking place in the civic-political space impacting upon local people.

The somewhat inadequate and hackneyed term 'challenge' and the barely supportable, nonsensical cliché 'making a difference' barely begin to address the magnitude of the task. Nor do these phrases adequately express the moral and civic dimensions of the professionalised duty, and the complexity of negotiating compassionately, sagaciously and skilfully both the bounded territories and those areas of 'no man's land' that are made up of diverse peoples and multiple identities, representing numerous communities in need.

In the first edition of *Islam and Social Work* (Ashencaen Crabtree *et al.* 2008), the relative socio-economic underprivileged status of Muslim communities living in Britain was considered in terms of access to employment, housing and education. The national picture has altered somewhat since then, with growing numbers of Muslims (albeit subject to gender differences) attaining university education and professional employment at a comparable rate to the general population and where unemployment of Muslims stands at 7.2 per cent compared to 4.0 per cent of the general population (Muslim Council of Britain [MCB] 2015). Despite these socio-economic changes, the MCB notes:

> Just under half (46% or 1.22 million) of the Muslim population lives in the 10% most deprived and 1.7% (46,000) in the 10% least deprived, Local Authority Districts in England, based on the Index of Multiple Deprivation measure. In 2001, 33% of the Muslim population resided in the 10% most deprived localities.
>
> (MCB 2015: 46)

Disadvantageous life circumstances combined with other negative and pejorative experiences create a toxic mix of perceived discrimination marring and deforming victims and perpetrators alike. In respect of Muslims this phenomena is often classified as conforming to Islamophobic prejudice.

Islamophobia

Discrimination arises in part through the assumption of the existence of an essentialised Muslim identity, immutable and alien, which is encapsulated in the concept of 'Islamophobia'. This is another contested term, differing from other determinants of discrimination in being neither solely prejudice against ethnicity nor religious affiliation but situating itself somewhere between the two (Hussain and Bagguely 2012; Lorente 2010).

The definition of Islamophobia, which first appeared in the UK in 1997 in *Islamophobia: A Challenge for Us All*, remains in currency, summing up a portrayal of Islam as:

1   Monolithic and static
2   Separate and 'other' – not sharing other values
3   Inferior to the West
4   An aggressive enemy
5   Muslims as manipulative
6   Critical of the West
7   Patriarchy and sexism are implicit to Islam.

(Runnymede Trust 1997)

Taras (2013) has since then added other characteristics of Islamophobia: Muslims as irrational and aggressive; Islamic ideologies as used for political and military agendas (we assume, Taras means predominantly assumed, rather than used at all, which would be an untenable position). Islamophobia for Taras includes an assumption of intolerance towards Western critiques, as then deserving of exclusion and thereby making anti-Muslim hostility natural and normal (Taras 2013). Other examples that have been given of Islamophobic attitudes include not serving halal food in institutional settings (Bloul 2008), and banning of headscarves in school settings (Haque 2004).

In exploring the ambiguous construction of the concept of 'Islamophobia' as a problematic and somewhat incoherently defined all-inclusive concept, Lorente (2010: 117) concludes that it acts as a 'universal container of social practices and meanings regardless of the contextual conditions upon which those built until present have been based'.

Fleischmann *et al.* (2011) consider the social repercussions of disaffection among Muslim youth, who are deemed more likely to react towards perceived Islamophobia by constructing a stronger religiously-based identity, which may also be linked to political action, than the reaction of the previous (migrant) generation. The authors articulate that the European mission in consequence must be based on achieving social and political integration for Muslim minority groups. Richards (2013) offers an interesting analysis of the cyclical nature of reaction through an examination of a series of 'tit-for-tat' clashes between extremist groups in Britain: Islamist and British supremacist nationalists; duly hypothesising on the symbiotic dynamics of this destruction interplay.

Parenting, youth and counter-terrorism

The overall national picture of a young Muslim population has remained reasonably consistent over the past decade, where 33 per cent of British Muslims are aged 15 years old or under (MCB 2015). This carries important implications in terms of the overlapping factors of potential underprivileged conditions relating to child poverty, inadequate housing and the nature of the community infrastructure. In respect of children other factors such as education form important considerations, whether in relation to mainstream schooling or the new British social policy initiative of Free Schools, enabling faith groups (among others) to set up their own schools for specific purposes.

Parenting in Britain and many other countries of the West is no longer assumed to be a dependable domain of personal expertise. Increasingly that private domain is now viewed as subject to social policy strategies and surveillance by professionals as part of a risk prevention approach (Fathi and Yakak in press). The context of extremism provides the tense backdrop to the issue of parenting and the begetting of normative citizens. The London bombings of 2005 were notably carried out by what was described in the media as 'four home-grown suicide bombers' (Campbell and Laville 2005). Chillingly, the Madrid Jihadist bombers of 2004 were also assumed to be successfully socially integrated into Spanish society, albeit in their case Maghrebian migrants (Jordan *et al.* 2008).

Accordingly, in response to the conversion of a few Britons to violent Islamist causes, the domain of Muslim parenting has come under general scrutiny. This is tacitly subject to the suspicion that such families are insufficiently inculcating the necessary social values and conduct for children to smoothly acquire normative citizen values. Concerns have also been raised in the political and media arena at a perceived lack of a coherent and strongly articulated moderate Muslim voice protesting against Islamist propaganda, implicating the role of imams and where some mosques are viewed as potential sites of radicalisation.

In response to the so-called threat of global terrorism, the 'Prevent' strategy is an important plank in CONTEST, the British government's counter-terrorist strategy. Prevent is aimed at tackling the radicalisation of Muslim youth and works across a wide range of community and statutory provisions. Controversially, British schools and institutions of higher education are required to engage with the Prevent strategy, to identify conspiratorial conversion of young people while promoting 'British values', a contested notion in itself and previously considered tacit rather than explicit, but is now defined in a predictable list as including tolerance, democracy, individual liberty and the supremacy of the rule of law (Citizenship Foundation 2015). This strategically organised approach attempts to steer the impressionable minds of young people away from perceived malign, socially disruptive influences, but in so doing adds a heavily politicised policing role to that of educator, which continues to generate deep disquiet within those professions (Parker in press).

In addition to the perceived dangers of an 'enemy within', the recruitment of a number of Britons, including the absconding of a few British schoolgirls, to the notorious ISIS cause has created a wave of concerns of the hazards facing disaffected young Muslims. The increasing awareness of ISIS' very sophisticated and vicious use of social media to recruit as well as advertise its latest atrocities has been noted. The possible infiltration of Jihadists smuggled into Britain camouflaged among groups of legitimate refugees is a perturbing threat to many, however unlikely; escalating public anxiety and serving to obscure the plight of the real victims of ISIS in the Middle East, both Christians and Muslims. It also acts as superb propaganda for such groups and unwittingly plays into their agendas.

Regrettably, therefore, perceived Islamist threats and responses to these threats do not create a particularly auspicious environment to closely scrutinise and challenge counter-terrorist strategies and the potentially damaging consequence of these. Prevent, for example, is in danger of creating a controversial conceptualisation of democratic dissent in citizenry of crude polarised proportions (Parker in press). In so doing, concerns are raised that these strategies may actually be fostering a deepening sense of alienation and grievance in Muslim communities. The latest counter-extremist strategy by the British government is to place the responsibility of policing young people upon their parents, who are now expected to apply to have their child's passport confiscated by the State, if they are concerned that the minor may abscond to join terrorist groups. Failure to take due precautions will in turn rebound upon such parents as constructed within a discourse of responsible citizenship. However, a sense of proportionality is also required to put the threat of Islamist radicalisation among the British public into proper context, where we learn from that of 2.7 million Muslims in the UK, official estimates are that around 700 individuals have travelled to Syria, which amounts to 0.026 per cent of the self-identifying Muslim population (BBC News 2015).

To bridge a widening gap between vulnerability as a classified criteria for social work intervention and vulnerability as requiring social work support in consequence of State intervention, Surinder Guru's (2012) illuminating study offers some powerful insights. Here she focuses on the impact of counter-terrorist surveillance on the families of suspected terrorists in the UK, revealing how terrifying the State response can be to families subjected to sudden police raids:

> The kids were frightened—crying ... screaming. They even wet themselves standing. They were so scared when they saw their father on the floor ... Even the older ones urinated themselves because they were so scared. I tried to reassure them that he would be back soon ... but I could not stop them crying...
>
> (Guru 2012: 1166)

Guru draws essential connections between the personal and political ramifications bearing down on individual families. In so doing she urges that social workers need to engage with the political sharp-end of these forms of vulnerability and to draw the links between individual circumstances and macro policy enacted at meso-level community intervention (Ashencaen Crabtree 2014).

Gender normativity

In respect of Muslim families, MCB (2015: 68) note that there is a 'surprisingly high' number of lone parents with dependent children, standing at 77,000 compared to 260,000 cohabiting couples with such dependents. How far lone parenting constitutes an actual social problem is highly debatable, and where religious, cultural and politicised opinions will be formative in putting forward a range of social constructions and associated polemics.

Lone parenting is often used as a short-hand for parenting by a majority of lone mothers, which in itself is laden with socio-religio-cultural and political constructions. Ashencaen Crabtree and Husain (2012) argue, however, that the issue of representation of women as the embodiment of culture and religion is a general patriarchal device that seeks to appropriate or reject, but in both cases serves to objectivise and control women as bearers of cultural values. Representations of Muslims are conventionally conveyed by images of Muslim women in enveloping dress, head covering and veil. Macdonald (2006) dismisses this stereotype as serving to metaphorically obscure more important areas of relevant debate. By contrast, Mernissi (1992) disagrees, in viewing dress as a quintessential signifier of social representation of Muslim womanhood, within a socio-historical context (Ashencaen Crabtree and Husain 2012). Zine (2004) asserts that the projected image of the hijab-covered women in itself represents global terrorism, fanaticism and sexist oppression – and indeed one can see such conflict-worn images of idealised Muslim womanhood as intentionally visibly invisible – and thus inevitably an image also adopted by ISIS.

The iconography is complete in Moallem's (2008) discussion of the symbolised figure of 'Muslimwoman' as a site of contested discourses between the 'imperialist West' and Islamist groups, replete with the struggle to take ownership of the right to speak on her behalf. It would be easy to construe in consequence that feminism, for want of a better term, has but a very tenuous hold in the Muslim world. While the term 'feminist' may resurrect a number of assumed political and identity positions particularly resonant in the Northern hemisphere, Muslim women's emancipatory struggles for recognition and rights within Islam are to the fore among such activist bodies as Malaysia's Sisters in Islam. However, similar action groups do not necessarily reject Islam as such but rather seek to deconstruct masculine interpretations of the Holy Qur'an by stripping text back to its original empowering content, uncontaminated by subsequent gender politics (Ashencaen Crabtree and Husain 2012).

Ageing

In consideration of life span issues the elderly minority ethnic population of the UK is increasing, where the majority of such elders are likely to be first generation migrants to the UK. This is also true for the UK's Muslim elders, whose access to appropriate services may be compromised by English language proficiency, dietary requirements, together with inhibitions concerning receiving care away from the family context. In the Holy Qur'an can be found numerous injunctions urging filial respect and care of ageing parents:

> Your Lord has enjoined you to worship none but Him, and to show kindness to your parents. If either or both of them attain old age in your dwelling, shown them no sign of impatience, nor rebuke them: but speak to them kind words. Treat them with humility and tenderness and say: "Lord, be merciful to them. They nursed me when I was an infant."
>
> ('The Night Journey', Holy Qur'an: 17)

Guided by these readings many families may well feel conflict regarding acceptance of external help. Additionally, assumption behind the notion that 'they care for their own' has been implicated in the failure of social services and other welfare groups to offer sufficient levels of services to ME groups, beyond the issue of potential client groups not opting to become service users (Ashencaen Crabtree et al. 2008).

Gender norms governing social interactions are other important considerations in relation to offering appropriate services, where female- or male-only groups may be viewed as essential, but often run counter to the mixed-sex groups operated in many services. These socio-religio demarcations of gender can also extend to the use of transport to services, preventing some elders from reaching day services from the outset. Yet increased longevity and age-related decline in combination with individual health, cultural and faith-based suggests huge systematic challenges (Ashencaen Crabtree *et al.* 2017).

In respect of how old age is constructed in Islam, this provides a portrait that is both unvarnished, stark even, and yet dignified in its stoic acceptance of the inevitable. The Qur'anic verse, 'Al Asr' uses the familiar metaphor of old age as constituting the late afternoon of life descending into night. This is no golden time but one where loss is acknowledged as cumulative and inevitable. Al Asr is austerely cast and in so doing rebukes the mythology and pursuit of eternal youth, long associated with the West, as a desperate flight from reality. Decrepitude of body and even of mind is to be expected and it is no dishonour at all to recognise that – in some senses quite the reverse. For the pious Muslim, the ultimate destination and *goal* of human life is death, where judgement awaits and believers will be admitted to Paradise (Ashencaen Crabtree 2014; Moody 1990).

As described, uneasy tensions gripping British society equally enmesh Muslim migrant elders, particularly those from the Middle East, where both the events of 9/11 and the later London Islamist bombings of 7 July 2005, and resultant social attitudes of Islamophobia, generate a troubling sense of vulnerability and exposure among Muslim communities (Fiddian-Qasmiyeh and Qasmiyehm 2010), which bears down across all generations.

Concluding remarks

An expansive area has been traversed in critically examining the current socio-political context surrounding British Muslims as a problematised community within a tense multicultural discourse, which does not implicate other ME British groups to any similar degree. A highly complex and indeed fraught confusion of intertwined positionings requires cautious unravelling and here we return to the useful metaphors pertaining to the known and the unknown, the seen and unseen. It is difficult to imagine any contemporary, and well-established organised religious group to which are attached so many contradictory messages and so much inflamed debate. This can well be viewed as deplorable, where the impact of this legacy is likely to fall heavily on individual families and their immediate ecological network, with much damage done in consequence.

That which remains less seen and thus less known pertains to the Islam of the Abrahamic traditions, a religion fundamentally of peace and tolerance, although this message is increasingly drowned out by the volley of discordant voices competing for dominance. The credibility of this ancient message, however, is greatly undermined by the conflagration of harmful and dangerous messages and discourses emanating from many quarters, projecting destructive images of both Muslims and non-Muslims that contorted and deformed though they are, are received as accurate depictions by the receiver. The right to speak of what Islam is appears to have been wrested and usurped from ordinary Muslim citizens, whose voice requires orchestration and amplification for reasoned exchange in the civil forum of multicultural debate, and by so doing decentralises immoderate and prejudiced voices and thereby destabilises the centrifugal axis of threatened extremist violence.

Note

1 A convention often used as a mark of respect and frequently shortened to (PBUH).

References

Al-Krenawi, A. (2012) 'Islam, human rights and social work in a changing world', in S. Ashencaen Crabtree, J. Parker and A. Azman (eds) *The Cup, The Gun and The Crescent*, London: Whiting & Birch.

Ashencaen Crabtree, S. (2014) 'Islamophobia and the Manichean constructions of the "other": a contemporary European problematic', in S. Ashencaen Crabtree (ed) *Diversity and the Processes of Marginalisation and Otherness: giving voice to hidden themes – a European perspective*, London: Policy Press.

Ashencaen Crabtree, S. and Husain, F. (2012) 'Within, without: dialogical perspectives on feminism and Islam', *Religion and Gender*, 2(1): 128–49.

Ashencaen Crabtree, S., Husain, F. and Spalek, B. (2008) *Islam and Social Work: debating values, transforming practice*, 1st edn, Bristol: Policy Press.

Ashencaen Crabtree, S., Husain, F. and Spalek, B. (2017) *Islam and Social Work: culturally sensitive practice in a diverse world,* 2nd edn, Bristol: Policy Press.

BBC News (2015) 'Who Are Britain's Jihadists?' *News*. Online. Available HTTP: www.bbc.co.uk/news/uk-32026985 (accessed 19 July 2015).

Bloul, R.A.D. (2008) 'Anti-discrimination Laws, Islamophobia, and ethnicization of Muslim identities in Europe and Australia', *Journal of Muslim Minority Affairs*, 28(1): 7–25.

Campbell, D. and Laville, S. (2005) 'British suicide bombers carried out London attacks, say police', *The Guardian*, 13 July 2005. Online. Available HTTP: www.theguardian.com/uk/2005/jul/13/july7.uksecurity6 (accessed 27 October 2015).

Citizenship Foundation (2015) *Doing SMSC*. Online. Available HTTP: www.doingsmsc.org.uk (accessed 18 October 2015).

Fathi, M. and Hakak, Y. (in press) 'Muslim parenting in the West: a review article', *Sociology Compass*.

Fiddian-Qasmiyeh, E. and Qasmiyehm Y. (2010) 'Muslim asylum-seekers and refugees: negotiating identity, politics and religion in the UK', *Journal of Refugee Studies*, 23(3): 294–314.

Fleischman, F., Phalet, K. and Klein, O. (2011) 'Religious identification and politicization for political Islam and political action among the Turkish and Moroccan second generation in Europe', *British Journal of Social Psychology*, 50(4): 628–48.

Furness, S. and Gilligan, P. (2010) *Religion, Belief and Social Work*, Policy Press: University of Bristol.

Grossfoguel, R. and Mielants, E. (2006) 'The long-durée entanglement between Islamophobia and racism in the modern/colonial capitalist/patriarchal world-system: an introduction', *Human Architecture*, 5(1): 1–12.

Gündüz, Z.Y. (2010) 'The European Union at 50: xenophobia, Islamophobia and the rise of the Radical Right', *Journal of Muslim Minority Affairs*, 30(1): 36–47.

Guru, S. (2012) 'Under siege: families of counter-terrorism', *The British Journal of Social Work,* 42(5): 1151–73.

Haque, A. (2004) 'Islamophobià in North America: confronting the menace', in B. van Driel (ed) *Confronting Islamophobia in Educational Practice*, Stoke on Trent: Trentham Books.

Hussain, Y. and Bagguley, P. (2012) 'Securitized citizens: Islamophobia, racism and the 7/7 London bombings', *The Sociological Review*, 60(4): 715–34.

Jordan, J., Mañas, F.M. and Horsburgh, N. (2008) 'Strengths and weaknesses of grassrootJihadist networks: the Madrid bombings', *Studies in Conflict and Terrorism*, 31(1): 17–29.

Jikeli, G., (2013) *Young Muslims in Europe: Islamic identity and hostile attitudes*. Online. Available HTTP: http://research.allacademic.com/index.php?click_key=1&PHPSESSID=8ieeqp11au7u52i1ohmb4rirl3 (accessed 8 August 2016).

Lorente, J.R. (2010) 'Discrepancies around the use of the term "Islamophobia"', *Human Architecture: Journal of the Sociology of Self-Knowledge*, VIII(2): 115–28.

Macdonald, M. (2006) 'Muslim women and the veil', *Feminist Media Studies*, 6(1): 7–23.

Mernissi, F. (1992) *A Feminist Interpretation of Women's Rights in Islam*, Reading: Berkshire Addison Wesley Publishing Company.

Moallem, M. (2008) 'Muslim women and the politics of representation', *Journal of Feminist Studies in Religion*, 24(1): 106–10.

Moody, H.R. (1990) 'The Islamic vision of aging and death', *Generations*, 14(4): 15-19.

Parker, J. (in press) 'Students and *Prevent*: towards new models of citizenship?', *Sociology*.

Parker, J. and Doel, M. (2013) 'Professional social work and the professional social work identity?', in J. Parker and M. Doel (eds) *Professional Social Work*, London: Learning Matters/Sage.

Richards, B. (2013) 'A case study in community conflict', unpublished paper presentation, Bournemouth University, *Festival of Learning*, June, 2013.

Runnymede Trust (1997) *Islamophobia: a challenge for us all*, London: Runnymede Trust.

Taras, R. (2013) '"Islamophobia never stands still": race, religion and culture', *Ethnic and Racial Studies*, 36(3): 417–33.

The Muslim Council of Britain [MCB] (2015) *British Muslims in Numbers*, London: MCB.

Zine, J. (2004) 'Creating a critical faith-centered space for antiracist feminism', *Feminist Studies in Religion*, 2(2): 167–87.

14

Religious and spiritual perspectives of social work among the Palestinians

Alean Al-Krenawi

Religion and spirituality

This chapter will examine religiosity and spirituality in the context of social work. Religiosity has been roughly defined by Hill and Hood (1999: 5) as 'phenomena that include some relevance to traditional institutionalized searches to acknowledge and maintain some relationship with the transcendent', while spirituality is defined as 'that most human of experiences that seeks to transcend self and find meaning and purpose through connection with others, nature, and/or a Supreme Being, which may or may not involve religious structures or traditions' (Buck 2006: 289).

Research in Europe and North America has shown that religiosity and religious identity are both positively correlated with psychological wellbeing (e.g. Francis and Katz 2002; Hackney and Sanders 2003; Lewis *et al.* 2005). Abu-Rayya and Abu-Rayya (2009a) presented a similar case examining the Muslim population, where they found a positive relation between religious identity and psychological wellbeing. Abu-Rayya and Abu-Rayya (2009b) found the same connection among Palestinians, and expounded that ethnic identification is not the only factor relevant here, but that religious identification is also important for the wellbeing of minority populations. Defining oneself as religious was related to higher levels of positive affect and social relations, as well as higher self-esteem levels.

Religion and spirituality are also used as mechanisms to help cope with difficulties such as trauma and bereavement. Religious coping refers to the act of using religious activities, such as additional praying or attending additional religious services, in response to a stressful event, thus using the religious/spiritual activities and beliefs to cope with the stress (Abeles *et al.* 1999). Ano and Vasconcelles (2005) examined religious coping strategies and discovered that there is a positive relationship between using religion to cope with psychosocial difficulties and having good psychological adjustments and positive outcomes to stressful events. Religious coping strategies, such as benevolent religious reappraisals, collaborative religious coping and seeking spiritual support act as adaptive functions.

Religious coping strategies also help those coping with the loss of a loved one, and are associated with better adjustment to adverse events (Mattlin *et al.* 1990). For example, mothers who lost a twin cited a better ability to cope when they believed there was a higher purpose to the loss (Swanson *et al.* 2002) and recently bereaved parents who reported perceived spiritual support had lower depression scores (Maton 1989). In the case of Islam, Muslims are told to focus on religious beliefs and religious practices when they experience a loss; the Qur'an states that even in these circumstances, the main focus should always be God. Muslims believe that by renewing their acceptance of the will of God, the bereaved will be able to cope with their loss by drawing strength from the link to God and their religion. In addition, Islam has specific mourning rituals and behaviours that are meant to help the bereaved (Rubin and Yasien-Esmael 2004).

Islam

Islam is a monotheistic religion believing in one God, Allah, and in the Prophet Mohammad, the messenger of Allah. Islam has two main streams: Sunni and Shiite. Sunnis comprise approximately 90 per cent of Muslims worldwide, with Shiites making up the remaining 10 per cent. Sunni Islam privileges an unmediated relationship between the worshipper and God, whereas in Shiite Islam a hierarchical interpretive structure is salient (Hodge 2005).

The Qur'an, the canonical text of Islam, is understood to be the word of God (*Allah*) as revealed to the Prophet Mohammad. 'Qur'an' in Arabic means 'recitation'. The Qur'an is the primary source of Islamic Law (*shari'a*) that comprehensively regulates life for pious Muslims (Al-Krenawi 2012). Observant Muslims may believe in the existence of angels and the devil as well (Al-Krenawi 2012; Hodge 2005). Nonetheless, generalisations are out of place in that individuals who identify as Muslim express all behaviours and beliefs.

Islamic law stipulates that five 'pillars' must be observed by its devotees. The first pillar of Islam is the recitation of '*Shahadah*', which affirms a belief in one God, whose final prophet was Mohammad. This affirmation can be understood not only as a declaration of faith, but also as a socio-political statement implying that a single deity governs the world. The second pillar of Islam is the prayer referred to as '*Salah*'. It is incumbent upon male Muslims to recite these prayers five times per day, and to prostrate in the direction of their holy city of Mecca. The prayers may be recited individually or congregationally, either in a mosque or anywhere else. The third pillar is '*Zakah*', which means 'charity'. This pillar is multi-ethnic, in that the money is intended for the needy among Muslims and non-Muslims alike. '*Zakah*' is construed as a corrective to social inequalities. The fourth pillar is '*Siyam*', or the month-long fasting of Ramadan, where Muslims refrain from eating, drinking and sexual relations during daylight hours while continuing with their daily activities. The goal of the fast is to establish an emotional tie with the poor. Ramadan concludes with a three-day festival referred to as the feast of '*Eid Al-Fitr*'. The fifth pillar is the pilgrimage to Mecca, the '*Hijj*,' to be undertaken at least once in one's lifetime, providing one has the financial, emotional and physical abilities necessary to undertake the journey (Al-Krenawi 2012).

Three foundational values, in addition to the five pillars, are widely affirmed by Muslims globally: family, community and the ultimate rule of God. These notions may be seen as interwoven tenets reflecting an integrated Islamic worldview (Hodge 2005).

Muslim society

Societies in the West are usually low-context societies where the individual is prized over the collective. These societies are fast-paced and always in a state of transition (Hall 1976). On the other hand, Muslim societies are high-context societies, where the collective is considered to be of more importance than the individual. Society is slow to accept change, social peace is sought after and social stability is thought to be one of the highest achievements. Emphasising the collective is another form of social peace, one endorsed in the Qur'an, with the mutually responsive collective following the ways of the Qur'an: 'Help each other in the acts of goodness and piety and do not extend help to each other in sinful acts or transgression behaviours' (Qur'an 5: 2). The Prophet Mohammad advised Muslims to help other Muslims in need, whether they are the oppressor or the oppressed. The Hadith adds to this idea and says that each person is a shepherd who is responsible for his flock (Nagati 1993). This sense of collective responsibility is further reinforced by how the Muslim views his or her place within society. Islam, it should be emphasised, is not concerned with the welfare of the individual alone, but rather it seeks to achieve a wider societal wellbeing. While ensuring the individual's freedom, it places equal stress on mutual responsibility.

Family

The sense of collective responsibility naturally extends to one's family. The welfare of the family is valued over the welfare of the individual, and thus identity is constructed according to family (Wasfi 1964). In Palestinian society, family is treasured, as are extended family members, because families have an important role according to Islam. Muslims live according to the traditional, patriarchal family structure, which defines the familial roles, status and obligations (Hall 2007). The Qur'an states that one must consider their family in every decision, a concept that serves to enforce the importance of the collective being over an independent, individual one. Religious spiritualism of an individual is not important, but rather the spiritualism of the family, as well as the role of the family in the community as a whole (Hall 2007).

The Palestinian case

Palestinians are a minority group within Israel. Over 700,000 Palestinians are Muslim, roughly 150,000 are Christian and almost 100,000 are Druze, Circassian or other groups. The vast majority reside in all-Arab towns and villages located in three main areas: the Galilee in the north, the 'Little Triangle' in the centre and the West Bank (Statistical Abstract of Israel 1998). The West Bank is the largest area of Palestine, and its population is 75 per cent Muslim, 17 per cent Jewish, and 8 per cent Christian (Al-Krenawi et al. 2009). The Palestinian Territories of Gaza, the West Bank, and east Jerusalem consist of approximately 4.6 million people (Halevy 2015). The sociopolitical situation for Palestinians is one full of trauma and bereavement. Due to poor relations with the Israelis, both sides have suffered from poor economic activity, a lack of political rights, social dislocation, as well as a multitude of psychological stress. There were many socioeconomic effects as well, such as the loss of land and orchards, and men losing their jobs due to road closures caused immense poverty. Both the West Bank and Gaza experienced considerable economic decline in both the first and second Intifada, violent Palestinian uprisings against the Israelis (Al-Krenawi et al. 2009).

Many damaging psychosocial effects have also been noted. The Intifada affected the entire Palestinian population, who suffered from anxiety, fear, shock and sadness, and worried that schools would shut down. Palestinians living near Israeli villages were most affected, with many highly apprehensive at the prospect of houses being demolished. In August 2004, the Palestinians Center Bureau of Statistics conducted a psychological health survey of children and youth aged 5–17 years, which reported that 11 per cent of the sample suffered from nervousness, 10 per cent showed a different kind of fear, 9.9 per cent lacked concentration and 5.8 per cent exhibited aggressive behaviour. Additionally, 30.8 per cent of the respondents had been exposed to violence. In December 2004, a similar study was conducted by Giacaman and colleagues (2004) in the West Bank, which showed that 73 per cent of the population felt insecure and 80 per cent expressed fear of continued Israeli occupation of the West Bank. Both Israelis and Palestinians reported fear and emotional stress over the safety of themselves and family members (Ramon *et al.* 2006). Support was required in order to cope with physical trauma and with the death of loved ones. In comparison to the first Intifada, the second Intifada caused less of an impact as the violence was already fast becoming an everyday occurrence and there was more support and cohesion among the people.

The Arabs in Israel also experienced stress stemming from being part of a minority group. Many perceive themselves as suffering from systematic economic, educational and cultural discrimination. Such social inequity has been identified as a risk factor for psychological distress, feelings of worthlessness, helplessness and powerlessness, of being regarded with disdain, as well as sadness and fear (Al-Krenawi 2005). This insecurity was reinforced by the increased rate of domestic violence. Al-Ashhab (2005) reported that 11.3 per cent of Palestinians reported they were victims of household violence, a rate that had doubled since 1996, and 29.5 per cent of the population reported being targets of an aggressive act or assault.

Underutilisation of social work services by Palestinians

Research has shown that help-seeking behaviours differ depending on ethnicity, gender, nationality, religion and socioeconomic status (Al-Krenawi *et al.* 2004). With regard to Islam and social work, problems arise for Palestinians because Islam's worldview contradicts some of the main viewpoints and practices of social work. The first contradiction is that Muslims look at Islam as providing complete guidance in all one's needs in life, with spirituality referred to in all points of life, while social work views Islam as a single component of religion that one must consider while making a treatment plan (Barise 2005). A second inconsistency is found in how one views the concept of helping behaviour. In Islam, one asks for help from God and sees the subsequent help as coming from God. In social work, the social workers provide the help and the help comes from them. A third discrepancy is the nature of human need; Islam believes that spirituality is the most important human need, while social workers believe that needs are only as important as people think they are. The fourth contradiction is that Muslims believe that when faced with a hardship, one needs to respond by turning to religion, to God, and not to a social worker. They believe that suffering makes a person stronger and is necessary in order to have one's sins be forgiven (Barise 2005). Another reason for the underutilisation of social workers stems from the society's attitude towards them. When a problem arises in the Arab community, advice is usually sought out from friends and family. A social worker is only turned to as a last resort, as they are perceived as an outsider that the family does not trust (Al-Krenawi and Graham 2000). Finally, Palestinians view the help-seeking services as contradicting their religious values, as the social workers are seen as having discarded religious values.

Mosque

Traditionally, help-seeking services have been provided at the mosque, as the mosque is not only a place of prayer, but also a venue for the provision of educational, welfare and conflict resolution services for Palestinian groups, families, couples and individuals. The congregation can turn to the Imam, the mosque's clergy analogous to priests and rabbis, who assumed his role within the community by virtue of being knowledgeable with the laws and ways of Islam. The position of Imam is a central role in the spiritual and communal life of Muslims, and the congregation displays a great deal of respect towards and trust in the Imam (Siddiqui 2004). The Imam's duties consist of leading prayers and providing advice and assistance to the community.

In all religions, congregants tend to turn to their religious communities when help is needed, regardless of whether clergy are the ones best suited to help. Thus, clergy often serve as the first line of mental health care for members of their communities, particularly in minority communities. A study by Wang and colleagues (2003) discovered that clergy provide more mental health care than psychiatrists, including treating people with serious mental illness. Leavey and colleagues (2007) conducted a study about the functionality of clergy as a resource for mental health. They discovered that Muslim and Jewish clergy reported that in many cases the mosque and synagogue were the first stop for families when a member of the family experienced emotional and psychiatric problems. These studies help illustrate the great importance placed on the function of the mosque within Islam and why it is crucial for social workers to have a greater understanding of the culture and practice of Muslims. Social workers will be able to connect with and assist Muslim clients only once they fully understand their culture, as the social worker's response has to take into account the wholeness of the client, which in this case includes the culture of the individual Muslim, the group and the community, and how they each relate to the religion of Islam.

Traditional healers

Palestinian society has traditionally relied upon the services of traditional healers. In this practice, healer and client share a common worldview that stresses the importance of their joint origin and helps them understand the problem, its sources and the best ways of relating to it. The healer directs, advises, guides, instructs and suggests practical courses of treatment. In addition, the client believes that the healer has supernatural powers (El-Islam 1982), as the healers are meant to be intervening in the spiritual world.

Arab healers are called Sheiks or Moalj Bel-Quran in Arabic, and they base their healing on the Qur'an and Hadith (Mohammad's sayings). One type of healer, Qur'anic healers, have healing clinics among the Palestinians in the Gaza Strip, central Israel, and the West Bank. The healers in these clinics share many similarities with social workers; they both use assessment procedures, implement theory learnt at universities and believe in proper training, consultation and supervision. The traditional healers use the client's belief in their knowledge and techniques in order to ensure success (Murphy 1973). These healers practice healing that is in accordance with Islamic values and agrees with the concept of a patriarchal society.

Traditional healers tend to have good relationships with the clients and their families, which is important as engaging the client's family is a large part of the healing and treatment process. The healer tends to rely on the family in order to ensure that the client is following the instructions, as well as to receive reports on the condition of the client. In addition, family is used as a support network (Al-Krenawi and Graham 1997). The healer relies on the dominant person in the client's family to help bring client change and to mobilise the family and the community.

The role of traditional healer is now being occupied by social workers, though Palestinians are slow to make the switch. For social workers to begin to work with the Muslim community, they need to understand all the religious and cultural details involved. Qur'anic healers have a strong foothold in helping Arab society, so it can be helpful for social workers to learn from them how to help this population. Such knowledge is necessary in order to enable dialogue between the social workers and the healers and Muslim society, as well as to appreciate cultural and religious sensitivities towards Muslim society.

Cultural differences and cultural stigma

Many cultural differences can be found between Palestinian society and social workers; consequently it can be difficult for them to work together. The Arab culture prizes building a trusting relationship over solving the initial problem, while the social worker wants a professional relationship maintained with a focus on solving the actual problem. Here, the cultural difference seen is in regard to interpersonal, professional relationships. Miscommunication stemming from cultural differences between the client and social worker can occur as well, though this difficulty is partially attributed to the social worker's lack of knowledge about Arab culture (Al-Krenawi *et al.* 1994). An additional problem is likely to arise when clients comprehend the social worker according to their own cultural code, thereby misunderstanding the social worker's intention.

Another barrier for the Palestinian society regarding help-seeking behaviour is the stigma of shame attached to seeing a social worker. Both Palestinian and Israeli Arabs reported having higher levels of perceived stigma attached to using mental health services than their other national counterparts (with no significant differences between Arab Israelis and Arab Palestinians). Several scholars point to the association between stigma and seeking mental health services (Al-Adawi *et al.* 2002; Al-Krenawi and Graham 1999, 2000; Savaya 1995).

Implications for social work practice

Social workers working with the Palestinian population are beginning to understand that this population has specific nuances that affect their help-seeking behaviours. As the majority of Palestinians are Muslim, the social worker needs a good understanding of Islamic culture. However, they also need to be able to acknowledge that Palestinians from other religious traditions may have other issues and there is a need to be culturally sensitive to those matters as well. When creating an intervention for the majority Muslim population, the social worker must take into account that Muslim society is characterised by the emphasis on the collective over the individual, the slow pace of societal change and a great sense of social stability (Al-Krenawi and Graham 1996). In accordance with the collective society, all of the family members will be concerned about anything that affects one family member and thus all will wish to intrude on the treatment. Because of the importance of family in the society, when a social worker comes to the community, they are not just speaking to the individual but rather to the entire family.

The social worker must acquire religious knowledge and include spirituality in the treatment plan in order to be able to appropriately help the client. This is one way to help the Palestinian population to embrace social workers; by having the social workers learn about Arab spirituality and the Arab population. This will put the social workers in an advantageous position and enable them to help and be allowed to help the Arab families. While social workers may not share the Palestinian religion and spirituality, it is important to acknowledge their clients' spirituality, as well as their values and belief systems.

After learning about the importance of the mosque and Imam, it would be beneficial to form a relationship with the Islamic clergy, in order to learn from them. While some Arabs would rather have fellow Islamic social workers, others prefer to speak to someone outside of the community. Someone outside the community is also preferred in the case of a religious problem, so the client can have a neutral space to explore their feelings. Palestinians place great importance on traditional healers and religious leaders, so it is therefore very important for the social worker to consider how religion impacts clients and to use this as a helping tool. The social worker must leave space for religious rituals and ceremonies, as they have a large psychosocial impact on the lives of Palestinians.

The need for clinicians to exercise cultural sensitivity in treating clients of a different ethnic or religious group than their own is a commonplace factor of the helping professions. Clinicians are expected to be familiar with and accept their clients' cultures and to take the cultures' norms and values into account. The social worker must develop a culturally appropriate model of intervention, which acknowledges global and local knowledge within spirituality and religion.

References

Abeles, R., Ellison, C., George, L., Idler, E., Krause, N., Levin, J., Ory, M., Pargament, K., Powell, L., Underwood, L. and Williams, D. (1999) *Multidimensional Measurement of Religiousness/Spirituality for Use in Health Research*, Kalamazoo, MI: Fetzer Institute Publication.

Abu-Rayya, H.M. and Abu-Rayya, M.H. (2009a) 'Acculturation, religious identity, and psychological wellbeing among Palestinians in Israel', *International Journal of Intercultural Relations*, 33(4): 325–31.

Abu-Rayya, H.M. and Abu-Rayya, M.H. (2009b) 'Ethnic identification, religious identity, and psychological wellbeing among Muslim and Christian Palestinians in Israel', *Mental Health, Religion and Culture*, 12(2): 147–55.

Al-Adawi, S., Dorvlo, A. S. S., Al-Ismaily, S. S., Al-Ghafry, D. A., Al-Noobi, B. Z., Al-Salmi, A., Burke, D.T., Shah, M.K., Ghassany, H., Chand, S.P. (2002) 'Perception of and attitude towards mental illness in Oman', *The International Journal of Social Psychiatry*, 48(4): 305–17.

Al-Ashhab, B. (2005) 'An update on mental health services in the West Bank', *The Israel Journal of Psychiatry and Related Sciences*, 42(2): 81–3.

Al-Krenawi, A. (2005) 'Socio-political aspects of mental health practice with Arabs in the Israeli context', *The Israel Journal of Psychiatry and Related Sciences*, 42(2): 126–36.

Al-Krenawi, A. (2012) 'A study of psychological symptoms, family function, marital and life satisfactions of polygamous and monogamous women: the Palestinian case', *International Journal of Social Psychiatry*, 58 (1): 79–86.

Al-Krenawi, A. and Graham, J.R. (1996) 'Tackling mental illness: roles for old and new disciplines', *World Health Forum*, 17(3): 246–8.

Al-Krenawi, A. and Graham, J.R. (1997) 'Spirit possession and exorcism in the treatment of a Bedouin psychiatric patient', *Clinical Social Work Journal*, 25(2): 211–22.

Al-Krenawi, A. and Graham, J.R (1999) 'Social work and Koranic mental health healers', *International Social Work*, 42(12): 53–65.

Al-Krenawi, A. and Graham, J.R (2000) 'Culturally sensitive social work practice with Arab clients in mental health settings', *Health and Social Work*, 25(1): 9–22.

Al-Krenawi, A., Graham, J.R., Al-Bedah, E.A., Kadri, H.M. and Sehwail, M.A. (2009) 'Cross-national comparison of Middle Eastern university students: help-seeking behaviors, attitudes toward helping professionals, and cultural beliefs about mental health problems', *Community Mental Health Journal*, 45(1): 26–36.

Al-Krenawi, A., Graham, J.R., Dean, Y.Z. and Eltaiba, N. (2004) 'Cross-national study of attitudes towards seeking professional help: Jordan, United Arab Emirates (UAE) and Arabs in Israel', *International Journal of Social Psychiatry*, 50(2): 102–14.

Al-Krenawi, A., Maoz, B. and Reicher, B. (1994) 'Familial and cultural issues in the brief strategic treatment of Israeli Bedouins', *Family Systems Medicine*, 12(4): 415–25.

Ano, G. G., and Vasconcelles, E. B. (2005) 'Religious coping and psychological adjustment to stress: a meta-analysis', *Journal of Clinical Psychology*, 61(4): 461–80.

Barise, A. (2005) 'Social work with Muslims: insights from the teachings of Islam', *Critical Social Work*, 6(2): 73–89. Online. Available HTTP: www1.uwindsor.ca/criticalsocialwork/social-work-with-muslims-insights-from-the-teachings-of-islam (accessed 8 August 2016).

Buck, H.G. (2006) 'Spirituality: concept analysis and model development', *Holistic Nursing Practice*, 20(6): 288–92.

El-Islam, M.F. (1982) 'Arabic cultural psychiatry', *Transcultural Psychiatry*, 19(1): 5–24.

Francis, L.J. and Katz, Y.J. (2002) 'Religiosity and happiness: a study among Israeli female undergraduates', *Research in the Social Scientific Study of Religion*, 13: 75–86.

Giacaman, R., Husseini, A., Gordon, N.H. and Awartani, F. (2004) 'Imprints on the consciousness: the impact on Palestinian civilians of the Israeli Army invasion of West Bank towns', *The European Journal of Public Health*, 14(3): 286–90.

Hackney, C. and Sanders, G. (2003) 'Religiosity and mental health: a meta-analysis of recent studies', *Journal for the Scientific Study of Religion*, 42(1): 43–55.

Halevy, D. (2015) 'Just how many Arabs are in Israel?', *Arutz Sheva*, 10 July 2015. Online. Available HTTP: www.israelnationalnews.com/News/News.aspx/197944#.Vguy7OxVhHx (accessed 22 November 2015).

Hall, R.E. (1976) *Beyond Culture*, New York: Doubleday.

Hall, R.E. (2007) 'Social work practice with Arab families: the implications of spirituality vis-a-vis Islam', *Advances in Social Work*, 8(2): 328–37.

Hill, P.C. and Hood, R.W. (eds) (1999) *Measures of Religiosity*, Birmingham, AL: Religious Education Press.

Hodge, D. R. (2005) 'Social work and the house of Islam: orienting practitioners to the beliefs and values of Muslims in the United States', *Social Work*, 50(2): 162–73.

Leavey, G., Loewenthal, K. and King, M. (2007) 'Challenges to sanctuary: the clergy as a resource for mental health care in the community', *Social Science and Medicine*, 65(3): 548–59.

Lewis, C.A., Maltby, J. and Day L. (2005) 'Religious orientation, religious coping, and happiness among UK adults', *Personality and Individual Differences*, 38(5): 1193–202.

Maton, K.I. (1989) 'The stress-buffering role of spiritual support: cross-sectional and prospective investigations', *Journal for the Scientific Study of Religion*, 28(3): 310–23.

Mattlin, J.A., Wethington, E. and Kessler, R.C. (1990) 'Situational determinants of coping and coping effectiveness', *Journal of Health and Social Behavior*, 31(1): 103–22.

Murphy, H.B.M. (1973) 'Current trends in transcultural psychiatry', *Proceedings of the Royal Society of Medicine*, 66(7): 711–6.

Nagati, M.A. (1993) *The Tradition of the Prophet and Psychology*, Cairo: Dar AlShorok Press.

Ramon, S., Campbell, J., Lindsay, J., McCrystal, P., and Baidoun, N. (2006) 'The impact of political conflict on social work: experiences from Northern Ireland, Israel and Palestine', *The British Journal of Social Work*, 36(3): 435–50.

Rubin, S.S., and Yasien-Esmael, H. (2004) 'Loss and bereavement among Israel's Muslims: acceptance of God's will, grief, and the relationship to the deceased', *OMEGA: Journal of Death and Dying*, 49(2): 149–62.

Savaya, R. (1995) 'Attitudes towards family and marital counseling among Israeli Arab women', *Journal of Social Service Research*, 21(1): 35–51.

Siddiqui, S. (2004) *A Professional Guide for Canadian Imams*, Winnipeg, Canada: Islamic Social Services Association Inc.

Statistical Abstract of Israel (1998) *No. 49, Tables 2.1, 12.7, 5*, Jerusalem: Central Bureau of Statistics.

Swanson, P.B., Pearsall-Jones, J.G. and Hay, D.A. (2002) 'How mothers cope with the death of a twin or higher multiple', *Twin Research and Human Genetics*, 5(3): 156–64.

Wang, P.S., Berglund, P.A. and Kessler, R.C. (2003) 'Patterns and correlates of contacting clergy for mental disorders in the United States', *Health Services Research*, 38(2): 647–73.

Wasfi, A. (1964) *Dearborn Arab-Moslem Community: a study of acculturation*, East Lansing, MI: Michigan State University.

Part IV
Faith-based service provision

15

Partners in service and justice

Catholic social welfare and the social work profession

Linda Plitt Donaldson

Introduction

The commandment to love God and thy neighbour has inspired Christian communities over the centuries to organise countless efforts to care for poor and vulnerable members of society. Since its inception, the Catholic Church has made caring for the poor one of its central activities as lay and religious men and women have organised charity through Catholic parishes throughout the world. As a global institution, the Catholic Church's charitable and social welfare functions have touched nearly every corner of the world, and in doing so, it has influenced and been influenced by many other faith-based and secular partners in addressing human need, including the profession of social work.

This chapter will begin by giving an overview of the Church's global engagement in social welfare, including examples of its mutual and reciprocal influence on the social work profession. Next, the chapter will describe the core principles that guide the social mission of the Catholic Church. The chapter will conclude with some reflections on the papacy of Pope Francis and its potential influence on the social work profession.

Overview of the Catholic Church's global engagement in social welfare

The Catholic response to poverty and human suffering has been made manifest for centuries by countless men and women, lay and religious, who have dedicated their lives to serving the poor. Early responses to poverty and human need were typically organised at the parish-level on a voluntary basis. Parishes are the basic unit of the Catholic Church, comprising Catholic families who typically live within a particular geographic area and attend the church within those boundaries (Joseph and Conrad 2010). Providing opportunities for parishioners to care for their neighbours through their parish has been and remains a central way for pastors to facilitate the participation of their parishioners in Christ's ministry. Over time, as the Catholic population increased along with the needs of parish families and surrounding communities, the approach to meeting those growing needs required a more organised and structured response. Today, organised Catholic responses to poverty vary in terms of their founding, structure, level of oversight by Catholic bishops and integration with non-Catholic and/or state-sponsored social welfare. Some Catholic social welfare emerged from the *charisms* of men and women religious and their particular calling as the hands and feet of Christ. Other Catholic responses to need were created through faith-inspired lay movements or emerged through the Catholic bishops and coordinated through national bishops conferences. Each is briefly described as follows.

Most religious orders were founded a century or more ago by men and women who identified a particular gift of the spirit or *charism* around which they carried forth the ministry of Jesus Christ in service to the Church and the world. Examples of such men and women are St. Francis and St. Claire of Assisi (Franciscans), St. Teresa of Calcutta (Mother Teresa) (Missionaries of Charity), St. Ignatius of Loyola (Jesuits), St. Vincent de Paul (Vincentians) and St. Louise de Marillac (Daughters of Charity). Considering themselves the hands and feet of Christ, the majority of religious congregations are engaged in alleviating the suffering and needs of people who are poor throughout the world whether through social services, social development, education, health care, child welfare and/or contemplative practices. As a consequence, men and women religious have helped establish many of the basic institutions of society to care for human needs. For example, in 2009, the United States House of Representatives passed Resolution 411 recognising that 'Catholic sisters have played a vital role in shaping life in the United States' (United States House of Representatives 2009: para 1), especially in their contributions to education, health care, social services and advocacy for peace and justice.

In addition to men and women religious, many Catholic lay men and women have founded movements to give expression to their commitment to people who are poor and vulnerable. Dorothy Day, founder of the Catholic Worker Movement in 1933, was committed to nonviolence and solidarity with the poor (Klement 2011). Most people associate the Catholic Worker Movement with their 'Houses of Hospitality', of which there are currently 236 in the US and abroad (Catholic Worker Movement 2016). Catholic workers living in the community commit to voluntary poverty and to extending the works of mercy (e.g. food, shelter, clothing, hospitality) to people in need. Many Catholic worker communities are also engaged in advocating and speaking out for social and economic justice.

Another organised response to poverty started by a lay Catholic is the St. Vincent de Paul Society [SVDP] founded in 1833 by Frederic Ozanam. Mr Ozanam mobilised laymen[1] to provide charity and support to people who lived in the poorest neighbourhoods of Paris, France. By 1840, the society had grown to over 1,000 members, including establishing its first international conference (local associations were referred to as conferences) in Rome in 1836 (McColgan 1951). Over the next 50 years, the Society grew its international presence to over 26 countries, including in Europe, the United Kingdom, Australia, North America, Africa and Asia. Currently, St. Vincent de Paul Societies are in 149 countries with over 800,000 members addressing the needs of 35 million people who are poor and vulnerable (SVDP 2016).

The most far-reaching and well-known international/national Catholic social welfare organisation is Caritas Internationalis, which has over 160 member agencies located in seven regions around the world, including Africa, Asia, Europe, Latin America and the Caribbean, the Middle East and North Africa, North America and Oceania (Caritas Internationalis 2016). Member agencies from each country operate autonomously under their national bishops conferences and take a particular form based on the needs of the local community. Programmes could include social services, child and welfare services, social development, emergency and disaster assistance, or refugee resettlement. All Caritas agencies share the same overall purpose: to end poverty, promote justice and restore dignity. In the United States, the Caritas agencies are Catholic Charities USA [CCUSA] and Catholic Relief Services [CRS]. CCUSA, with its 177 member agencies, is one of the largest social service providers in the US, employing over 60,000 staff members many of whom are professional social workers.

In 2014, CCUSA served nearly 9 million people in the form of providing housing, shelter, health care, food, day care, adoption, refugee resettlement, prisoner re-entry services, employment and other services (CCUSA 2014). Catholic Relief Services, founded by the US Catholic bishops in 1943 to address the suffering and displacement of World War II survivors, remains active today in over 100 countries on five continents on numerous humanitarian initiatives to promote health, human development and peace (CRS 2016).

Catholic social welfare and professional social work

The relationship between Catholic social welfare and the development of the social work profession varies by country and its individual historical and socio-political contexts. A rich analysis of the historical, political, social and economic context for the Catholic Church's involvement in the development of social work in each country across the world warrants a book-length volume. This chapter will provide a few examples.

In the United States, the Catholic Church, through the St. Vincent de Paul Society, was influential in the development and professionalisation of Catholic social welfare in the late nineteenth and early twentieth century. At that time, Catholic parishes continued to be important mechanisms for addressing the material, social and spiritual needs of the growing communities in the United States. Volunteers from Catholic parishes cared for women, men and children who were poor and frail, and they welcomed and supported newly arriving immigrants (Joseph and Conrad 2010); the St. Vincent de Paul Society supported such efforts, having been established in the US during 1845. However, the growing rates of immigration, particularly Catholic immigration, strained the resources of parish communities and the Society. Between 1850 and 1906, the Catholic population grew from 5 per cent to 14 per cent of the total population (Byrne 2000). Arriving to urban centres with few resources and skills in urban trades, many of the newly arriving immigrants, largely Catholic, contributed to the worsening humanitarian conditions of the cities.

For example, in 1852, 'the Association for Improving the Condition of the Poor (AICP) [in New York City] reported that three-quarters of its assistance went to Catholics' (Brown and McKeown 1997: 2), and ten years later, the AICP reported that Catholics comprised the majority of people in public almshouses, and half of New York City's criminal population. The US bishops publicly acknowledged the extent of poverty experienced by Catholics in their 1866 pastoral letter, writing, 'it is a melancholy fact, and a very humiliating avowal for us to make that a very large portion of the vicious and idle youth of our principal cities are the children of Catholic parents' (cited in Brown and McKeown 1997: 2).

The dire condition of families and communities in the early twentieth century created a need for Catholic social welfare to transition from a local 'parish-based ministry of charity to a more professionally organised diocesan-wide ministry' (Hehir 2010: 34). Consequently, in 1910 members of the Society of St. Vincent de Paul and several Catholic clerics founded the National Conference of Catholic Charities [NCCC] (now known as Catholic Charities USA or CCUSA) to harness and coordinate knowledge and resources from the experiences of local agencies to improve and standardise their 'professional social work practices' (Conrad and Joseph 2010: 52). The founders also felt that a national organisation would facilitate the Church's effort to speak with a stronger voice on social legislation, and some argued that a national association of Catholic charities agencies would situate Catholic relief efforts in the mainstream of social work and better position them for state and federal funding (Hehir 2010).

The early founders of the National Conference of Catholic Charities believed that the complex nature of poverty alleviation required professional training for social workers. Monsignor

William Kerby, first Executive Secretary of NCCC and a sociology professor at Catholic University of America [CUA], strongly endorsed the emerging models of social work practice referred to as 'scientific charity' (Kerby 1921), and helped establish the National Catholic Service School, founded in 1918 to train Catholic women to help with the war effort (Hartmann-Ting 2008). When the war ended, the bishops recognised a continuing need for Catholic involvement in social welfare and professional education so they, through the National Catholic Welfare Council, made the training school for women a permanent institution and renamed it the National Catholic School of Social Service [NCSSS] (Hartmann-Ting 2008). It became a co-educational institution when it merged with the male-only CUA School of Social Work in 1947.

Monsignor John O'Grady succeeded Kerby as Executive Secretary for NCCC, and held that position from 1920 to 1961. He also served as Dean of the CUA School of Social Work from 1934 to 1938 and oversaw the growth, influence and professionalisation of Catholic social services during his tenure.

In addition to educating American social workers for professional practice, NCSSS has educated a number of Catholic social workers that became pioneers in their home countries. For example, in 1928, NCSSS trained Australia's first professional social workers, Norma Parker and Constance Moffitt, who, upon returning to their home country, established medical social work in St. Vincent's Hospital in Melbourne and Sydney as well as the Catholic Social Services Bureau in Melbourne (Crisp 2010). The number of Catholic agencies in Australia blossomed in the 1970s, and now Catholic agencies are one of the largest providers of social welfare services in Australia (Crisp 2010).

The development of professional social work in Ireland was challenged by the tension between perspectives that viewed social work as a voluntary versus professional endeavour. Catholics felt strongly about the voluntary and spiritually-based nature of charity, and felt that professionalising social work reflected a more Protestant approach to charity provision (Skehill 2000). As opportunities for professional social work training began to emerge in the United Kingdom, the Catholic Church resisted sending their volunteers for more professional training. Irish Catholic women who wanted to pursue advanced training in family welfare casework needed to obtain a dispensation from their bishop to attend Trinity College, Dublin, a 'protestant' institution. However, by the 1960s, the Catholic Church became more supportive of professionally-trained workers, and the professionalisation of the social work profession expanded and solidified in the late twentieth century (Skehill 2000).

During the 1960s, the Catholic Church also fostered social work education and the development of the profession in other countries. For example, in 1964, the Jesuits established a school of social work in Harare, Zimbabwe, which grew into a full bachelor's degree programme offered at the University of Zimbabwe (Chogugudza 2009). In Central America, 'the Catholic Church played a major role in promoting social work education' (Julia 2008: 5), whose curricula was largely influenced by the established programmes in the United States. Consequently, the universities were largely based on Western ideals, values and individually-based models that often clashed with the collectivist and macro-oriented approaches to poverty of the Central American people. However, at the grassroots, local church authorities were reading, interpreting and preaching the gospel in light of the experience of the poor, referred to as *liberation theology*. Liberation theology coincided with the reconceptualisation movement in Latin America, which rejected capitalism and American influence, and for a time, 'social work became more political, more radical, and more focused on political consciousness' (Healy 2008: 156). These are just a few examples of how the Catholic Church influenced, for better or worse, the global development of the social work profession.

Overview of Catholic Social Teaching: guiding principles for the service and justice dimensions of the Catholic social mission

That body of work that provides the theological foundation and inspiration for Catholic action for service and justice is referred to as Catholic Social Teaching [CST]. CST is rooted in the life and teachings of Jesus Christ who was sent by God to 'bring good tidings to the poor ... to proclaim liberty to the captives ... and to let the oppressed go free' (Luke 4:18). Jesus identified the two greatest commandments as loving God and loving one's neighbour (Matthew 22: 37–40). When asked who is our neighbour, Jesus responded by telling the story of the Good Samaritan (Luke 10:29–37), which demonstrates that everyone is our neighbour regardless of race, ethnicity, political affiliation or economic status. Jesus also said that we would be judged by how we cared for the poor and vulnerable among us (Matthew 25: 31–46). Through word and deed, Jesus identified with people who were poor and marginalised and challenged leaders and structures that oppressed the poor, sustaining himself through prayer.

Modern Catholic Social Teaching traces its beginnings to 1891, when Pope Leo XIII wrote the first papal encyclical, *Rerum Novarum*, to respond to the harsh living and working conditions of industrialised Europe. By issuing this encyclical, he set in motion a tradition of preparing papal and church documents that address social issues thought to be of great significance during a particular time in history. *Rerum Novarum* is the first of a set of official church documents that comprise the 'body' of Catholic Social Teaching. The *Compendium of the Social Doctrine of the Church* (Pontifical Council for Justice and Peace 2004) is an overview of CST that draws from the body of CST until its publication in 2004 but does not include some of the important documents since issued by Pope Benedict XVI or Pope Francis. Donaldson and Belanger (2012) include an abbreviated list of some of the earlier church documents that may be of most interest to social workers.

Several core principles are associated with Catholic Social Teaching. These principles serve as important guideposts for discerning right action in a particular situation. These core principles are described as follows.

- The **Life and Dignity of the Human Person** holds that all human beings have inviolable dignity and worth because they were created in the image and likeness of God. 'The Church sees in men and women, in every person, the living image of God himself' (Pontifical Council for Justice and Peace 2004: n105). CST reminds us that all human beings are the temple of God and the spirit of God dwells within them (1 Corinthians, 3:16). Our ability to see the face and presence of Christ in all people should compel us to treat everyone with tenderness, care and justice, and to act in a manner that reflects our own dignity.
- The **Common Good** is the 'sum of all social conditions which allow people, either as groups or as individuals, to reach their fulfillment more fully and more easily' (Pontifical Council for Justice and Peace 2004: n164). Conditions for the common good include 'commitment to peace ... a sound juridical system, the protection of the environment, the provision of essential services to all ... food, housing, work, education ... transportation, basic health care, freedom of communication and the protection of religious freedom' (Pontifical Council for Justice and Peace 2004: n166).

  Social conditions that are just enable people to participate in family, community, spiritual, economic, political and social spheres of life. One's ability to participate in those spheres of life is directly proportional to one's capacity to exercise and fully realise one's sacred dignity. Catholic action for justice has often been directed at creating conditions where people can reasonably participate in all spheres of life, particularly family and community life (e.g. advocacy for living wages, worker protection, child care, affordable housing and/or safe communities).

Important for the common good is the condition of labour and the rights of workers. Modern CST began with an encyclical on the condition of labour, speaking to the rights and duties of employers and workers including the right to form unions and be paid just wages to support a family and attend to spiritual needs. Subsequent encyclicals have deepened and clarified the Church's understanding of the relationship between work and labour, underscoring that 1) work is for the person, not the person for work; 2) labour has priority over capital; and 3) industry should neither oppress humanity nor compromise the health of the planet.

- **Solidarity** is 'a firm and persevering determination to commit oneself to the common good' (Pontifical Council for Justice and Peace 2004: n193). At a deep level, solidarity recognises the interdependence of all, and is found in 'a commitment to the good of one's neighbor with the readiness to lose oneself for the sake of the others' (Pontifical Council for Justice and Peace 2004: n193).
- **Subsidiarity** offers a vision for the ordering, functioning and governance of a society where people or institutions closest to a situation should have the autonomy to exercise their proper role in that situation. For example, families should not do for an individual, what an individual can do for him or herself. Communities should not do for a family, what a family can do for itself. Governments should not do for an individual, family or community, what each of those can do for itself. However, CST allows that certain situations require action by governments, such as when there is 'a serious social imbalance or injustice where only the intervention of the public authority can create conditions of equality, justice, or peace' (Pontifical Council for Justice and Peace 2004: n188).
- **Preferential Option for the Poor** refers to the Church's view that those who are poor or vulnerable deserve our priority and special consideration. 'A basic moral test for any society is how it treats those who are most vulnerable' (USCCB 2015 n53). Jesus made this clear through his life example, and also through his teachings, particularly his teaching on the Judgment of Nations:

> I was hungry and you gave me food,
> I was thirsty and you gave me drink,
> A stranger and you welcomed me,
> Naked and you clothed me,
> Ill and you cared for me,
> In prison and you visited me …
> What you did for the least of these brothers of mine you did for me.
>
> (Matthew 25: 35–40)

Catholic Social Teaching provides a lens for viewing the world and framing a set of questions around a particular social condition. The See-Judge-Act model created by Belgian priest Cardinal Joseph Cardijn in the early twentieth century (Zotti 1990) is one social analysis model that invites us to observe current conditions, analyse contemporary situations in light of their historical and structural context, assess them against our values (e.g. human dignity, common good, impact on the poor and vulnerable), and take action. Action could take the form of services and social support for an individual or family, action to address the structural causes of human suffering, or both. Catholic social teaching invites us to 'walk with two feet of love in action' (USCCB 2012) and engage in direct service *and* social justice activities to respond to human needs.

The 'Pope Francis Effect' and social work

Pope Francis has had a galvanising impact on people across the world. In 2015, he was the second most followed world leader on Twitter, nearing 20 million followers, and is considered the most influential world leader based on an average 9,929 retweets of his postings as compared to the nearest contender at 4,419 (Lüfkens 2015). A Pew Research poll posted his favourability ratings among American Catholics at 90 per cent, all Americans at 70 per cent and those claiming no religious affiliation at 68 per cent (Masci 2015). Pope Francis' popularity is linked to his authentic and radical commitment to living and teaching the gospel values rooted in the life and teachings of Jesus Christ. People first glimpsed his radical embrace of the gospel in the moments after his election when he took the name Francis after St. Francis of Assisi, whom he described as 'the man of poverty, the man of peace, the man who loves and protects creation' (Staff Reporter 2013). Throughout his papacy, Pope Francis' words and deeds have reflected the spirit of his namesake.

Themes from Pope Francis' papacy could be conceptualised as the four Ps: People, Poverty, Planet and Peace (O'Loughlin 2015). Like Jesus, Pope Francis has emphasised the importance of mercy, compassion and care of people, particularly the poor. He often uses the word 'encounter' and its importance for our physical, intellectual and spiritual growth. 'We come from others, we belong to others, and our lives are enlarged by our encounter with others' (Pope Francis 2013: n38). He urges all people of good will to encounter people who are poor:

> We have to learn to be on the side of the poor and not just indulge in rhetoric about the poor! Let us go out to meet them, look into their eyes, and listen to them. The poor provide us with a concrete opportunity to encounter Christ himself and to touch his suffering flesh … the poor are not just people to whom we can give something. They have *much to offer us and to teach us.* How much we have to learn from the wisdom of the poor!
> (Pope Francis 2014: n3)

And it is not only through the corporal works of mercy (e.g. feeding, clothing, visiting) that we are called to encounter the poor. Pope Francis urges people to restore 'solidarity to the heart of human culture' (Pope Francis 2014: n3), to recognise our interdependence, and to organise for social justice. 'The future of humanity does not lie solely in the hands of great leaders, the great powers and the elites. It is fundamentally in the hands of peoples and in their ability to organize' (Pope Francis 2015a: n3).

In his encyclical *Laudato Si: on care for our common home*, Pope Francis (2015b: n10) highlights the 'inseparable bond … between concern for nature, justice for the poor, commitment to society, and interior peace'. He repeatedly states that 'everything is connected', and throughout he underscores the 'intimate relationship between the poor and the fragility of the planet' (2015: n16). He also writes explicitly about the impact of pollution and dangerous waste producing 'a broad spectrum of health hazards, especially for the poor, [that] cause millions of premature deaths' (2015b: n19). In particular, Pope Francis addresses the warming effects that compromise 'their means of subsistence [which] are largely dependent on natural reserves and economic systemic services such as agriculture, fishing, and forestry' (2015b: n19) and adds that the suffering of the poor is compounded because they have no financial resources to help them adapt to the effects of climate change. Pope Francis also takes to task multinational corporations who 'do [in developing countries] what they would never do in … the so-called first world … leav[ing] behind great human and environmental liabilities' (2015b: n51).

The four themes of Pope Francis' papacy coincide with the general mandates of the social work profession found in many of the Codes of Ethics of national associations of social work. Many country social work codes speak to the inherent dignity of human beings, and the importance of community and social relationships that are related to the Pope's call to *encounter* those who are poor, vulnerable and marginalised. The International Federation of Social Workers [IFSW] and the International Association of Schools of Social Work [IASSW] define social work as a profession that 'promotes social change and development, social cohesion and the empowerment and liberation of people' (IFSW 2014). Many country Codes of Ethics speak to having a special concern for vulnerable populations, including those who are poor. The preamble of the Code of Ethics of National Association of Social Workers in the United States says:

> The primary mission of the social work profession is to enhance human well-being and help meet the basic human needs of all people, with particular attention to the needs and empowerment of people who are vulnerable, oppressed, and living in poverty.
>
> (NASW 2008: 1)

While there is tremendous convergence between Pope Francis' words and deeds and the social work profession, there remain areas of dissonance as well. For example, the social work profession generally supports a full range of human rights including reproductive rights, and the right to marriage for same-sex couples. Many in the international social work community also view the use of condoms as an important public health strategy and that efforts to curb the incidence of HIV and other diseases are adversely impacted in developing countries with large Catholic populations because of the ban on condom use. While Pope Francis has not changed Church teaching on these topics, he is encouraging dialogue and bridge building, recognising there is much work that can be done in areas where stakeholders share common ground. Perhaps the leadership of Pope Francis may create space for greater dialogue and increasing partnerships between Church officials and a wider range of stakeholders who share a desire to address human needs and suffering.

Despite disagreements one has with the Catholic Church, no one can deny its far-reaching impact in meeting human needs and promoting social development throughout the world. Social workers of all stripes have been inspired by the wisdom and courage of Pope Francis, who has demonstrated that he is not afraid to walk in solidarity with the poor and outcast members of society. Standing on centuries of Catholic Social Teaching, Pope Francis provides a challenge to social workers everywhere to once again prioritise the central tenets of our profession.

Note

1 The Ladies of Charity was the counterpart association for women.

References

Brown, D.M. and McKeown, E. (1997) *The Poor Belong to Us: Catholic Charities and American welfare*, Cambridge, MA: Harvard University Press.

Byrne, J. (2000) *Roman Catholics and Immigration in Nineteenth Century America*. Online. Available HTTP: http://nationalhumanitiescenter.org/tserve/nineteen/nkeyinfo/nromcath.htm (accessed 1 January 2016).

Caritas Internationalis (2016) *Governance*. Online. Available HTTP: www.caritas.org/who-we-are/gov ernance/ (accessed 5 February 2016).

Catholic Charities USA [CCUSA] (2014) *2014 Catholic Charities Annual Survey Summary*. Online. Available HTTP: https://files.catholiccharitiesusa.org/files/publications/2014-Annual-Survey_Summary.pdf?m time=20150828143835 (accessed 1 January 2016).

Catholic Relief Services [CRS] (2016) *About*. Online. Available HTTP: www.crs.org/about (accessed 5 February 2016).

Catholic Worker Movement (2016) *Directory*. Online. Available HTTP: www.catholicworker.org/com munities/directory.html (accessed 5 February 2016).

Chogugudza, C. (2009) 'Social work education, training and employment in Africa: the case of Zimbabwe', *Ufahamu: A Journal of African Studies*, 35(1): 1–9.

Conrad, A.P. and Joseph, M.V. (2010) 'The rise of professionalization: Catholic charities and social work', in B. Hehir (ed) *Catholic Charities USA: 100 years at the intersection of charity and justice*, Collegeville, MN: Liturgical Press.

Crisp, B.R. (2010) 'Catholic agencies: making a distinct contribution to Australian social welfare provi sion?' *The Australasian Catholic Record*, 87(4): 440–51.

Donaldson, L.P. and Belanger, K. (2012) 'Catholic social teaching: principles for the service and justice dimensions of social work practice and education', *Social Work and Christianity*, 39(2): 119–27.

Hartmann-Ting, L.E. (2008) 'The National Catholic School of Social Service: redefining Catholic wom anhood through the professionalization of social work during the interwar years', *US Catholic Historian*, 26(1): 101–19.

Healy, L. (2008) *International Social Work: professional action in an interdependent world*, New York: Oxford University Press.

Hehir, B. (2010) 'Theology, social teaching and Catholic Charities', in B. Hehir (ed) *Catholic Charities USA: 100 years at the intersection of charity and justice*, Collegeville, MN: Liturgical Press.

International Federation of Social Workers [IFSW] and International Association of Schools of Social Work [IAASW] (2014) *Global Definition of Social Work*. Online. Available HTTP: http://ifsw.org/get-involved/global-definition-of-social-work/ (accessed 3 August 2016).

Joseph, M.V. and Conrad, A.P. (2010) 'The parish comes full circle and beyond: the role of local parishes in the work of Catholic Charities', in B. Hehir (ed) *Catholic Charities USA: 100 years at the intersection of charity and justice*, Collegeville, MN: Liturgical Press.

Julia, M. (2008) 'International social work and social welfare: Central America', *Encyclopedia of Social Work*. Online. Available: HTTP: http://socialwork.oxfordre.com/view/10.1093/acrefore/97801999 75839.001.0001/acrefore-9780199975839-e-567 (accessed 24 February 2016).

Kerby, W. (1921) *The Social Mission of Charity*, New York: MacMillan Company.

Klement, A. (2011) 'Dorothy Day and Caesar Chavez: American Catholic lives in nonviolence', *US Catholic Historian*, 29(3): 67–90.

Lüfkens, M. (2015) *Twiplomacy Study*. Online. Available HTTP: http://twiplomacy.com/blog/twiplo macy-study-2015/#section-intro (accessed 1 January 2016).

Masci, D. (2015) *Pope Francis' Popularity Extends Beyond Catholics*. Online. Available HTTP: www.pewre search.org/fact-tank/2015/03/13/americans-of-different-religions-and-even-those-without-embrace-pope-francis/ (accessed 1 January 2016).

McColgan, D. (1951) *A Century of Charity: the first one hundred years of the Society of St. Vincent de Paul in the United States*, Milwaukee: The Bruce Publishing Company.

National Association of Social Workers [NASW] (2008) *Code of Ethics*, Online. Available HTTP: www. socialworkers.org/pubs/code/code.asp (accessed 1 January 2016).

O'Loughlin, M. (2015) *The Pope in Philly: crowds, tweets, money, and … Latin?* Online. Available HTTP: www.cruxnow.com/church/2015/08/29/the-pope-in-philly-crowds-tweets-money-and-latin/ (accessed 1 January 2016).

Pontifical Council for Justice and Peace (2004). *Compendium of the Social Doctrine of the Church*, Washington, DC: United States Conference of Catholic Bishops.

Pope Francis (2013) *Lumen Fidei*. Online. Available HTTP: http://w2.vatican.va/content/francesco/en/encyclicals/documents/papa-francesco_20130629_enciclica-lumen-fidei.html (accessed 1 January 2016).

Pope Francis (2014) *Message of Pope Francis for the Twenty Ninth World Youth Day 2014*. Online. Available HTTP: http://w2.vatican.va/content/francesco/en/messages/youth/documents/papa-francesco_2014 0121_messaggio-giovani_2014.html (accessed 1 January 2016).

Pope Francis (2015a) *Speech at World Meeting of Popular Movements*. Online. Available HTTP: http://en.radiovaticana.va/news/2015/07/10/pope_francis_speech_at_world_meeting_of_popular_movements/1157291 (accessed 1 January 2016).

Pope Francis (2015b) *Laudato Si: on care for our common home*. Online. Available HTTP: http://w2.vatican.va/content/francesco/en/encyclicals/documents/papa-francesco_20150524_enciclica-laudato-si.html (accessed 1 January 2016).

Skehill, C. (2000) 'An examination of the transition from philanthropy to professional social work in Ireland', *Research on Social Work Practice,* 10(6): 688–704.

Staff Reporter (2013) 'Pope Francis reveals why he chose his name', *Catholic Herald*. Online. Available HTTP: www.catholicherald.co.uk/news/2013/03/16/pope-francis-reveals-why-he-chose-name/ (accessed 1 January 2016).

St Vincent de Paul Society [SVDP] (2016) *Annual Report*. Online. Available HTTP: http://en.ssvpglobal.org/Documentation (accessed 27 January 2016).

United States Conference of Catholic Bishops [USCCB] (2012) *The Two Feet of Love in Action: facilitator's guide*. Department of Justice, Peace and Human Development, United States Conference of Catholic Bishops. Online. Available HTTP: www.usccb.org/about/justice-peace-and-human-development/upload/Two-Feet-of-Love-in-Action-Facilitator-s-Guide.pdf (accessed 1 January 2016).

United States Conference of Catholic Bishops [USCCB] (2015) *Forming Consciences for Faithful Citizenship: a call to political responsibility from the Catholic Bishops of the United States with introductory note*. USCCB: Washington, DC. Online. Available HTTP: www.usccb.org/issues-and-action/faithful-citizenship/upload/forming-consciences-for-faithful-citizenship.pdf (accessed 1 January 2016).

United States House of Representatives (2009) *Resolution 411*, 111th Congress, 155 Cong. Rec. E2345 (2009) (enacted).

Zotti, M.I. (1990) 'The young Christian workers', *US Catholic Historian*, 9(4): 387–400.

16

Residential childcare in faith-based institutions

Mark Smith

Introduction

Much of the history of social welfare can be traced back to Church involvement in care provision deriving from a monastic tradition. The post-Reformation period witnessed the growth of different kinds of religious congregations that were not monastic but sought to provide an active religious presence in the towns and cities that began to emerge with industrialisation. In moving away from a contemplative ideal, this new form of religious presence challenged the previous Church order. Much of it was expressed through educational action on behalf of the urban poor, which saw education as both a means to instill moral probity but also as a route out of poverty. Indeed, until the later nineteenth century most education, especially of the poorer classes, was reliant on the work of religious orders or religiously-inspired philanthropists and often involved residential provision. In this sense, the focus of the emerging orders on the education of the poor might be contrasted with the role of more traditional Catholic Orders such as the Jesuits, Dominicans and Benedictines in providing schools for a Catholic elite.

This chapter sketches some of that movement of religiously-inspired involvement in social care and education through identifying some of the main congregations involved in this mission. The outline is neither comprehensive nor systematic and does not claim academic or theological expertise in this area. I write from personal experience of having worked as a lay social care worker for a Catholic teaching order, the De La Salle Brothers in a residential school in Scotland, over the course of the 1980s. While I recognise the international reach of the religious congregations, my focus is primarily the UK and Ireland. My perspective is that of a critical Catholic, but one whose experience in working for the Brothers was formative to my understanding of child care and is one I have taken with me into my subsequent career in child care and as a social work academic. Contrary to the picture that has come to the fore in recent decades (see Chapter 23 by Philip Gilligan), I found the Brothers I worked for to be humane and generous men who created a culture of discipline but also of fun and forgiveness and whose pastoral mission extended to their care of staff. This generally positive experience of working for them has made it hard for me to recognise some of the reports of abuse that have subsequently emerged, including in relation to the school I worked in, and of the assumptions in the press and in wider policy communities about regimes within which abuse was systemic and entrenched.

The disjunction between personal experience and popular account has led me to take a particular interest in the vexed issue of historical abuse and I offer some reflections on this.

Some of the main orders

De La Salle Brothers

I begin this brief tour of religious orders with the De La Salle Brothers, one of the earliest teaching orders. John Baptist de La Salle (1651–1719) was born to wealthy parents at Reims in France. He was ordained a priest in 1678 and two years later received a doctorate in theology. During that period he became involved with a group of young men, themselves having only an elementary education, in order to establish schools for poor boys. He undertook to use his own education for the service of the poor; he abandoned his family home, moved in with his group of teachers, renounced his position as Canon of Reims Cathedral and his wealth, and formed the community that became known as the Brothers of the Christian Schools.

Although himself a priest, De La Salle decided that members of the Order of Brothers should not be ordained, but should dedicate themselves exclusively to the education of youth. His method represented a new form of religious life, a community of consecrated laymen with a mission to provide free schools. Members of the order take vows of chastity, poverty, obedience, stability in the institute and association for the educational service of the poor and are required to give their services without any remuneration. Lasallian spirituality was built around a spirit of community, a spirit of faith, a spirit of zeal and a 'practical' spirituality (Rummery 2012). Unlike traditional education, which was still largely delivered in Latin, students were taught in the vernacular. Other features of the Lasallian method included grouping students according to ability and achievement, integration of religious instruction with secular subjects, well-prepared teachers with a sense of vocation and mission, and the involvement of parents. The vernacular and practical core of their mission, the fact that many of the Brothers came from relatively poor backgrounds themselves and their lack of theological education led Voltaire to call them by the nickname '*Frères Ignorantins*' (Ignorant Brothers). More generally, the relatively poor educational background among some of those attracted or sent to the religious orders remained a persistent feature of their work (Crisp 2014).

Nevertheless, De La Salle and his Brothers created a network of schools throughout France, which included programmes for training lay teachers, Sunday courses for working young men, and one of the first institutions in France for the care of delinquents. Their work provided the foundation of modern popular education and the teaching profession. De La Salle wrote text books and guidelines for teachers. His work quickly spread through France and, after his death, continued to spread internationally. The order was approved by Pope Benedict XIII in 1724. In 1900 John Baptist de La Salle was declared a Saint and in 1950 was made Patron Saint of all those who work in the field of education. The Order has gone on to operate in nearly every country of Europe, America, Asia and Africa, becoming the largest Catholic lay religious order of men exclusively devoted to education.

Following the restoration of the Catholic hierarchies in England (1850) and Scotland (1878) the Order expanded in the UK, establishing a number of grammar schools in England, thus contributing to the growth of a Catholic middle class. They made a particular contribution to the provision of Reform or Industrial Schools (brought together under the title Approved School in 1933). It is their work in such schools that has retrospectively become the focus of so much negative publicity, an issue I return to.

Salesians of Don Bosco

Another of the great teaching orders is the Salesians of Don Bosco. John Bosco (1815–88) was born in Piedmont in Italy. His early years were spent as a shepherd until, in 1835, he entered the seminary. On his ordination, he went to Turin to embark on his ministry. One of his duties there was to accompany another priest on prison visits. The conditions of the children held in prisons resolved him to devote his life to their care and education. In the course of his parish duties he struck up a relationship with a street urchin, Bartolomeo Garelli, and began instructing him in prayer and education. Bartolomeo's companions joined him in the parish 'Oratory' and within a few years numbers had grown to over 400 (Saxton 1907).

In the autumn of 1844, Don Bosco was appointed assistant chaplain to the *Rifugio*, where another priest, Don Borel, joined him in his work. The members of the Oratory now gathered at the *Rifugio*, and numbers of boys from the surrounding district applied for admission. About this time, too, Don Bosco began night schools and once factories had closed for the day, boys made their way to his rooms where he and Don Borel offered them a rudimentary education. The evening classes grew and gradually dormitories were provided for many who wanted or needed to live there.

The municipal authorities came to recognise the importance of Don Bosco's work and he began a fund for the erection of technical schools and workshops. In 1868, to meet the needs of the Valdocco quarter of Turin, Don Bosco built a large church. Fifty priests and teachers who had been assisting him formed a society under a common rule that was approved by Pope Pius IX, in 1874. The organisation was called 'Salesians' after St. Francis de Sales, the Bishop of Geneva in the sixteenth and seventeenth centuries, who was renowned for his kindness and humanity.

Don Bosco's educational philosophy was largely set down in a brief treatise entitled *The Preventive System in the Education of the Young*. He was a practical educator rather than an educational theorist, although many of his educational methods resonate with later educational theory (Morrison 1979). His educational philosophy was based on 'reason', 'religion' and 'kindness'. His method was largely free of external discipline, being based on intrinsic measures of guidance, correcting and counselling. A Circular to Salesian Schools, 1883, advised against the use of general and corporal punishment and stated that any punishment administered ought to be based on justice and the hope of pardon. He wrote that as far as possible, teachers should avoid punishing but should try to gain love before inspiring fear. Great emphasis was placed on the importance of play and of music.

Although largely eschewing punishment, the Salesian Method was not permissive. In his rules Don Bosco identified frequent Confession and Communion and Daily Mass among the pillars of his educational method, the chief object of which was to form the will and to temper the character. In one of his books, he has discussed the causes of weakness of character, which he claimed derived largely from a misdirected kindness in the rearing of children. Discipline was maintained through what might nowadays be called relationship-based practice. Teachers were expected to act as 'loving fathers' or brothers. The preventative method was based on presence and assistance offered at the opportune moment, through personal encounter. Outside of the classroom, teachers were encouraged to mingle freely with pupils, breaking down age barriers and generation gaps.

At the time of Don Bosco's death in 1888 there were 250 Salesian houses worldwide, working in hospitals, asylums, prisons and nursing the sick. The founder was beatified by Pope Pius XI in 1929 and canonised in 1934.

Christian Brothers

The Irish Christian Brothers were founded in Waterford in 1802, by a local merchant, Edmund Rice. At that point in Irish history, it was illegal for Catholics to educate their children as Catholics or for a teacher to do so. In 1802 Rice devoted his fortune and future life to opening his first school, assisted for a time by a few teachers. Soon after, some young men, drawn by Rice's example, joined him and in 1803 the citizens of Waterford built a monastery for them. As the work of the Brothers became known they were approached to open houses in Cork and in Dublin. In 1820 the Vatican accepted the Brothers as a religious institute of the Church, the first Irish Order to be so approved.

The Brothers' work in Ireland grew to encompass primary and secondary schools but also orphanages and industrial schools. The Institute spread to the UK and the first of what was to reach around 50 Australian communities was opened in 1868. Another establishment was opened in St John's Newfoundland in 1875 and the Order's reach later extended to India and the United States. It had a clear aim of providing an education that would otherwise have been denied them to clever boys, irrespective of their social class.

Daughters of Charity

It was not only male orders that responded to the needs of the urban poor. From the mid nineteenth century, the Company of the Daughters of Charity of St Vincent de Paul identified the UK as a potential mission field and its presence grew rapidly over the second half of the century. The Daughters' mission was based on a Vincentian theology of poverty, which sees those who are poor and despised by the world as representing Jesus Christ. The Daughters took annual renewable simple vows.

After an abortive attempt to open a house in Salford, Manchester, the Daughters established bases in Drogheda in Ireland in 1855 and in the industrial northern English town of Sheffield. Between 1857 and 1900, 48 houses were opened across England and Scotland with a further eight being established in Ireland (O'Brien n.d.). By 1900 the Daughters had grown to be amongst the largest religious institutes in Britain, becoming a new Province of Great Britain (encompassing Ireland) in 1885. They undertook a range of social welfare functions including parish visiting of the sick poor, the distribution of food and clothing, crèches for the children of working mothers, night schools for working men and women, hostels for working girls and prison visiting. The Daughters also became responsible for the management and staffing of a wide range of institutions for those in poverty: children's homes and industrial schools, homes for those with disabilities, reformatory schools for young people in the criminal justice system, and mother and baby homes (O'Brien n.d.). So while the focus of most religious congregations was primarily educational, the Daughters assumed a broader social welfare function with education being one among many roles.

Residential care took several forms: the orphanage was the most common, but there were also Industrial Schools and Reformatories for young offenders and residential schools for poor children with disabilities, which became something of a specialism for the Daughters in Britain. In Scotland, the Daughters' orphanage and Poor Law School near Lanark took sight and hearing-impaired children from across Scotland until a separate specialist residential school was established by them in 1911:

> By 1884 two thirds of the Daughters' houses in Britain were dedicated to residential care of poor and neglected children or to those with some kind of disability making them unique

in their concentration of effort on welfare with children from impoverished backgrounds and children with disabilities.

(O'Brien n.d.: 6)

One of the unusual features of the Daughters' work was that it extended to working with destitute boys and young men, an area that was unusual among women teachers or indeed among other women's religious congregations. In 1862 the Daughters took over the running of St Vincent's Industrial School for Boys' in Liverpool, which had been struggling under lay management. Under their management, the school was returned to disciplinary and financial control within three years. The management committee applied successfully in 1868 to have it registered as a Home Office Industrial School and St Vincent's was approved to receive 210 boys under the age of 14. By 1900 the Daughters were responsible for running and staffing nine boys' industrial schools and orphanages.

The discovery of abuse

Over the course of the latter half of the twentieth century, the role of religious orders in residential care began to decline for several reasons; at a general level the state(s) began to assume greater responsibility for education and care. In addition, vocations began to fall off as the demands of religious life became less attractive than they might once had been, in terms of the security and status it had provided and when considered alongside the growing number of opportunities opening up in secular life.

A particular body blow for the congregations, however, came with revelations of historical abuse, which emerged over the course of the 1990s. Although early complaints of abuse did not involve Church schools or homes, when the floodgates opened they quickly went on to engulf just about every religious congregation that had been involved in education and care across the Western World. One of the first and largest scandals centred around the Mount Cashel Boys Home in St John's Newfoundland, operated by the Christian Brothers of Ireland in Canada. Over the late 1980s and 1990s, more than 300 orphanage residents claimed to have been physically and sexually abused by staff there. When revelations emerged, it was claimed that earlier attempts to raise concerns had been subject to the by now all too familiar charge of having been covered up.

From the early 1990s onwards just about every jurisdiction in the developed world has faced allegations of historical abuse carried out by religious congregations. In Canada and Australia, in particular, the policy of removing indigenous children from the influence of their families and culture and placing them in residential schools in order to assimilate them into dominant Christian cultures has come under particular scrutiny. In Australia, this population has become known as the 'Stolen generation'.

The easy way to interpret this and the way this period in history has been presented is such that abuse was understood to have been 'systemic, pervasive, chronic, excessive, arbitrary, (and) endemic' (Bunting 2009) in Church-run institutions. Undoubtedly, the Irish Commission to Inquire into Child Abuse (also known as the *Ryan Report* 2009) provides ample evidence of practices that broach little dissent or defence. A visceral urge to condemn, however, has largely prevented a more considered reflection on events that are still very raw.

Part of the difficulty in coming to a measured position on the subject of historical abuse is that the historiography of residential schools is, according to Maguire (2009), largely non-existent, and for the most part reliant on non-scholarly media sources, the credibility and objectivity of which she regards as questionable. One of the flaws Maguire identifies in this approach is what she identifies as an uncritical reliance on the accounts of those who claim to have been abused and the failure to set such accounts alongside other sources of evidence.

One attempt to inject some broader perspective into the *Ryan Report* and its impact on Irish society is provided in Fr Tony Flannery's edited volume (2009), *Responding to the Ryan Report*. The starting point of the book is to acknowledge some of the abuses that took place but to try and understand some of the conditions that might have allowed this to happen. A number of contextual factors are raised, not least what Sean Fagan (2009) identifies as the 'bad theology' at the heart of Catholicism and especially Irish Catholicism, in matters of sex. In this aspect it had failed to move beyond St Augustine's personal angst regarding sex and its association in his mind and writings with mortal sin. This has left a legacy, reinforced over the centuries, of attitudes towards sex that have not been healthy.

Yet, while it is an easy target, it is probably too simple to make a direct link between repressed sexual feelings and sexual abuse. In fact, Philip Jenkins' (2001) work suggests that priests and religious individuals are no more likely to sexually abuse than the population as a whole and indeed the problem of child abuse is one that affects every denomination. Marie Keenan (2009) in the Flannery book tellingly advises that we need to move beyond a search for individual pathology and blame. Nevertheless, the abuse scandals have undoubtedly cast a spotlight on the difficulties with the Church's views on sex; even if celibacy and all that goes along with that in terms of the mortification of the body did not directly lead to sexual abuse, it must, in some cases, have contributed to a sense of sexual tension and resentment, which may on occasion have manifest in other less than healthy ways in attitudes and relationships from the religious towards those they cared for.

Another structural feature of the Church that perhaps allowed abuse to continue involved internal Church hierarchies. Orders such as the Jesuits, Dominicans or even Diocesan clergy often drew recruits from a different social class to the Religious who ran the schools. These may have been regarded within the Church, as well as by literary commentators such as Voltaire, as *Frères Ignorantins*; as a result, Church hierarchies did not pay too much attention to the day-to-day work of the Orders. A further aspect to this class dimension, Coldrey (2006) argues, is that the working-class origin of many of the religious congregations might bring with it a relative class affinity to children in care. He claims that this could lead to a clash of the solid, respectable values of the religious Brothers and Sisters being set against the seemingly indigent and delinquent behaviours of children in care, the result of which could be resistance and (over) reaction.

At another level still, the work of the Orders perhaps lost much of the charism of their founders as the roles they were expected to fulfil became institutionalised in compulsory and state provision, with all that entailed in terms of the 'dirty work' of daily caring for often badly behaved youngsters in difficult circumstances. Wardhaugh and Wilding (1993: 5) outline a number of dimensions by which residential care of children becomes contaminated, but note that, above all: '(t)he essential element (of corruption) … is that it constitutes an active betrayal of the basic values on which the organisation is supposedly based.' This perhaps happens when initial moral impulse becomes institutionalised and reified.

A backcloth to all of these developments was that the Orders were confronting broader societal trends, which included growing secularism. With the growth in Freudian psychology from the 1920s onwards the focus of social interventions shifted from the soul to the psyche (Hacking 1995). And, while some religious Sisters and Brothers embraced some of the growing psychological discourse (for example, in the work of the Notre Dame Clinic in Glasgow), the primary work of the religious orders remained practical and spiritual (and indeed structural in the sense of consolidating Catholic communities). This practical/spiritual foundation could begin to appear anachronistic within an increasingly secular and therapeutic world.

Butler and Drakeford (2005) in their book on scandal in social work note that scandals occur, not when political and social structures are solid and successful, but rather when they are in crisis, when society's tectonic plates are shifting. Young (2011) goes on to argue that when societies are in crisis, personal and social unease is displaced onto a scapegoat; scapegoated groups are not chosen by accident, but are closely related to the source of anxiety (Young 2007: 141). In some respects, what we have witnessed over the past few decades is not merely a reaction to some of the undoubted scandals that have engulfed the Orders but the deflection of wider social anxieties around losing erstwhile moral certainties onto the institution that sought to assure us of these.

Discussion

When the dust settles on (relatively) recent scandals, there may be the opportunity to consider the role of the religious Orders in social care provision with some sense of perspective. This will surely involve recognising their many and massive achievements. The breadth and scope of their work over the course of the nineteenth and twentieth centuries in particular have spanned every area of social welfare provision but, in the case of a majority of Orders, with a particular focus on education. Their concern was not just direct care but extended to teacher training colleges and writing educational manuals, many of which have continued resonance today.

The Orders brought a sense of mission and purpose that could rarely be matched by lay organisations. The work of the Daughters of Charity, for instance, reflected a Vincentian spirit of *caritas* or 'indiscriminate charity'. Contrary to most secular institutions of the time, they recognised no distinction between the deserving and undeserving poor. In their London *maisons de charite*, they imposed no admissions criteria, unlike those operated by better-known foundling hospitals run by Victorian philanthropists such as Thomas Coram. Additionally, unlike the foundling hospitals where once an infant was admitted it could not be taken back by the mother (Ramsland 1992), the Daughters allowed the mother free access to the child (O'Brien n.d).

In the UK, the Orders' educational mission reflected the priority of the Catholic hierarchy, priests and leading laity to enhance and consolidate the role of the Catholic community in the face of an often hostile Protestant majority. The Catholic hierarchy was clear that poverty and ignorance must be tackled if individual and community status was to be lifted. In the UK, this involved some fairly sophisticated negotiation with state structures and expectations for funding, requiring accommodation to the state's demands at one level, while resisting cultural norms and practices that the Orders perceived as being at odds with a Catholic understanding of poverty, charity and the practice of care. In the Catholic state of Ireland, the Orders worked hand-in-glove with the state. It is this relationship that, arguably, allowed some of the less acceptable practices that have since come to light to continue for so long.

In moving towards a conclusion to this chapter, I am drawn to David Webb's (2010) article 'A Certain Moment' in which he reflects on the life and work of a great aunt who had been matron of a Church of England children's home. He contrasts earlier certainties about the moral order and carers' consequential obligations towards children, with the confusion, ambiguity and doubt that characterises much present day child care. I am writing this chapter in the aftermath of recent scandals in Northern English towns, in which young girls, many of them in state care, were identified as being sexually abused by groups of men in the community. Residential care workers in such cases are accused of adopting what Webb (2010) identifies as a free-floating and laissez-faire approach to welfare. It is clear that we have still not got the balance right in the care of troubled children. As Webb concludes, in contrasting a religiously-inspired version of care with present day provision; 'the drawing of any invidious comparisons with what takes place today in "corporate care" might invite a brief reflection on the parable of the mote and the beam' (Webb 2010: 1400).

In all of this, there is a sense of looking back in time. The care and education offered by the religious congregations was 'of its time'. At its best it was fluid, dynamic and responsive. Like all religious provision, once institutionalised, it could become complacent and resentful. But it has, largely, fulfilled its mission. In developed countries, the state has rightly taken on responsibility for the provision of social welfare and education. The religious orders might justifiably reflect that their job is done in such societies and that the focus of ongoing mission work is in the developing world.

References

Bunting, M. (2009) 'An abuse too far by the Catholic church', *The Guardian*. Online. Available HTTP: www.theguardian.com/commentisfree/belief/2009/may/21/catholic-abuse-ireland-ryan (accessed 5 February 2016).

Butler, I., and Drakeford, M. (2005) *Scandal, Social Policy and Social Welfare*, Bristol: BASW/Policy Press.

Coldrey, B. (2006) '"The extreme end of a spectrum of violence": physical abuse, hegemony and resistance in British residential care', *Children and Society*, 15(2): 95–106.

Commission to Inquire into Child Abuse (2009) *Commission to Inquire into Child Abuse Investigation Committee Report*. Online. Available HTTP: www.childabusecommission.ie/rpt/pdfs/ (accessed 6 February 2016).

Crisp, B.R. (2014) *Social Work and Faith-Based Organizations*, London: Routledge.

Fagan, S. (2009) 'The abuse and our bad theology', in T. Flannery (ed) *Responding to the Ryan Report*, Dublin: Columba Press.

Flannery, T. (ed) (2009) *Responding to the Ryan Report*, Dublin: Columba Press.

Hacking, I. (1995) *Rewriting the Soul: multiple personality and the sciences of memory*, Princeton: Princeton University Press.

Jenkins, P. (2001) *Paedophiles and Priests: anatomy of a contemporary crisis*, New York: Oxford University Press.

Keenan, M. (2009) 'Them and us: the clergy child sexual offender as "other"', in T. Flannery (ed) *Responding to the Ryan Report*, Dublin: Columba Press.

Maguire, M. (2009) *Precarious Childhood in Post-Independence Ireland*, Manchester: Manchester University Press

Morrison, J. (1979) *The Educational Philosophy of St. John Bosco*, New Rochelle, NY: Don Bosco Publications.

O'Brien, S. (n.d.) *The Daughters of Charity and Vincentian Charity in Victorian Britain*. Online. Available HTTP: https://cambridge.academia.edu/SusanOBrien/Papers (accessed 5 February 2016).

Ramsland, J. (1992) 'The London Foundling Hospital and its significance as a child saving institution', *Australian Social Work*, 45(2): 23–36.

Rummery, G. (2012) *Lasallian Spirituality*. Online. Available HTTP: www.lasalle.org/wp-content/uploads/2012/02/lasallian_spirit_en.pdf (accessed 5 February 2016).

Saxton, E. (1907) 'St. Giovanni Melchior Bosco', in *The Catholic Encyclopedia*, New York: Robert Appleton Company. Online. Available HTTP: www.newadvent.org/cathen/02689d.htm (accessed 6 February 2016).

Wardaugh, J. and Wilding, P. (1993) 'Towards an explanation of the corruption of care', *Critical Social Policy*, 13(37): 4–31.

Webb, D. (2010) 'A certain moment: some personal reflections on aspects of residential childcare in the 1950s', *The British Journal of Social Work*, 40(5): 1387–401.

Young, J. (2007) *The Vertigo of Late Modernity*, London: Sage.

Young, J. (2011) *The Criminological Imagination*, Cambridge: Polity Press.

17

The background and roles of The Salvation Army in providing social and faith-based services

Michael Wolf-Branigin and Katie Hirtz Bingaman

Introduction

At the beginning of the annual Christmas season in the United States and many other Western countries, red kettles appear at shopping areas, sporting venues and other places where people gather. To most, these kettles are the face of The Salvation Army [TSA] and provide their initial introduction to some charitable work as their cash donations will provide gifts and meals to families (Zavada 2015). To others, they view TSA as a place to donate old clothing and furniture for resale in the thrift stores operated by the adult rehabilitation centres (Hazzard 1998). What the majority of these people do not realise is that these are simply two popular and ubiquitous services of a world-wide religious and charitable movement that has been underway for 150 years.

This chapter discusses the religious orientation of The Salvation Army. It explains their organisational structure; highlights the major services it provides; explains in-depth one field of services, substance misuse, as an example of their faith-based service provision; and discusses two controversies relating to Lesbian, Gay, Bisexual and Transgender (LGBT) people and the privatisation of services in which The Salvation Army has been involved over the past two decades.

Founding of The Salvation Army

The Salvation Army was founded in London, England in 1865 under the leadership of General William Booth, a Methodist minister who was concerned about the effects of rapid urbanisation. The beginnings of this evangelical movement in Victorian England parallel similar efforts in addressing and alleviating the troubles of rapid industrialisation and emergence of social insurances found in Northern Europe and North America (Walker 2001).

William Booth and his wife, Catherine, left the New Methodist Connection Church in London when they would not allow him to minister to those the Booths believed were in the most need and to whom they were dedicating their lives. Booth's perspective was further influenced by his observation that the cab horses in London, which were used to pull carriages and carts, were treated better than some people (Booth 1890). Booth began the Christian Mission, which eventually became The Salvation Army, funded by money he raised from donations from bar patrons and others (Walker 2001). While many thought this to be improper, Booth was noted as justifying the efforts by stating 'Once the money is cleansed by the tears of the widows and orphans, it was blessed in God's eyes'.

While Booth began providing services in the East End of London in the 1860s, his more formal framework for service delivery was outlined in his book *In Darkest England and the Way Out* (Booth 1890), which remains an essential or recommended reading in many higher education programmes of social work and human services. This visionary book took what is now considered an early holistic approach, consistent with social work and environmental values. This was accomplished by realising the need to view the mind, body and spirit when working with individuals, families and communities that had become disenfranchised by the lack of concern from the government and other citizens.

Just as contemporary social work values the role of biology, psychology, sociology and spirituality (NASW 2008), Booth was astute in his stance that understanding the overall needs of people arises from addressing the needs of the soul as well as their body. Booth took the approach that there were certain aspects of improving the quality of life of others that governments and societies were not well equipped to accomplish. He had an early awareness that without feeding the stomachs of persons in need, he and his followers would not be able to feed their souls (McKinley 1995).

Because of Booth's strong belief in providing direct services to marginalised individuals, his organisation has been at the forefront of social services since it was founded, despite being primarily a religious organisation (Hazzard 1998). The religious basis under which TSA operates is revealed in its motto, 'Blood and Fire', in which the red signifies the blood shed by Jesus Christ and the yellow represents the fire of the Holy Spirit (Eason and Green 2012).

The Salvation Army's organisational structure

The religious orientation of The Salvation Army highlights the major services it provides, and explains the organisational structure. Booth liked the perceived efficiency of a military structure in mobilising forces and addressing emergent human need (Winston 2000). Since its beginning, uniformed officers, including both men and women, have been ordained ministers. A similar organisational structure is followed throughout the world.

Although it has a hierarchical structure, service provision is very decentralised as local corps programmes respond to local needs. The TSA is lead by one General (William Booth being the first). International Headquarters is based in London, England because of its founding there in the 1860s. Territorial Headquarter (THQ) offices are located worldwide with several countries having more than one THQ (e.g. the United States has four THQs) whereas in other countries THQs may be combined (e.g. Canada and Bermuda share a THQ). At a more local level, programmes and corps services typically report to Divisional Headquarters (DHQ), which in turn are accountable to their THQ. It is at the THQ that Commissioners elect the General; THQs are also where governmental and foundation contracts are signed, and from where monitoring of social services is organised. TSA's mission statement reflects these principles, and states:

> The Salvation Army, an international movement, is an evangelical part of the universal Christian Church. Its message is based on the Bible. Its ministry is motivated by the love of God. Its mission is to preach the gospel of Jesus Christ and to meet human needs in His name without discrimination.

> (The Salvation Army 2016)

The stated mission to serve the human needs of vulnerable and impoverished populations underscores The Salvation Army's range of services. Among these services are disaster relief, international development, women's ministries, anti-human trafficking efforts and schooling. Services are provided in the form of material and financial provisions, education, coordination of resources and on-the-ground support.

On a global scale, the delivery of international healthcare is TSA's core service element. These programmes are usually funded through donations, and operate out of the World Services Office. The prioritisation of healthcare is an extension of the Christian healing mission as modelled by Jesus Christ, who was believed to have cured those with chronic illnesses, those with disabilities and helped the families of the deceased. The Salvation Army believes that the most effective healthcare, particularly in poor communities where individuals are more prone to preventable diseases, is done within homes and families (The Salvation Army 2015c). From this perspective, especially in the global South, there is a focus on community-based healthcare interventions wherein trained local corps members empower community members to take ownership of their health. The Salvation Army rejects what they believe is a secular approach to healthcare in which expert providers wait for the sick and suffering to come to them for healing. Instead, TSA uses an egalitarian 'covenant partner' approach to healthcare in which they move services 'out of the building and into the communities to meet people where they are'.

Although The Salvation Army is firm in its stance that healthcare is most effective when it can be brought into homes and communities, much of their ministry occurs in war-torn, deeply impoverished societies. Because of this, TSA has established institutional bases that act as anchors in the communities. Across the more than 120 countries, these bases include 20 general hospitals; 45 maternity hospitals; 123 health clinics; 440 hostels for the homeless; 228 children's homes; 116 homes for the elderly; 60 homes for the disabled; 12 homes for the blind; 57 reprimand and probation homes; 41 homes for street children; 41 mother and infant homes; 77 care homes for vulnerable people; and 104 homes for refugees. In addition, The Salvation Army has 2,286 educational outreach institutions. TSA conservatively estimates that between seven and eight million workers are currently involved in healthcare programmes and community development. Addiction treatment and recovery services are a particular focus of healthcare service efforts since Booth made this one of his focus populations. Worldwide, The Salvation Army has established 204 residential recovery centres for addiction and substance misuse (The Salvation Army 2015d).

Despite this large international infrastructure, local Salvation Army corps programmes are the foundation upon which spiritual activities including Bible study, fellowship meetings, religious services, music programmes, youth activities and pastoral counselling are provided. Spiritual services are available to, but not mandatory, for social service programmes and treatment clientele and the centres' surrounding neighbourhoods or communities. TSA services and programmes typically evolve via local advisory mechanisms and the input of various community stakeholders. Local administrative units have community advisory boards and committees composed of residents and concerned citizens, who provide guidance on the specific needs of the community. An important concern is whether the increasing centralisation of management impedes the ability of local units to organise when responding to the expressed needs in a community. This issue will become even more critical as TSA continues to increase its programmatic activities by creating new agencies while continuing to support many existing ones (Weinberg 2001).

Salvation Army social service provision in the United States

When The Salvation Army first came to the United States, it arrived in a country in which Christian social activists had, since before the American Revolution, played significant roles in shaping egalitarian views for the equitable distribution of resources (Wallis 2008). Since then, The Salvation Army has played a vital role in shaping contemporary social service delivery. It marshalled resources to develop a system of addiction treatment centres, particularly in the substance misuse and addictions arena with its establishment of adult rehabilitation centres (designed as work rehabilitation services) and Harbour Light programmes specifically for the treatment of addiction. These were developed in response to the period's societal conditions using TSA's spiritual, organisational and financial resources.

The backbone of service provision is the delivery of emergency services that have been historically known as 'soup, soap, and salvation'. These services take many forms and include disaster relief, homeless shelters, emergency food services and utility payment assistance. Not all services are provided at all locations as the menu of service options remains based on demonstrated local need, the level at which the organisation's workers can provide services and availability of financial resources. Many locations have limited financial resources and are therefore unable to hire professional social work personnel. These locations most likely provide basic support services.

Throughout the evolution of their history in the United States, The Salvation Army has adapted to local and national trends (Taiz 2001). For example, during the Progressive Era of the late nineteenth and early twentieth centuries, The Salvation Army expanded their corps programmes and focused more closely on immigrant groups such as Chinese and Scandinavians (McKinney 1995). As the Great Depression arrived, responding to basic needs, including providing food and shelter, required greater attention. Despite the fact that The Salvation Army in the US contracted during the post-World War II era because of white flight from urban cores (Reed 1981), Harbour Light programming grew following World War II and the Vietnam War as more service personnel returned home with addictions. An upward trend appeared in programme use and funding following major US military involvement as service personnel returned to the US. Social programme planners must ask whether this surge in interest reflected a greater ability to fund such programmes, or if it is due to the result of increased need demonstrated by service personnel exhibiting indicators of post-traumatic stress or some other disorder.

The Salvation Army currently operates a variety of programmes including shelters, thrift stores, adult rehabilitation programmes, orphanages, camp programmes for children, gift giving for the children of those who are incarcerated, day care, re-entry programmes for ex-offenders, choirs and brass bands, and Sunday church services. Given that it is one of the world's largest charitable organisations, in addition to contracts with various governments and foundations, it relies heavily on individuals to give money. Nevertheless, the costs of service provision remain comparatively low given that ordained ministers, who have taken a vow of poverty, are the primary operators of social services. An example can be found in the provision of ex-offender services that operate with only a 3 per cent overhead (Drucker 1989).

As The Salvation Army is primarily a religious organisation, services are viewed as secondary to their spiritual mission. This is an important distinction as the United States Constitution mandates a strong separation between church and state. Therefore, social services provided through governmental funding, whether it be federal, state or local, cannot require participation in religious activities as a basis for receiving those services.

In order to provide a more concrete and sophisticated example, we will discuss briefly The Salvation Army's comprehensive array of treatment services in several North American cities. These are named Harbour Light programmes, in which detoxification, residential, outpatient and other services are provided. Similar to other TSA programmes, these services are provided within a religious setting in which the clientele may choose to participate in spiritual services. A similar organisational structure is followed throughout the world (The Salvation Army 2015b). These Harbour Light Centres provide a range of no/low-fee, holistic recovery services to those with substance misuse and addictions, as well as offering residential (including detoxification services) and transitional housing, group and individual therapy, vocational training and leisure activities. In response to the need to provide treatment services to adults (primarily men), TSA developed their network of substance misuse treatment facilities beginning in Detroit in 1939 that then spread throughout the United States and Canada. Charitable donations and private funding from foundations to serve a predominately white alcohol-abusing population initially funded these Harbour Lights facilities.

Since the 1960s, these programmes and services have sought and received large amounts of governmental funding to treat a more racially and ethnically diverse population with multi-substance misuse problems (Wolf-Branigin 2009). While focused initially on men in recovery when first initiated, in recent decades TSA has increasingly provided services to women that address their unique needs. For example, in Detroit, Michigan, for the past 20 plus years, TSA has operated a programme specifically for women with addictions and are pregnant and/or have children under the age of three years within a residential treatment service.

Given The Salvation Army's fundamentalist orientation in the Christian religion, their substance misuse treatment services typically have applied Alcoholics Anonymous [AA] principles to supplement their daily regime. Spirituality relating to the belief in a higher power, in approaches such as AA and other self-help movements (Alcoholics Anonymous 2007), remains instrumental in some approaches to addiction treatment. While several early leaders of Harbour Light programmes became sober through their involvement in The Salvation Army and self-help movements, current programme directors tend to have advanced academic degrees in social work and human service related fields. As it has been since TSA's beginnings, the continued role of spirituality in clients' belief systems and whether these clients choose to participate in treatment services demonstrates the clients' desire to enter and successfully complete treatment (Wolf-Branigin and Duke 2007).

Most Harbour Light treatment schemes have options that can last for approximately six months, with typically a 55–60 per cent programme completion rate (Wolf-Branigin 2009). This length of time includes involvement in both residential and outpatient treatments as funding sources over the past two decades prefer briefer periods in the more expensive residential services. All of the programmes have an optional religious component, which cannot be required if a programme receives any governmental funding from the local, state/provincial or federal level. In 2014 alone, The Salvation Army served over 148,000 individuals with substance misuse issues. Because of the relatively advanced and formalised level of services, many of the Harbour Light services receive external accreditation from organisations such as Commission on Accreditation of Rehabilitation Facilities [CARF] International or The Joint Commission. These accrediting bodies are voluntary international bodies that provide a review of the organisation's operations and, if successful, assure that minimum standards are met. This allows for the programmes to obtain additional funding from specialised contracts and insurance companies. All services abide by local/state licensing standards.

Recent controversies

Given the plethora of areas in which TSA operates and its fundamentalist Christian roots, it is no surprise that it has met occasional controversy. This is most apparent in respect of the rights of LGBT individuals and some contracts into which the organisation has entered. Although the officers, soldiers and employees are expected not to discriminate in service provision since the late twentieth century, controversy has stirred regarding The Salvation Army's fundamentalist views on the civil rights of LGBT individuals. This has impacted on several governmental funding contracts in the United States, United Kingdom, New Zealand and other parts of the world.

Representatives of TSA state that there is no scriptural basis for discrimination against LGBT individuals, and they have publically stated that they do not discriminate in their hiring practices or in their services. However, there has been some discrepancy between the various Territorial Headquarters' agreeing and signing service contracts as local, state and federal anti-discrimination policies. This includes some highly publicised actions and stances taken by the organisation both at a Territorial Headquarters level, and in some national and local chapters (Jones 2013).

In their position statement on 'Marriage and Family' that was available on the organisation's website until 2012, TSA stated that the Bible both directly and implicitly condemns homosexuality. The statement noted that any attempts to 'establish or promote such relationships as viable alternatives to heterosexually-based family life do not conform to God's will for society'. These views have been evident in TSA's political fight against LGBT civil rights in various chapters.

Numerous public scandals regarding what some might call their dated views on LGBT rights has forced TSA to commit to examining their official stances and their political activism. In 2008, the organisation made a public statement noting, 'The Salvation Army remains focused on building bridges of understanding and dialogue between itself and the gay community'. In 2013, the organisation removed links to ex-gay conversion therapy providers from their website. As of now, The Salvation Army emphasises its official 'no discrimination' policy in both its hiring and service practices; however, the organisation has yet to express full support for equal civil rights for LGBTQ individuals (The Salvation Army 2015a).

In recent decades, a different concern has arisen as state governments in the United States have contracted services to TSA in order to shed responsibility for their provision and reduce costs. One example is the former General Assistance programme in the state of Michigan that provided a monthly financial stipend to single adults (Sherman 1995).

The emergence of the *Charitable Choice* movement in the United States in the late 1990s has highlighted tensions within TSA as to who it employs and what services it provides. *Charitable Choice* was a federal initiative encouraging the contracting of governmental funds to faith-based organisations in order to provide direct services to children, adults and families (Carlson-Thies 2001). Under this programme, TSA received governmental funding while discriminating against the employment of LGBT workers (Blackwell and Dziegielewski 2005).

Conclusion

The Salvation Army provides a spectrum of social services worldwide in order to address and alleviate need. Local Salvation Army corps and programmes are often viewed by social workers as last resorts for placing their clients with diverse financial and other human service needs. While those working in the social services field appreciate this approach, recent controversies in the areas of LGBT rights and the TSA's role in receiving governmental funding in order to privatise services will be problematic to many. Social workers will rightfully feel some conflict with their past positions on LGBT and neo-liberal positions; however, at the local social service provision level, these views tend to be non-existent.

References

Alcoholics Anonymous (2007) *The Big Book*, 4th edn, New York: Alcoholics Anonymous World Services.
Blackwell, C.W. and Dziegielewski, S.F. (2005) 'The privatization of social services from public to sectarian', *Journal of Human Behavior in the Social Environment*, 11(2): 25–41.
Booth, W. (1890) *In Darkest England and the Way Out*, London: The Salvation Army.
Carlson-Thies, S. (2001) 'Charitable Choice: bringing religion back into American welfare', *Journal of Policy History*, 13(1): 109–32.
Drucker, P.E. (1989) 'What business can learn from non-profits', *Harvard Business Review*, July–August 1989.
Eason, A.M. and Green, R.J. (2012) *Boundless Salvation: the shorter writings of William Booth*, New York: Peter Lang.
Hazzard, J.W. (1998) 'Marching on the margins: an analysis of The Salvation Army in the United States', *Review of Religious Research*, 40(2): 121–41.
Jones, Z. (2013) 'The Salvation Army's History of Anti-LGBT Discrimination', *The Huffington Post*, 11 December 2013. Online. Available HTTP: www.huffingtonpost.com/zinnia-jones/the-salvation-armys-histo_b_4422938.html?ir=Australia (accessed 1 December 2015).
McKinley, E. (1995) *Marching to Glory: the history of The Salvation Army in the United States 1880–1992*, Grand Rapids: Eerdmans Publishing.
National Association of Social Workers [NASW] (2008) *Code of Ethics*, Washington, DC: NASW Press. Online. Available HTTP: http://socialworkers.org/nasw/ethics/default.asp (accessed 23 November 2015).
Sherman, A.L. (1995) 'Cross purposes', *Policy Review*, 74: 58–63.
Taiz, L. (2001) *Hallelujah Lads and Lasses: remaking The Salvation Army in America 1880–1930*, Chapel Hill, NC: University of North Carolina Press.
The Salvation Army (2015a) *The Salvation Army and the LGBT Community*. Online. Available HTTP: www.salvationarmyusa.org/usn/nodiscrimination (accessed 1 December 2015).
The Salvation Army (2015b) *Harbor Light Centers*. Online. Available HTTP: www.salvationarmyusa.org/usn/harbor-light (accessed 1 December 2015).
The Salvation Army (2015c) *International Health Services*. Online. Available HTTP: www.salvationarmy.org/ihq/health (accessed 1 December 2015).
The Salvation Army (2015d) *Statistics*. Online. Available HTTP: www.salvationarmy.org/ihq/statistics (accessed 1 December 2015).
The Salvation Army (2016) *International Mission Statement*. Online. Available HTTP: www.salvationarmy.org/ihq/Mission (accessed 24 February 2016).
Walker, P.J. (2001) *Pulling the Devil's Kingdom Down: The Salvation Army in Victorian England*, Berkeley, CA: University of California Press.
Wallis, J. (2008) *The Great Awakening: reviving faith a politics in a post-religious right America*, New York: Harper Collins.
Weinberg, B. (2001) *A Limited Partnership: the politics of religion, welfare, and social service*, New York: Columbia University Press.
Winston, D. (2000) *Red-hot and Righteous: the urban religion of the Salvation Army*, Cambridge, MA: Harvard University Press.
Wolf-Branigin, M. (2009) 'The emergence of formalized Salvation Army addictions treatment', *Journal of Religion and Spirituality in Social Work*, 28(3): 327–37.
Wolf-Branigin, M. and Duke, J. (2007) 'Spiritual involvement as a predictor to completing a Salvation Army substance abuse treatment program', *Research on Social Work Practice*, 17(2): 239–45.
Zavada, J. (2015) 'Salvation Army's red kettles turn coins into compassion', *About Religion*. Online. Available HTTP: http://christianity.about.com/od/Salvation-Army/a/Red-Kettles.htm (accessed 1 December 2015).

18

South Asian gurus, their movements and social service

Samta P. Pandya

Introduction

The figure of the guru has shown itself to be one of the most enigmatic features of the Hindu religious world, originating from the Indian context. Recent literature places them in the context of their multiple roles in South Asian society more generally. The focus is on the domaining effects and the expansibility of the gurus, a discourse that has further been enhanced by their Diaspora presence. Popular modern guru organisations in India own and manage vast institutional and financial empires, command an international presence and, within India, attract followers largely from educated, urban, 'middle class' sections of the country's population.

Social welfare activities belong to a common repertoire of social service engagements undertaken by a wide range of guru-led movements. One could say that such activities are at once emblematic, and a furtherance, of the guru's multiple societal entanglements. Social service is essentially seen as one core strategy of proliferation and world affirmation across guru-led movements and hence a legitimising trope. There is in effect a 'guru governmentality' through this social service, where the state borrows from or harnesses the guru-devotee relationship in order to fulfill certain governmental ends (Copeman and Ikegame 2012). However, at times, guru-led movements' ideologies of social service often foreshadow and support a more radical, political Hindutva doctrine (Mehta 2008). This is in a doctrinally non-confrontational way, camouflaged by what Zavos (2001) calls *sanatana dharma* (universal religion), as an unmediated reactionary force. Service is directed towards building a society complying with Hindu nationalism's agenda of revolutionary nationhood (Basu and Bannerjee 2006). Remembrance of the guru is a catalyst for social action and demonstrates a preference for principles such as human rights, peace and justice.

Drawing from and based on the basic premise that the South Asian guru is multifaceted, uncontainable, a domain crosser par excellence and a total social phenomenon (Jenkins 2010), I discuss through a few illustrations and a general meta analysis drawing from field insights, how these guru-led movements interplay social action and service and thereby build their legitimacy in society. Towards deploying social service as a legitimising trope, guru-led movements cultivate it through the following architectures: unique visions on society, ideas on social ethics, on social action and on social service and work. Further, how this guru faith manifests in practice, through tangible social services and an interplay of memory and oblivion, thereby evolving their unique style, is the crux of this chapter.

The architecture of guru-led movements' social service: visions on society, social ethics, social action and service

Visions on society

Guru-led movements' visions of society stem from the doctrine of 'belonging'; that the real practical world belongs to the Absolute and the ethereal. They innovatively reconfigure the social space, discursively shaping community notions coalesced around sets of faith-oriented lenses and resonating differentially in a complex network of 'public spheres'. For instance, for the Ramakrishna Mission, one of the oldest guru-led movements, society is generally viewed as a macrocosm, a larger existential and tangible yet ephemeral reality on which the divine play or *lilaprasangas* are undertaken (Dhar 2006). Human beings are actors and the larger administration rests with the higher power. In the binary scheme of things, society comprises the material world 'out there' vis-à-vis the spiritual world within. For a more contemporary guru-led movement such as the Art of Living Foundation, started by the charismatic teacher Sri Ravi Shankar in Bengaluru, India in 1982, society is viewed as the basic existential domain, a composite of beings that are supposed to be in quest of the Absolute. Society in the Art of Living terms is effectively 'matter', the reality that is attainable, knowable and should eventually be on the path of transcendence (Sri Sri Publications Trust 2007).

On social ethics

Guru-led movements have peculiar views on deontological and teleological ethics. The deontological dimensions of guru-led movements' ethics are moral religious sentiments, containing notions of divine nature and their attributes. The teleological dimensions of guru-led movements' ethics are perceptions, i.e. ways of taking/understanding the world and differential theological sentiments as expressions of reflective/reflexive acts on the part of the faith commune.

For instance, the Brahmakumaris World Spiritual University, a millenarian Hindu sect, proposes a set of 'deontological' codes including strict adherence to the Raja Yoga (a Hindu philosophy of consecration) regime. There is a stoic belief in the 'world tree' theory, which proposes the Brahmakumari souls alone are the embodiment of 'truth' and 'light' and hence located on the highest branch. Therefore, there is a calculated 'othering' of non-Brahmakumari souls or beings, an erasure of their very existence, mentally first, and then believed to be physically inevitable in the apocalypse (which is also considered inevitable).

The teleological forms of Brahmakumaris' ethics are seen in their 'assimilative and world affirmative' paradigm, wherein Brahmakumaris's repertoire is instrumental, both at the level of epistemology as well as praxis. The epistemological instrumentalism emerges from its shift in focus and teachings from pure metaphysical soul discourses to the ethnography of everyday living. Apart from the regular course and advanced meditation course for the spiritually enlightened and ready to receive, Brahmakumaris also conduct tailor-made courses on areas of 'material success' and 'worldly relationships', all garnished with the Raja Yoga apotheosis. The praxis instrumentalism then emerges in the shaping of the metaphysical Raja Yoga to a tailored form, non-Brahmakumari souls not being apocryphal but perceived by Brahmakumari souls as in need of an anchor, which they supposedly provide (Walliss 2007).

For another guru-led movement, Chinmaya Mission, social ethics entail the Chinmaya

Mission version of Hindu ethnocentrism, operating wherefrom is the tripartite social connectivity of 'love, harmony and service' (Tejomayananda 2001). The social and teleological ethics are attributed to the 'action' component of Vedanta, to which are attached twin aspects: 1) a dynamic vision of life and worldview, which is totalitarian, and 2) this-worldly-spirituality through work sans attachment to fruits of labour (Central Chinmaya Mission Trust 1989), a spiritual alienation of sorts that would accumulate transcendental benefits for the individual, and hence through synergy, for society at large. Therefore, in certain ways a Hindu utilitarian ethical vision prevails: Hindu ideals of oneness, equity, harmony, service and spiritual attitude in work (Chinmayananda 1980; Emir 1994), ensuring the greatest good for the greatest number.

Thus, in terms of social ethics, guru-led movements can be said to address 'framework questions' as well as to some extent 'application questions' (Dalmiya 2009). They essentially examine social ethics or ethical subjectivity not from the point of the moral agents, but from the point of view of the objects/persons that are recipients of the ethical concerns of guru-led movements, thereby forwarding two dimensions: moral considerability (which is the framework question demanding a criterion of having standing in the ethical domain), and moral weight (or the application question of adjudication or judgement as to who should obtain the benefits most).

Guru-led movements' stance on social ethics proposes that all 'beings' as part of the Infinite are worthy of moral consideration. This is an ethically expansive move, as it invites all socially ostracised groups squarely back to the moral table. On the application question, the guru-led movements' stance is that of universal care, but not devoid of the politics of power and privileges, which willy-nilly enter the discourse. Basically, what comes to the foreground with respect to guru-led movements' social ethics is the duty of 'beneficence': notions of moral/social duty and a generalised ethical subjectivity.

On social action

Guru-led movements' stance on social action emerges from a distinctively indigenous cosmovision and cosmology. The quest for social justice is effectively a de-colonial effort in which the mantle of Hindu-derived spirituality is utilised by the guru-led movements to dethrone colonial hegemonies. The mandate operates within a field determined by colonial and post-colonial formations of meaning: guru-led movements signify a cultural production of sorts, in which the sphere of the socio-religious is re-articulated.

For instance, Ramakrishna Mission posits itself as a crucial religio-spiritual actor responsible for emancipation. Action here essentially transcends self – the motto and aphorism of 'selfless action' prevail. According to Bhajanananda (2006) and Smarananda (2006), there are four broad types of action, or what is called in Indic literature, *karma yoga*, existing in the Ramakrishna Mission: *nishkama karma* or work without motive; *bhagawatpritikama karma* or work done with the desire of pleasing the Lord; *prapatti* or total self-surrender to the Lord; and work as participation in divine *lila*.

Action for Vivekananda Kendra (a service-based, Vivekananda ideology-driven mission and spiritual organisation) is emancipation, for which the antidote is spiritualism. Further, this action, according to Vivekananda Kendra's ideals, is associated with attributes of dispassion, detachment, oneness of the other and service (Parameswaran 2004) as the modus operandi. The Mata Amritanandamayi Mission (started by devotees of the hugging saint Mata Amritanandamayi or Amma) stance towards action is universalistic, involving tackling multiple systems geared towards the clientele, in a spiritual way, with Amma's teachings as showing the right way.

The Art of Living-defined social action has the following qualifications: spiritualised, dialogic, devotional and dispassionate. The concept given for action is *ishwarapranidhana*; i.e.

recognition of the divine in all, and hence all beings as worthy of devotion. *Tapa* (penance), *swadhyaya* (self-study undertaken for pure knowledge) and *ishwarapranidhana* (seeing the divine in all) are all called *kriya yoga* or the yoga of action (Sri Sri Publications Trust 2007).

On social service and work

On service and social work, Sri Ramakrishna emphasised the importance of selfless action: Ramakrishna's gospel of service is based on the spirit of practical Vedanta. The summum bonum here is to work simultaneously for one's own liberation and for the good of the world (Adiswarananda 2006). Three forms of understanding service and social work emerge – the 'normative', through the dictum '*sivajnanejivaseva*' (i.e. serving beings as manifestations of Godhead); the 'ideational', through the adage '*atmanomoksarthamjagathitaya ca*' (meaning for one's own liberation and good of the world); and the 'epistemological', where there is a theistic notion of service a theistic existential appropriation of social work is undertaken. Theistic existential appropriation basically implies the given-ness of this worldly existence; sufferings as a natural outcome of existence; the imperative of transcendence; the existence and proof of God and Divine being posited later as the Divine Mother; and Ramakrishna Mission's endeavours as playing a critical role in alleviating this-worldliness to divinity, by accepting divinity of beings. The modus operandi of those endeavours, i.e. the way social service is carried out, is the theistic existential appropriation of service.

Guru-led movements' stances on service and work also re-enforce the link between community development and spirituality. Spiritual teachings of guru-led movements are generally placed at the top of the hierarchy of service (to body, mind and soul) (Beckerlegge 2007), with variations on political engagement policies. Further, one peculiarity of the guru-led movements' stance on service/work is that the general delivery of *seva* or service is dependent more on the interior disposition of the performer and less on the inner transformation of the recipient. Service position is more as a 'religious *sadhana*', a means to spiritual realisation, which resembles historical religious forms of charitable action rather than featuring objective service. In some way, the derivation and appeal to traditional Hindu stances to support the service rhetoric also makes the guru-led movements prisoners of the past history, historiography and hagiography determining what service should be and how it is defined.

The core of service/work proclaims more of ultimate goals, i.e. transformation, recognition of divinity in beings, supramental manifestation, and less of proximate goals such as inequality and poverty alleviation. However, it is more a matter of degree, the focus not being exclusively on consciousness raising. In contrast to the secular service sector where philosophies draw from different sources and epistemes, in the guru-led movement contexts, the philosophy of service/action/work is derived solely from its core faith-oriented ideational stances. The service/work positions of guru-led movements eventually resemble an 'experiential realism', where although secular and faith-based approaches deal with the same reality, faith inserts the divine mandate in the service. It challenges the secular to acknowledge the transcendent frame of reference and moral accountability. The secularist insight and presence, on the other hand, challenges the faith orientation to reconceptualise general assumptions on God, creation and eschatology, so as to integrate secularist ingredients in service.

Faith in practice: the tangibility of social service

Faith manifests in practice in guru-led movements through tangible social service. The genesis of social service for the guru-led movements has been initially serendipitous and later systematised, or apriori streamlined for translation of charisma and faith. The initiation and streamlining of social services in guru-led movements has been through a coalition of charisma power and devotees' and followers' interest in perpetuation. Nevertheless, a need to create a world of shared meanings and practices has also been recognised, resulting in a paradigm shift in guru-led social services from the traditional 'privatised' role of faith, with a focus on the spiritual–sacred, towards the 'public' role, which embodies multidimensional social capital.

The idea/mandate is to bring faith to the public realm in a visible way, beyond rituals, towards a community orientation. This mandate also entails a kind of 're-authoring', the guru-led movements being the navigator of the process; the reconfiguration is derived from guru-led movements' faith and spiritual knowledge. Ideologically, faith is essentially seen as providing a moral base on which to re-build a deterritorialised global culture, transcending economics and essentially dealing with the essence of humanity and what is right. The portrayed governing idea of guru-led movements is to serve the cause of social integration by re-creating bonds of solidarity in an imagined commune. The question nevertheless remains in terms of whose commune and what nature of integration. The service ideology of guru-led movements is not of the nature of armchair prophecy, but mediated actively by religious and civil practices – philanthropic giving, collective prayer and rituals. Habitual practices of *seva*, *sadhana* and *yoga* within the guru-led movement context, rather than simple espousal of beliefs, have been responsible for the service repertoire. Within this practice-driven ideational account, there is a relationship between faith, affiliations to guru-led movements and philanthropic engagements of concerned stakeholders. Faith discerns certain meaning systems of self–other exchange within which the tradition of service and also norms of community organising around the faith principle are created.

The scope encompasses the core social sectors of development such as education, health and livelihood as well as certain customised programmes. The mission is inevitably 'social', through the prism of faith. The mandate is 'service' through which to eventually realise twin transcendental ideals of spiritual–material upliftment and proliferate the 'message'. Both of these are derivatives of the mission – the guru-led movements' mission-ideals then seep into the social canvass through the projects either in an apriori, parallel and/or retrospective manner. The management of these institutionalised efforts have a 'missionary consciousness'; there is an order ministration of evangelical nature.

Social services and guru-led movements

The engagement of guru-led movements in core sectors of development such as education, health and livelihoods describe the scope of guru-led social services at one level. At another it also projects the guru-led movements' assertion/partnership in development goals in a resource limited setting, by simultaneously factoring in culture. The mission is to respond to a religious calling, and cultivate a faith-informed vision of care using faith resources. All the guru-led movements use some form of religious imagery in their mission statements to communicate their faith-basedness in the 'public face'. In fact, for guru-led movements, the service as a part of the mission is also considered as a practice of faith, not too distinct from other expressions of faith. Discourse is an important tool by which guru-led movements' missions are highlighted, through which the guru-led movements' stance is projected comprising of social practices and enabling the construction of meanings and identities. Mission statements of guru-led movements, with their 'social' and 'faith' amalgam, are culturally patterned for determining relevance for their public. In realising the service mandate through the social initiatives, guru-led movements establish a middle ground between the secular and sacred – focusing on the faith community efforts in influencing/effecting change.

In terms of practicalities in the management of social services, guru-led movements' 'public face' is characterised by religious phraseology in their mission statements and religious symbolism in their logos. Headed by the charismatic guru, the members of the order are in charge and the adherent base forms a volitional second line supported by paid staff with a fair degree of formalisation in recruitment. 'Faith' nevertheless remains the overarching raison d'etre for engagement at all levels. Finance generation is through modes of exchange beyond market logics, 'philanthropy' being one core source. In terms of social service goods delivered, guru-led movements provide flexible services involving relational programmes, with faith-oriented services also being a part of the package. The organisational culture is imbued with 'faith' as the overarching and underlying tenet. There is a certain kind of reliance on secular expertise, but not sans the spiritual veto power in information processing and decision-making. Hence, the secular/profane is not discounted in managerial aspects; faith is an important and un-negotiable add-on.

In the management of guru-led movements' projects there is an engagement of leadership, use of structures and resources and practical amendments in guru-led movements' functional policies to aid intervention. There is an inbuilt understanding in the management of the importance of providing a faith-based context for service. The guru-led movements' financial status and the orientation of the monastic order also influence the policy and management issues of social projects. Management entails an involved mediation process, with media, environments and networks through which symbols and expressions of faith are circulated and coalitions/partnerships built. Certain programmatic and systemic effects result from the infusion of guru-led movement players having consequences for the profile of services and who gets served. This, in effect, influences the transferability of guru-led movement interventions across religious and secular applications in order to satisfy constitutional issues of equity and public choice.

Further, the affirmative relationship of the guru-led movements with the legal system is an exercise in practiced legitimacy, a way to consolidate their stand as reasonable social actors. Guru-led movements' amicability with political and local governance is also a result of the state policy to view the guru-led movements as 'communities of character' (see Kennedy and Bielefeld 2006) that can generate social capital, which in turn contributes to social change and development. Sometimes, this falls in the realm of post-Enlightenment ethics discourse that dominates contemporary public policy discussions; guru-led movements are becoming crucial actors in local/translocal politics. Essentially, they have demonstrated potential in service outreach, partnering or assisting the state welfare agenda and rights mandate. The guru-led movements' relationship with state also signifies a policy shift from government to governance, emphasis put on the way in which discourses and traditions shape service delivery while simultaneously drawing attention to beliefs and worldviews that shape public choice (see Biebricher 2011; Ikegame 2012). The amicability is most defined in state policies of externalisation, wherein guru-led movements have managed to circumvent state imposed restrictions through the faith rhetoric and emerge as dominant transnational actors.

While complying with state mechanisms, the signature teachings of the gurus actually become the principal rhetoric supporting service. Not satisfied with simply delivering the goods, they also add the faith and morality ingredients into the basket. Even though state compliance may be a political act, for guru-led movements it is an act of applying faith to 'this world' and connecting to the roots.

Within the economic system there are relationships beyond market exchange as guru-led movements essentially deal with religious goods that are acquired or received through charisma and/or transcendental forces. Charisma and/or transcendental forces provide charismatic gifts in the form of meditation or spiritual and life skills techniques, which have become signature goods of guru-led movements. Even though these goods involve certain rational actions in terms of demand and supply, the market model does not adequately describe the tactics resulting in guru-led movements relying on philanthropy as the main source of funding.

With the follower groups in civil society, guru-led movements tap into intrinsic–extrinsic religiosity–spirituality and tamper with the religio-spiritual orientations to then affect notions of self and cognitions of associates. Their beneficiaries are viewed as an imagined community of would-be followers, with guru-led movements' utilising their faith capital along with social service to reach out. They also extend, using Wilson's (2011) term, an ethics of hospitality towards potential service seekers, especially in situations where alternatives are limited. That way a combination of bonding–bridging social capital is generated.

The dynamics of guru-led movements' social service: memory, oblivion and style

Memory is the political economy of faith assertions: gurus' charisma and his/her organisational memory transferring onto public memory creation and recreating ideational stances. Oblivion is the non-transference of organisational memory to public memory. The service style is characterised by the antagonisms and contradictions derived through the correspondence between memory and oblivion.

Guru-led movements' memory is, thus, like a spiritual rationality wherein there is a shared inherent purpose to experience connectedness with the transcendental vision demonstrated by guru-led movements. The rationality element validates this worldly action – shared higher-level purposes being connectedness with the Absolute and others. Essentially, social conditions influence how memory acquires meaning through faith and related practices. Faith informs social practices of guru-led movements and remembrance of the charismatic guru lineage is a catalyst for social action. This memory then demonstrates a preference for principles of human rights, peace, solidarity and 'signs of the times' are considered as the basis for social analysis. Memory also very strongly shapes social imaginations – placing on the charismatic guru and teachings a kind of doctrinal responsibility to feed into the pragmatics and contextualities of social justice. Guru-led movements' memory is culturally loaded; they ensure a cultural continuity by preserving the 'knowledge' through mnemonics (practical Vedanta, Raja Yoga, Integral Yoga, Sudarshan Kriyatechniques being illustrations), rendering it possible for followers to reconstruct their cultural identities. Mnemonics interplay with social action through image creation of the charismatic guru as a 'socially aligned' figure, ceremonial practices that combine ritual prayer with service, narrative building of the embeddedness of service in the guru-led movement historiography and genealogy and inscriptions in its publics.

For guru-led movements the oblivion dynamics arise in the course of the movements' reflexive acts in re-defining and refining their own positions in relation to the larger socio-political environ. Oblivion has been further enhanced by neo–liberalisation, which has opened spaces for guru-led movements to enter into the public realm in newer ways and probably also to enter into mainstream 'secular' partnerships.

Guru-led movements' styles of service/action go beyond simple instilling/extolling of virtues, but rather portray themselves as vanguards of fulfilling social obligations. The operational ontology of guru-led movements contains communitarian notions of social citizenship. Essentially the immanence of the soul is emphasised. Other aspects are that of integrality of the human experience, commune as predominant and social justice notions as fertilising/impregnating aspects of charity/philanthropy. There is a stylised form of faith-based social logic, and the 'public good' factor in the guru-led movements ideals is the utopia towards which sociality is geared.

Faith and a collateral seepage of Hindu hegemony through service is the general political economy for the guru-led movements. This is manifested through service religiosity, staff religiosity and in general organisational faith. There is an institutional coupling of service with the resources, authorities and culture of guru-led movement ideas. Two analytical frames, drawing from Bradley (2009), define the political economy dynamics – one is the way faith shapes their perceptions of the world and their actions in development; and the other is the way this translates into practice.

Guru-led movements are particularly inclined towards engaging in services that promote wellbeing and are in line with their faith-based outlook. Contrary to being unblemished 'armies of compassion' (Kennedy and Beilefield 2006), guru-led movements have their intention of initiation/co-option spelt out in their mandate. This initiation/co-option is either a direct derivative of faith and/or truncated from the teachings-praxis calculus of the guru-led movements – the latter being more prominent. Faith-based services enumerate vulnerable populations and circumscribe their continued survival within bounded spatial realities. This process of 'emplacing', using Arif's (2008) concept, suggests a faith-coded bio-politics of the guru-led movements, i.e. a practice of governmentality that puts agents other than state, and thus the guru-led movements themselves, in a position of exerting power over continued social life.

Conclusion

The large-scale discharge/dissemination and conduct of social services is a driving force behind the guru-led movements' object-centred sociality. Here the object is the society and the cultures and subcultures that are not their own. The final purpose of this is the notion of integration. The fact that this normative consensus and the shared values and traditions that the movements' seek through this move of sociality is not possible in this growing and diverse cultural and ethnic consciousness, makes adequate room for the arguments of hegemony and domination that are a part and parcel of the guru-led movements' sociality.

Nevertheless, what guru-led movements manage on the social playground is a socio-culturally engineered consensus. Due to their resource endowments and partnering in the development goals in an essentially resource-limited setting, the metaphor of 'in thought collective' (with civil society, state and market) may be applicable. This kind of integration then gives the guru-led movements adequate grounding to be critical and powerful civil society actors in India and the Diaspora.

References

Adiswarananda, Swami (2006) 'Ramakrishna Mission: its gospel of service', in Swami Lokeswarananda, Swami Prabhananda, Swami Bhajanananda, Swami Purnatmananda, N. Chakrabarty and M. Sivaramkrishna (eds) *The Story of Ramakrishna Mission: Swami Vivekananda's vision and fulfilment*, Kolkata: Advaita Ashrama.

Arif, Y. (2008) 'Religion and rehabilitation: humanitarian biopolitics, city spaces and acts of religion', *International Journal of Urban and Regional Research*, 32(3): 671–89.

Basu, S. and Banerjee, S. (2006) 'The quest for manhood: masculine Hinduism and nation in Bengal', *Comparative Studies of South Asia, Africa and the Middle East*, 26(3): 476–90.

Beckerlegge, G. (2007) 'Responding to conflict: a test of the limits of neo-Vedântic social activism in the Ramakrishna math and mission?' *International Journal of Hindu Studies*, 11(1): 1–25.

Bhajananda, Swami (2006) *Selfless Work: its basis, methods and fulfilment*, Belur Math: Ramakrishna Mission Vivekananda University.

Biebricher, T. (2011) 'Faith-based initiatives and the challenges of governance', *Public Administration*, 89(3): 1001–14.

Bradley, T. (2009) 'A call for clarification and critical analysis of the work of faith-based development organisations (FBDOs)', *Progress in Development Studies*, 9(2): 101–14.

Central Chinmaya Mission Trust (CCMT) (1989) *Vedanta in Action*, Mumbai: CCMT.

Chinmayananda, Swami (1980) *Meditation and Life*, Mumbai: Central Chinmaya Mission Trust.

Copeman, J. and Ikegame, A. (2012) 'Guru Logics', *HAU: Journal of Ethnographic Theory*, 2(1): 289–336.

Dalmiya, V. (2009) 'Themetaphysics of ethical love: comparing practical Vedanta and feminist ethics', *Sophia*, 48(1): 221–35.

Dhar, S. (2006) 'Ramakrishna Mission and the total uplift of humanity: an overview of Ramakrishna Mission's contributions', in Swami Lokeswarananda, Swami Prabhananda, Swami Bhajanananda, Swami Purnatmananda, N. Chakrabarty and M. Sivaramkrishna (eds) *The Story of Ramakrishna Mission: Swami Vivekananda's vision and fulfilment*, Kolkata: Advaita Ashrama.

Emir, R. (1994) *Undoing: returning to simplicity*, Mumbai: Central Chinmaya Mission Trust.

Ikegame, A. (2012) 'The governing guru: Hindu mathas in liberalising India', in J. Copeman and A. Ikegame (eds) *The Guru in South Asia*, London: Routledge.

Jenkins, T. (2010) *The Life of Property: house, family and inheritance in Béarn, south-west France*, Oxford: Berghahn.

Kennedy, S.S. and Bielefeld, W. (2006) *Charitable Choice at Work: evaluating faith-based job programs in the states*, Washington DC: Georgetown University Press.

Mehta, R.B. (2008) 'The missionary Sannyasi and the burden of the colonized: the reluctant alliance between religion and nation in the writings of Swami Vivekananda (1863–1902)', *Comparative Studies of South Asia, Africa and the Middle East*, 28(2): 310–25.

Parameswaran, P. (2004) *Karma Yoga as Discussed by Swami Dayananda Saraswati*, Chennai: Vivekananda Kendra Prakashan Trust.

Smarananda, Swami (2006) 'The motto of the Ramakrishna Mission: "Atmanomoksarthamjagathitaya ca"', in Swami Lokeswarananda, Swami Prabhananda, Swami Bhajanananda, Swami Purnatmananda, N. Chakrabarty and M.Sivaramkrishna (eds) *The Story of Ramakrishna Mission: Swami Vivekananda's vision and fulfilment*, Kolkata: Advaita Ashrama.

Sri Sri Publications Trust (2007) *Spirituality: talks by H.H. Sri Sri Ravi Shankar*, Bangalore: Sri Sri Publications Trust.

Tejomayananda, Swami (2001) *Towards Greater Success*, Mumbai: Central Chinmaya Mission Trust.

Walliss, J. (2007) *The BrahmaKumaris as a reflexive tradition: responding to late modernity*, Delhi: Motilal Banarasidass Publishers Private Limited.

Wilson, E. (2011) 'Much to be proud of, much to be done: faith-based organisations and the politics of asylum in Australia', *Journal of Refugee Studies*, 24(3): 548–64.

Zavos, J. (2001) 'Defending Hindu tradition: sanatana dharma as a symbol of orthodoxy in colonial India', *Religion*, 31(2): 109–23.

19

Reclaiming compassion
Auschwitz, Holocaust remembrance and social work

John G. Fox

Introduction

[There are those] who will feel that the Holocaust, like the destruction of the Temple, belongs only to history—it won't affect their life. I think it's wrong because the Holocaust was not a Jewish problem ... I think the Holocaust was a universal problem

(Survivor testimony 0590 1995)

Religions and spiritualities have long been centrally concerned with the experience of suffering. For Judaism, this experience – and the endeavour to 'make sense' of and endure it – has had great prominence. Jewish history is replete with the experience of unearned suffering, often on a massive communal scale, with none more extreme or extensive than the Holocaust. Holocaust remembrance in the hope that such an event never be repeated is central to Judaism and undertaken through a range of Holocaust museums throughout the world, including the Jewish Holocaust Museum and Research Centre [JHC] in Melbourne, Australia.

Outside of Israel, Australia has the highest number of Holocaust survivors (per capita) (Paratz and Katz 2011) and the greater portion of these women and men settled in Melbourne. Since its establishment in 1984, the JHC has recorded the testimonies of over 1,500 of these survivors (JHC 2016a) as part of its commitment to 'combat anti-Semitism, racism and prejudice in the community and foster understanding between people' (JHC 2016b). These testimonies are supported by a wide range of artefacts that have been collected, archived and displayed by the Centre in its museum. The Centre also offers education programmes for primary, secondary and tertiary students – almost 21,000 students participated in those programmes in 2015 (Fineberg 2016). This work is not undertaken alone. The Centre is supported by an active, engaged community, both in its day-to-day operations and in the wide range of events and activities it facilitates.

The critical tradition of social work is also centrally concerned with unearned suffering – both in terms of assisting people to endure it and with its prevention. As a discipline, social work emerged out of the miseries of Industrial Revolution England, where so many people, displaced by unprecedented, far-reaching social and economic change, sought to 'make sense' of – and survive – those changes. Since that time, social work has expanded the scope of its concerns to understand and address the suffering often experienced with those who differ in terms of ability, age, class, gender, race and sexuality. Social work has sought to respond to the 'pain' suffered at the 'nexus with social structures' (Baines 2007: 191).

My work as a social work academic seeks to address those forms of thought that prevent the recognition of the personal impact of seemingly distinct, 'external' processes and structures. In my research, I have drawn on Marx (Fox 2015) to better comprehend how bodily experience affects agency and how a wealthy nation like Australia can dismiss the pain suffered by those experiencing poverty. That same question – how could bodily pain be so consistently ignored – led me to the works of the German social theorist Theodore Adorno, who considered that the devaluation of the body played a key part in enabling the Holocaust (principally through the suppression of compassion). As Scholar-in-Residence at the JHC, I am currently testing Adorno's ideas about compassion against the survivors' testimonies and considering how other aspects of Adorno's work might contribute to further collaborations with the Centre and similar organisations.

Adorno, social work and the Jewish Holocaust Centre

The JHC and the critical tradition of social work are both concerned with the cultural failure evidenced by the Holocaust and the need to promote a culture that, at the least, prevents its repetition. Testimonies and historical accounts of the Holocaust repeatedly refer to it as 'unimaginable' – that, in Germany, a place so deeply invested in so much that Western civilisation prized (and still prizes), culture could fail to prevent mass-murder on an industrial scale. One survivor, in his testimony recorded with the JHC, warns us against taking a similar comfort in the safeguards of our culture and political and legal systems today. He cautions others not to be complacent in a country like Australia 'because they are born here, and they've got all the rights in this country under the constitution'. He reminds us that 'We also had rights. We also had a constitution. We were also free people'. Germany and those countries it occupied in the Second World War, such as Poland, were also democracies and subject to the rule of law in the 1930s, with a rich public culture:

> That country [Germany], that intelligent nation, which gave the world the biggest philosophers. They gave us Beethoven and Mozart and Schubert and Schumann. We had Heine and Nietzsche. We had Karl Marx and Rosa Luxemburg and we had Adolf Hitler, and have had all these people who were prepared and ready in the name of their culture to murder innocent people.
>
> (Survivor testimony 0441 1993)

The failure of modern culture to prevent the Holocaust became one of the key concerns of the Critical School of Social Theory. The critical tradition of social work, like many philosophers, sociologists and psychologists, draws its roots from that school of thought, which originated in the 1930s in the Institute for Social Research at Frankfurt University, Germany. As both the time and place suggest, the Institute and its members were profoundly affected by the rise of Nazism and the Holocaust that followed. Theodore Adorno was a key member of that Institute and was forced to flee Germany after the Nazis banned the Institute, and his ability to work as an academic, given his Jewish heritage, but his influence after the Second World War was significant. He was then actively and prominently involved in public debates in Germany about collective responsibility.

Adorno was born in Frankfurt in 1903. He received his doctorate in philosophy in 1924 and then moved to Vienna to study Schonberg's revolutionary new approach to musical composition. In 1931 he joined the Institute and began the work for which he is famous. Adorno drew on both philosophy and music throughout his life. The manner in which his thought draws deeply on the intellectual and the artistic is a large part of what provides its richness and potential to contribute to both social work and the JHC.

Adorno regarded the Holocaust as evidence of Western culture's failure to achieve its central goal – the promotion of civil or civilised behaviour and the exclusion of barbarism. In his view, the Holocaust reflected long-standing features of Western society and required a radical revision of its foundations in order to prevent the recurrence of similar catastrophes. For Adorno, the Holocaust, as symbolised by the death camp Auschwitz, was not an historical aberration: it was 'not unique but, horrifyingly, exemplary' of Western civilisation (Bernstein 2001: 395). He saw the same tendencies reflected in other disasters or threats of his time, such as the colonial conflicts of the 1950s and 1960s (Adorno 1973, 2001a, 2003). He did not consider that Western society had progressed past these tendencies. Rather, like Max Horkheimer and Walter Benjamin, two other central figures in the Institute's founding work, he regarded the belief in progress as enabling past suffering to be forgotten, and even rationalised in the service of 'higher' goals (Adorno 2003: 23). Horkheimer (1995: 138–9) felt this so strongly that he said 'we are forbidden any such consolation about the world'. Instead, as Adorno (1973: 18) expressed it, we are obliged to make 'suffering eloquent' and look for its causes and their continuation in contemporary culture. So imminent was this threat in Adorno's eyes, he argued:

> The premier demand on all education is that Auschwitz not happen again ... Every debate about the ideals of education is trivial and inconsequential compared to this single ideal: never again Auschwitz. It was the barbarism all education strives against. One speaks of the threat of a relapse into barbarism. But it is not a threat – Auschwitz *was* the relapse, and barbarism continues as long as the fundamental conditions that favoured that relapse continue largely unchanged. That is the whole horror. The societal pressure still bears down, although the danger remains invisible nowadays.
>
> (Adorno 2003: 19)

Anti-Semitism, racism and Western thought

For Adorno, the Holocaust was enabled by what he called 'identity thinking' – the modern Western confidence that objects are 'identical' with our concepts of them (Jarvis 1998: 177). He argued that 'identity thinking' was always an incomplete account of its object and that it failed to consider what was outside its concepts, which Adorno called its 'residue' (Adorno 1973: 5). For Adorno, the treatment of an object in this way involved doing violence to its 'residue'. In his view, the Holocaust was founded on this violence: there 'identity thinking' enabled Jewish and other peoples to be solely considered in terms of narrow, incomplete stereotypes.

This 'identity thinking' reflects contemporary Western society and some of its long-standing approaches to the world: in particular, the conception of any thing – and, especially after the Enlightenment, the self as a thing existing-in-itself with an 'essence' or 'substance' without any dependence on any other thing. In everyday language, it is the idea that every thing has its 'nature'. We can trace the influence of this kind of thinking back over 2,500 years to pre-Socratic thought. However, 'notwithstanding ... changes in terminology, the emphasis [has] remained on some separate, unchanging quality that gave a being continuity and rendered that which is changeable ... emphemeral [and] inessential' (Fox 2015: 8). This approach to conceptualisation has been further promoted by capitalism's processes of commodification, which treat any thing, regardless of those involved in its production or use, as the absolute thing-in-itself and able to be exchanged without any reference to those relationships. Most recently, neo-liberalism has extended this alienated, atomistic approach to the world throughout much of public policy and public life.

This notion of an essence or substance is the grammar of Western thought, a structuring of how we form concepts of the nature of a thing – what we treat as part of its lasting nature (its 'essence') and what we treat as inessential or optional. This approach to conceptualisation, counting some aspects and not others, authorises the neglect of those other features or characteristics. It encourages a kind of hubris: in particular, it enables violence to be done, and not recognised (or, at least, not admitted). To treat a thing by reference to only some of its characteristics – especially if it is forced to conform to that limited vision – is to tear that thing apart. It is to hammer a square peg into a round hole – and to chop, bludgeon or tear away some vital part of that peg in order to make it fit.

This conceptual violence enabled anti-Semitism to characterise Jewish people (and others) with reference to some characteristics and ignore others, even when those characteristics, such as the shape of a person's nose, were repeatedly contradicted by experience. It is a violence that continues today. It enables asylum seekers arriving in – or even approaching – Australia to be considered as 'queue jumpers' and 'illegals' and the Australian government to claim that its actions in preventing them coming to Australia's shores are decent and humane.

Suppressing compassion

In Adorno's view, this violence was not only applied to others but to the very notion of the self. The West has long identified the human 'essence' with the mind, soul or other non-corporeal substance, and discounted, devalued and disciplined the body. So central has this view been that Adorno and Horkheimer (1997: 231) called it the 'underground' history of the West.

Adorno saw Western culture as built on the domination of our bodies, and of the balance of the physical or material world, with the essence of – the best of – our humanity then located elsewhere, in a thing we called reason. Over time the meaning of that term, and even where and how we discovered it, has varied, but since the Enlightenment, reason has been treated as something independent of our bodies, including our emotions. To be ethical, moral or just made the domination by reason an ideal: we secured our better selves (and better behaviour) through discipline, control or, to use Adorno's (1973: 363, 2005: 274) term, 'cold', reason.

Adorno was concerned that this emphasis on disciplining our non-rational selves – including our bodies – subtly enabled other kinds of violence, including that of the Holocaust. In part, that discipline might be seen to extend to the direct, physical violence meted out by the Nazis, both inside and outside the camps, but what Adorno was principally concerned with was the violence we first do to ourselves in disciplining our own bodies and reactions, especially those of compassion that might otherwise prompt us to reach out to those who are suffering.

'Never again': suffering and compassion

In the light of Western civilisation's failure to prevent the Holocaust, Adorno (2001a: 116) argued that 'Hitler has placed a new imperative on us; that ... Auschwitz should not be repeated'. The 'old' imperative was the philosopher Kant's 'categorical imperative': the unconditional obligation that human beings, as rational creatures, should only act in ways that could be universally accepted (Guyer 2006). Adorno (2001a: 116) insisted that it was 'impossible to found ... [the new] imperative on logic' as 'pure' or abstract thought lent itself far too easily to rationalisation, that is, to the circular reasoning that characterised 'identity thinking'. Instead, Adorno insisted that the West needed to revise its treatment of the human body. He (2001a: 117) thought that the only reliable foundation for ethical or moral conduct was the body, in particular our bodily or 'gut' reaction to others' suffering, and that 'the true basis of morality is to be found in bodily feeling' – that 'morality ... lives on in openly materialist motifs'.

Morality is fundamentally concerned with the just or fair treatment of others. It involves both the recognition that others are entitled to that treatment and that the obligation to do so applies to each of us in some unavoidable, undeniable way. In Adorno's view, that recognition is founded in our shared experiences of bodily pain. Within the materialist tradition of thought, the experience of bodily pain is the very basis for our experience of our selves as individuals (see Fox 2015 for a detailed consideration of this aspect of the materialist tradition). It is how we discover we are distinct from the world and begin to develop our consciousness and concept of our selves. It is an experience that precedes speech. From our earliest moments, bumping our heads on tables and chairs, we discover a world that is resistant to us, one that is distinct from us. It is an experience that is often revisited, if only through minor bumps and bruises, throughout the rest of our lives. It is a universal experience, a part of our humanity that all of us can recall and relate to. Adorno considered that we recalled this early, prelinguistic experience of pain when witnessing another's suffering. In his view, this recollection created an involuntary empathy. It provided a motive to care about the impact on the other person – and a connection with, and sense of common concern for, the other person.

One of the promotional posters for the JHC refers to 'history you cannot erase' and features an image of a person's forearm, on which a number had been tattooed. Tattooing prisoners was a common practice in the Auschwitz camp. Newly arrived men and women, already stripped of their humanity in many ways, were further reduced to mere 'specimens' (Adorno 2001a: 108), with the tattooed number thereafter being used instead of their names. It is an image of very personal, intimate, suffering. The image is followed by an invitation: 'To find out what really happened, visit our museum and ask a survivor.' The survivors' witness is central to the work of the JHC and like organisations: it provides the Centre's most compelling influence. As part of their education programme, survivors recount their experience of the Holocaust. They speak of their childhood, their families, the actions taken by the Nazis, their survival and their losses. They reflect on the causes of the Holocaust and the risks of its repetition. Often their accounts are vivid and painful, notwithstanding the years that have passed. For several years now I have brought social work students to hear the survivors' stories and the students consistently refer to this encounter as one of the most powerful experiences in all their studies.

'Never again': the role of art

However, the time fast approaches when the survivors will no longer be available to make this contribution, and the work to develop other influential forms of witness is a key concern of the Centre and similar institutions. Adorno's interest in the arts and aesthetic theory may be of relevance here. Adorno saw certain forms of art, particularly Modernist works with their emphasis on the combination of clashing images in the form of montages, as having a similar potential to the direct witness of suffering to 'shock' a person out of 'identity thinking'. This may appear to be contradicted by Adorno's (2000: 210) widely criticised statement that 'to write poetry after Auschwitz [was] barbaric'. However, as Adorno (2001a: 111) later stated, this was not a blanket condemnation of art, but only those forms that evaded confronting suffering.

Adorno drew these ideas from Walter Benjamin. Benjamin (1999: 2479) had reflected on the desensitising effects of modern life at the turn of the twentieth century, and considered how one could be 'shocked' – startled – into seeing the world afresh and experiencing it more fully. One of his most famous examples was the sight of someone in a crowd, and the frisson of recognition that lingers long afterwards. Adorno later wrote of the memories evoked by the names of places one had visited as a child. There was something potentially transformative about the juxtaposition of the familiar and desirable against the strange and unrelated. Both Benjamin and Adorno thought this same kind of productive shock could be made by works of art, particularly in the form of Modernist collages. They saw the promise of those collages residing in the way in which they could bring different, apparently unrelated, even clashing, images and ideas together – and thereby prompt the person viewing them to discover connections she or he had not previously seen.

In Adorno's view aesthetic experience could prompt involuntary change – that such experience was 'an involuntary adjustment to something extra-mental' (Adorno 2006: 213). He (1997: 331) defined this 'aesthetic comportment' in terms that shared an emphasis on the pre-linguistic experience that grounded his interest in reactions to witnessing others' pain. For Adorno, our aesthetic capacity was 'the capacity to shudder, as if goose bumps were the first aesthetic image…That shudder in which subjectivity stirs without yet being subjectivity is the act of being touched by the other'.

These strategies are already at work at the JHC and similar institutions. They form one's first encounter with the Centre, even before one enters its doors, through the Andrew Rogers' sculptured columns, the *Pillars of Witness*, which comprise 76 panels, each displaying images of the Holocaust, worked into the exterior fencing and gateway. One cannot enter the Centre without first passing by that imagery. That same kind of encounter also features within the JHC's museum. One prominent exhibit features a clear plastic tube containing small buttons in an amount representing the 1,500,000 children killed in the Holocaust. That shower of coloured buttons brings to mind the many clothes to which they were attached, and moments of ordinary, innocent, buttonings of shirts and blouses and coats – everyday acts of care and love – but its positioning, in the midst of the account of the murder of so many children, shouts the grief of loss. It makes 'suffering eloquent' (Adorno 1973: 18).

'Never again': rational analysis

This is not to say these collages – these artefacts and artworks – guarantee change. The 'gut' reaction to witnessing suffering or encountering a powerful artefact may prompt one to act, but does not ensure that one does so. That impulse can be, and often is, suppressed. The Holocaust is itself evidence of the extent and efficacy of that suppression. One survivor's account suggests that 'coldness'. She spoke of a German walking through a ghetto and finding some children on the street. She said:

> Very often Jewish children would come … to beg, and they … were just about dying. They would sit [in front of]…the houses, most of the time silent. Everyone saw them, but this time a German walked to them and said 'Oh, I can't look. It's inhuman, how you suffer.' Then he picked up a gun [and shot them].
>
> (Survivor testimony 0295B 1993)

Adorno was well aware of the limited potential of the experience of 'shock'. He believed that we could never do without 'the strength of the subject' (1973: xx) – that is, the power of critical analysis. For Adorno, aesthetic experience – even the experience of another's suffering – was necessary to prompt or open up the opportunity for different thought, but was never enough alone. It needed to be built upon by means of explanation and evidence – and some indication of a better response.

The JHC's education programme draws on the power of aesthetic experience, and then builds on that to engage participants in critical reflection. One of the first things presented in that programme is an image of the Melbourne Cricket Ground [MCG], a major local sporting venue with nation-wide recognition as the site at which many key events are held (and often televised). Given Australians' love of sport, the MCG is a very familiar, celebrated sight. JHC presenters use an image of the MCG with a capacity crowd (which is approximately 100,000 people), and then present multiple copies of that image to convey the magnitude of the Holocaust (60 pictures of the MCG, filled to capacity, represents 6,000,000 people). These images of the MCG – an ordinary and celebrated thing – are used with great impact to quantify the extent of the killings, and to demonstrate how truly comprehending that horror exceeds the grasp of numbers. It provides the kind of 'shock' Adorno believed aesthetic experience can offer. It opens up discussion.

The discussion that then follows centres on the presenter asking a relatively simple question: which race am I? That discussion, which begins with a simple concept, then proceeds to explore and critique it, concluding that there are no 'races', only the one human race. It is an example of just the work that I think Adorno had in mind for education after the Holocaust: taking an idea that suggests an essence or nature and deconstructing it so as to demonstrate, by reference to its own components, its insufficiency.

This kind of experience is one of the great potentials of Holocaust education. Confronting the suffering it involved, and discovering its connections to something so normal, so proximate, often leaves people lacking adequate words. Adorno suggests we need to build on that in order to overcome 'identity thinking': that we need to develop a sense of 'fallibility' (2001b: 169) in relation to our understandings of the world, and, as he put it, to give 'primacy to the object' (2008: 200). What he meant is that we should not presume to know the object of our attention – and, above all, to know each human being we encounter – but to try to see all their dimensions. To return to the metaphor of square pegs, it is to see its shape, and not just that it fits the loose category of being a peg.

This is very different to popular notions of reason or knowledge. It is not the confidence that, through observation and experimentation, we can discover objective, universally applicable knowledge (in other words, the positivist idea of knowledge). It is rather a consciousness of the inadequacies of our ideas, knowledge and classifications. It is to accept uncertainty, and a much less powerful, confident, convenient approach to the world and others.

This is not an easy perspective to grasp or act on. However, I think Adorno (Adorno 1973: 207) provides some guidance through his repeated references to the 'bilderverbot' – the Jewish prohibition of images of God. Within the Jewish tradition (and others) any such image would be inadequate to capture something that, by its very nature, transcends our world and our abilities. However, the absence of those images does not prevent one seeking to work toward the ideal of a good life, but presents it as an ideal that, even partially understood, is so meaningful as to encourage a lifelong striving to fulfil it.

Adorno's treatment of the bodily or 'materialistic motif' as the last foundation for morality presents a similar ideal: the elimination of bodily suffering. It presents an aim that, even though it only captures part of our humanity, goes so deeply to the quality of our lives – and the massive failure of our world to date – as to make a lifelong struggle to reduce it, however limited our understanding, a worthy goal.

Conclusion

Many of the West's most influential philosophers, including Kant, have devalued compassion as a guide to appropriate behaviour, yet valuing compassion has long been central to many religions and spiritualities. It is also a prominent part of Holocaust remembrance and research. Despite the failure of so many people to act to prevent the Holocaust, organisations like the JHC record the many instances in which some people did in fact intervene. Many survivors' accounts include at least one instance in which a stranger spontaneously sought to help them. The exceptional nature of these acts can prompt their treatment as a matter of character, as something founded in the 'essence' of those people. However, Adorno suggested that these acts were not solely a question of character, but cultural. He sought to explore the extent to which Western culture enabled or restrained those acts – and what might be required to make them more commonplace. This may seem unrealistic or naïve, yet the JHC and similar organisations have also celebrated those instances where whole communities acted to save other people. They celebrate the rescue of Jewish people by the Danes, who 'in a coordinated operation supported by the vast majority of the … population', transported most of their Jewish peoples to neutral Sweden (Friedlander 2007: 547). They hosted a major exhibition documenting the actions of the Muslim majority in Albania, who saved all the Jewish people who lived, or sought refuge, in that country (JHC 2016c). These collective acts suggest other, different, potentials, even within Western culture, and that those acts might be borne of everyday beliefs and their practice.

Adorno suggests that the limitation of collective compassion – solidarity – is closely connected with the effort to dominate the body. He also suggests that the very limits to that repression – the involuntary moments where we are prompted in other directions – remain with all their potential and locates that possibility not only in the direct expression of suffering but in its sensual representation. In the shared commitment to ensure the Holocaust and its like never happen again, critical social work and organisations like the JHC might best borrow from endeavours like the education programme at the JHC, with its promising combination of both aesthetic and intellectual engagement.

Acknowledgement

This research could not have been undertaken without the generous and thoughtful support of the Jewish Holocaust Museum and Research Centre (JHC) in appointing me as Scholar-in-Residence 2015/2016.

References

Adorno, T.W. (1973) *Negative Dialectics*, London: Routledge.
Adorno, T.W. (1997) *Aesthetic Theory*, Minneapolis: University of Minnesota Press.
Adorno, T.W. (2000) 'Cultural criticism and society', in B. O'Connor (ed) *The Adorno Reader*, Oxford: Blackwell Publishers.
Adorno, T.W. (2001a) *Metaphysics: concepts and problems*, Cambridge: Polity Press.
Adorno, T.W. (2001b) *Problems of Moral Philosophy*, Stanford: Standford University Press.
Adorno, T.W. (2003) 'Education after Auschwitz', in R. Tiedemann and T.W. Adorno (eds) *Can One Live After Auschwitz? A philosophical reader*, Stanford: Stanford University Press.
Adorno, T.W. (2005) *Critical Models: interventions and catchwords*, New York: Columbia University Press.
Adorno, T.W. (2006) *History and Freedom*, Malden: Polity Press.
Adorno, T.W. (2008) *Lectures on Negative Dialectics: fragments of a lecture course 1965/1966*, Cambridge: Polity Press.
Adorno, T.W. and Horkheimer, M. (1997) *Dialectic of Enlightenment*, London: Verso.

Baines, D. (2007) *Doing Anti-oppressive Practice: building transformative politicised social work*, Halifax: Fernwood Publishing.

Benjamin, W. (1999) *Illuminations*, London: Vintage Books.

Bernstein, J.M. (2001) *Adorno: disenchantment and ethics*, New York: Cambridge University Press.

Fineberg, W. (2016) *The Voice*, 17(2): 1.

Fox, J.G. (2015) *Marx, the Body, and Human Nature*, Basingstoke: Palgrave Macmillan.

Friedlander, S. (2007) *Nazi Germany and the Jews: 1939–1945 the years of extermination*, New York: Harper Perrenial.

Guyer, P. (2006) *Kant*, London: Routledge.

Horkheimer, M. (1995) 'A new concept of ideology?' in G.F. Hunter, M.S. Kramer, and J. Torpey (eds) *Between Philosophy and Social Science: selected early writings*, Cambridge, MA: MIT Press.

Jarvis, S. (1998) *Adorno: a critical introduction*, Cambridge: Polity Press.

Jewish Holocaust Centre (2016a) *Phillip Maisel Testimonies Project*. Online. Available HTTP: www.jhc.org. au/museum/collections/survivor-testimonies.html (accessed 20 March 2016).

Jewish Holocaust Centre (2016b) *Mission*. Online. Available HTTP: www.jhc.org.au/about-the-centre. html (accessed 20 March 2016).

Jewish Holocaust Centre (2016c) *New Exhibition from Yad Vashem: Besa, a code of honour*. Online. Available HTTP: www.jhc.org.au/news-and-events/news-from-the-jhc/item/423-besa-code.html (accessed 20 March 2016).

Paratz, E.D. and Katz, B. (2011) 'Ageing Holocaust survivors in Australia', *The Medical Journal of Australia*, 194(4): 194–7.

Survivor testimony 0295B (1993) Videorecording, Melbourne: Jewish Holocaust Centre.

Survivor testimony 0441 (1993) Videorecording, Melbourne: Jewish Holocaust Centre.

Survivor testimony 0590 (1995) Videorecording, Melbourne: Jewish Holocaust Centre.

20

At a crossroads

The Church of Sweden and its role as a welfare provider in a changing Swedish welfare state

Eva Jeppsson Grassman

Introduction

The aim of this chapter is to place the Church of Sweden within the contemporary ongoing discussion about the organisation and provision of welfare in Sweden.[1] The point of departure is the processes of changes that the Swedish welfare state has gone through in the past few decades, implying far-reaching deregulations and patterns of privatisation and contracting. On the other hand, the Church of Sweden has, since its separation from the State in the year 2000, taken on a new status that offers opportunities but also challenges, not least in the area of faith-based care provision. This chapter will discuss what characterises the changes that have taken place and how these changes affect the Church of Sweden, notably in the area of welfare and care provision. How has the Church, to date, contributed to welfare and care? What are the possible ways forward for the Church and its welfare work? Should the Church strengthen its role as a welfare and care provider in civil society through increased community work and through the creation of 'togetherness' and networks within the parishes? Should it strengthen its religious voice and its distinctive, religious character, not least through its traditional social work? Or should the Church launch itself into the contracted-out 'welfare market' as one among many contracted welfare providers that exist in Sweden today? The chapter elaborates on these different options, focusing on their prerequisites and consequences for the Church.

Background

Who should provide welfare in Sweden, what kind of welfare and how should it be provided? These are questions that have been focused on over the past couple of decades in Sweden, a country usually considered as a prime example of the Nordic welfare state model, yet characterised by important transitions in welfare organisation and provision in the past 25 years. Private welfare provision, pluralism and customer choice are ideologically-driven issues that have marked public discourse. The debate has engaged politicians, policymakers and the public. There were few private (profit/non-profit) contracted providers of welfare in Sweden 25 years ago. Today, around 20 per cent of all staff in publicly-funded elder care and service to people with disabilities, for instance, are employed by private for-profit companies that work on contracts and in a competitive market situation (Erlandsson *et al.* 2013). Similar patterns are found in other areas of welfare provision.

At the beginning of this transitional process (early 1990s) there were hopes that a deregulated welfare sector would give space and opportunity for involvement of voluntary, non-profit providers in welfare, not least in care provision. This has not taken place – it is mainly for-profit providers that have taken market shares. With these 25 years as background experience, the debate on how welfare provision should be organised now seems to have entered a 'phase 2', where, with various experiences of the drawbacks associated with for-profit solutions as a point of departure, once again, non-profit, voluntary, organisations in welfare have come onto the political agenda (Jeppsson Grassman 2014). The Church of Sweden and its role in welfare is an interesting case in this context. The Church has become increasingly visible in the past 20 years as an agent in welfare and care. This visibility takes on a particular significance for the Church at this time in history, since today, no longer a State Church and without the type of authority that came with that status, it is just one of many voluntary organisations that can act in the welfare market.

The Church of Sweden has gradually lost influence and authority over societal institutions and individuals. Sweden is generally considered to be a highly secularised country, as stressed in comparative literature (World Values Survey 2011). Yet the 'religious landscape' is more multi-faceted than that, not least due to extensive immigration of populations of various religious belongings. Sweden today is a society of religious pluralism (Sjödin 2011), but one in which the Church of Sweden is often not the religious body that attracts newcomers. The Church of Sweden, formerly a State majority Church with religious and administrative functions, dating back to the sixteenth century, has gradually lost members. This pattern of loss was accentuated by the deregulation of the State–Church relationship (2000), which has urged the Church to revise and partly redefine its role in Swedish society. It now constitutes the largest voluntary organisation in Sweden.

At the Church's separation from the State, it was explicitly underlined that the State's expectations – and financial prerequisites – for future support of the Church were that it should contribute to the solving of social problems in society (Swedish Government Official Report 1997). Today, with its gained freedom, the Church has the 'right' to pursue various social- and welfare-oriented projects more freely. It also needs to compensate for lost revenues, due to declining membership. The Church has a great wish and need to make itself useful – but how can this be achieved in a society where few people attend its religious services? Research in the past two decades has clearly illustrated how the Church struggles with contradictory expecta-tions, from society but also from within the Church organisation itself (Jeppsson Grassman 2001, 2014; Jeppsson Grassman and Whitaker 2009). In line with this pattern it is interesting to note that during the past two years, an investigation within the Church has been initiated to explore whether it should now take an important step forward and launch itself into a role as a regular contracted provider of core welfare services (The Official Reports of the Church of Sweden 2013).

In civil society

The described processes coincide with more general patterns of change in Swedish society, not least implying an increased focus on the role of civil society. This concept has received consider-able attention in social science in Sweden since the beginning of the 1990s. The research high-lights the increasing importance attributed to local voluntary organisations, civic participation, networks and local belonging, for 'voice' and democracy, but also for various dimensions of welfare (Jeppsson Grassman and Svedberg 2007; Trägårdh 2007). At the same time, in Swedish political discourse, a new ideological investment in civil society has taken place, based on at least two different interpretations of civil society and its role in welfare. The first discourse stresses the importance of local belonging, networks and civic participation for community and for welfare and care (Jeppsson Grassman 2001; Jeppsson Grassman and Whitaker 2009). Here, the concept is sometimes coupled with the concept of social capital, referring to networks and their attendant norms and trust, or addressing it as a personal resource of networks and belonging (Halpern 2005; Putnam 2000). Simultaneously, a second interpretation is connected with the previously described processes, i.e. the de-regulation of the Swedish welfare state, with new political expectations of pluralism and of voluntary organisations as actors in professional welfare provision, supported by volunteers and charity work. What is at stake is a development concerning civil society in another direction, based on a discourse with more distinct instrumental undertones. This way of interpreting civil society was rather unfamiliar to Sweden at the beginning of the 1990s. The country has an extensive voluntary sector, of a popular character, where membership is important and where around 50 per cent of the population is involved in volunteer work. However, it does not have its focus in social services (Jeppsson Grassman and Svedberg 2007). Church volunteering only represents a few per cent of all voluntary involvement.

What way in civil society?

The Church wants to play an important role in civil society – this is a clear pattern in the Church's discourse. How might this be achieved? Should it try to strengthen its voice as an agent of Christian faith, focus on local community and belonging in the parish, and thereby contribute to welfare and caregiving? Or should it develop its role as a professional welfare provider? Can it have more than one identity? The worry of not doing the right thing was a distinct pattern in Church discourse and actions, as expressed in the results from a study I conducted in the early 2000s of diaconal social work in all parishes in one middle-sized town (Jeppsson Grassman 2001). What is the traditional welfare role of the Church in the local context? What is there to build on and develop?

The parishes and their diaconal work

The Church has been – and still is – organised into parishes on the local level. In 2014, there were 1,364 parishes, each with its own local territory. The implication of this is that the notion of geography is an important dimension of the Church; one that has religious and social, but also administrative connotations in Sweden. The concepts of membership and belonging are equally multi-faceted in this context. Since 1996, there has no longer been any 'automatic adherence' to the Church of Sweden. Around 65 per cent of the Swedish population were still formal adherents to the Church in 2014. Of those, few were active members (around 7 per cent). 'The inner core' of the parish's religious life is probably even smaller. The traditional religious rituals of the Church (baptism, confirmation, marriage and funerals) still represent important links of belonging between the Church and the population, even if these links have also gradually weakened. Diaconal work, i.e. faith-based social work, is one of the cornerstones of the mission of the Church. Most parishes carry out such work, focusing on older parishioners, family carers and children, but also vulnerable groups such as asylum-seeking immigrants and the homeless (Engel 2006; Jeppsson Grassman 2001). The Church's diaconal work is not part of core welfare provision – it has a role as a 'supplement' to the services of the welfare state. Usually, deacons are employed for this work, i.e. specialised professional social workers.

The Church also conducts outreach work in hospitals, prisons and nursing homes, etc. However, it is the parish that is the site for most of the diaconal work. The need to broaden and deepen this work through community building in line with traditional theology, and the difficulty of achieving this, was pointed out by pastors and deacons in a study of the role of the Church of Sweden parishes in end-of-life care. A problem seemed to be that the local diaconal activities did not necessarily suffice to create networks and personal relationships within the parish (Jeppsson Grassman and Whitaker 2009). Yet such relationships ought to be a corner-stone of a Church anchored in civil society. The need and desire to be connected to a place and to a local context may take on a particular significance today, when the relationship between time and place is more fragmented than before, and the possibility of individuals freely choosing local contexts and belonging has increased (Jeppsson Grassman and Taghizadeh Larsson 2013). The Church of Sweden actually has a unique position in this respect, relative to other voluntary organisations, not least religious communities, through the parishes' local attachment (Jeppsson Grassman and Whitaker 2009; Sandberg 2009).

Welfare and care in parishes

The Church is just one of many organisations in civil society that are expected, in various ways, to offer fellowship and community as well as caring and social support. Caring relationships can meet different types of needs, including practical, physical, emotional, but also spiritual. How, then, is care and support pursued through diaconal social work in the parishes? This was the central question in the previously mentioned research where the diaconal work in all the parishes in one town was studied (Jeppsson Grassman 2001). The deacons in the parishes were interviewed. A common theme was that they stressed activities to promote 'social togetherness'. This seemed to imply social activities without constraints, where participants could meet, but were organised and structured by the deacons. Often, these gatherings seemed to be accompanied by some kind of programme, a speech or a film, etc. A very common ingredient was a meal to gather around – the Tuesday Soup, for instance. 'The Open House' was central in the narratives and it also illustrated the importance of the room – the premises where the gathering would take place. There seemed to be various forms of such activities. The results did not, however, really answer the question of whether 'social togetherness' was achieved, or how the participants themselves were involved in creating belonging and togetherness. Rather, it seemed to be that, most of the time, it was the deacons who staged and took responsibility for the 'togetherness-making'. Engel (2006), in her extensive analysis of the diaconal work of the Church of Sweden, makes a similar reflection. She argues that her research points to patterns where these open activities within the Church's diaconal work have a 'consumer-oriented' frame of reference, where ready-made programmes are offered to the participants, even in community-creating activities.

The second main orientation of the diaconal work, as illustrated by the results of the study, consisted of individual service to individuals. This was provided, on the one hand, by Church volunteers, for example in the form of visits to lonely parishioners who were old or disabled; on the other hand, this service was provided by the professional deacons. Counselling in stressful situations and in bereavement groups were situations where the deacons could use their skills, but also gave the diaconal work identity, the interviewed deacons maintained. Here, their role was service provision rather than activities in order to create belonging and community. These examples illustrate the issue of different care logics, which is further described in the next example.

The role as service provider seemed 'easier' for deacons and pastors to shoulder, than being actors in promoting community and belonging. The pastors and deacons did not person-ally know more than a fraction of their parishioners. The dilemma connected with this was illustrated in a study of spiritual support provided by the Church to parishioners and their families in end-of-life situations (Jeppsson Grassman and Whitaker 2009). The Church by tradition has an important role in spiritual care. The results indicated that, while the support offered to families in grief was very common, inclusive and well established, spiritual care given to parishioners at the end of their lives, surprisingly, turned out to be a rare and rather exclusive phenomenon in the Church of Sweden parishes. According to the results of the study, a vast majority of the parishes offered individual support to the mourners. Group support in the form of grief counselling groups was also very common. By contrast, a third of the respondents stated that their parish very seldom offered support to dying parishioners, and only 9 per cent said that their parish often offered such care or support.

How are these patterns to be understood? A key element in understanding these contrasting patterns seems to be the differences in what might be called 'care logic' and the prerequisites that underpin these patterns. The core element of the spiritual end-of-life care offered by the Church to the dying usually seemed to be a previously established long-standing relationship, usually built on shared religious values. Such relationships were rare to start with. This implies that a relational logic motivated the spiritual care process and seemed to be built on different elements, such as reciprocal relationships, belonging, shared values, trust and community. While most respondents maintained that an established relationship was a prerequisite for carrying out spiritual care for a dying parishioner, this did not seem to be the case in the grief counselling situation. Rather than following the relational logic that the end-of-life care situation is based on, it seemed to follow a 'service logic', characterised by provider–consumer positions where no previous relations were required. Support activities for those in grief actually appear to be a prime example of how the Church of Sweden took a role as a modern service provider.

The distinctive religious character

The same study illustrated another key issue: the important question of maintaining a distinctive religious character and individuality in the care and welfare services offered by the Church. What is it that the Church can offer that is special? There were significant contrasts in the character of the support offered and the language used in the two described care situations. The support offered at the end of life to parishioners had a religious character and the language that was used was based on the traditional theological repertoire. The support to the mourners, on the other hand, particularly in the 'bereavement groups', was formulated in a completely different language, rooted in typical theories about crisis and bereavement and with a psychodynamic approach. This approach seemed rather 'thin' and the language fragmented. No religious elements were allowed; 'they might scare the participants away'. While pastors and deacons who offered support to parishioners in end-of-life situations seemed well anchored in their capacity to give support with a distinctive religious character, those who provided support for the bereaved seemed vaguer about what was really the specificity of their contribution and uncertain if they really offered something that other professional groups could not provide just as well. One question that was fundamental to the study is the following: what is the significance of support and care provided by the Church if it has no religious particularity? This is a central question for the Church if it is to continue on into a professional provider's culture.

Customer choice and welfare

What would a full scale 'contracted provider role' imply for the Church of Sweden? As a provider of services within the core areas of welfare, the Church, through some form of non-profit provider organisation of its own, would take on contracts within the framework of the present rule of public sector outsourcing and within the Act on System of Choice in the Public Sector (LOV), which implies customer choice in welfare services. One of the ideas behind the deregulation of the welfare sector was to allow for alternative providers and customer choice. As already mentioned, far fewer voluntary organisations are involved in contracted provision than expected. One explanation for this has been that the legal requirements for procurement of contracts so far have favoured large, resourceful organisations, i.e. large, for-profit companies and their market logic. Another is that for most Swedish voluntary organisations, taking the step to becoming welfare providers has been too radical, due to the structure, values and culture of the organisations but also because they lack the ability to compete (Jegermalm and Jeppsson Grassman 2012).

The described privatisation processes in the welfare state have had ideological motivations. Now, after 25 years, Swedish society is in a situation where there are reasons to evaluate the results. The debate today seems permeated by a lack of trust in the providers in the welfare sector. In the past couple of years 'scandals' of different kinds connected to privatised, for-profit welfare have received great attention in the media: poor elder care, schools that have gone bankrupt, and not least enormous profits made by large companies in the welfare sector. Surveys conducted in recent years indicate that, while customer choice as an idea has gained strong support among Swedish people, a majority of people are opposed to profit-making in tax-financed welfare (Nilsson 2013). With this in mind, it seems reasonable to assume that in this present context of choice, non-profit solutions in welfare would be preferred by citizens, if they can present a trustworthy alternative. A recent survey conducted on demand by the Church of Sweden concerning welfare provision gave support to this argument (The Official Reports of the Church of Sweden 2013). This support means that now ought to be a perfect time for the Church of Sweden to develop its role as a welfare provider in certain areas. One of these areas is elder care – an area where, according to the opinion of the Swedish people, the Church of Sweden ought to extend its involvement.

The Church would then become a provider among other providers; but it is anxious to keep its own distinctive 'signature'. What would that imply in service provision? The Christian message? A diaconal frame of values? Is it possible to be a contracted provider of care and still keep one's 'signature'? Is it not precisely the theological and diaconal values that are the argument of the Church when it claims that it has something distinctive to offer as provider of welfare? The studies referred to earlier illustrate the dilemma connected with these questions.

The complications of being a welfare provider

Sweden is not the only European country to have deregulated welfare provision. Great Britain, for instance, implemented this type of process before Sweden. There, some of the consequences of this change for non-profit, voluntary organisations that carry out contracted welfare provision have been studied (Johnson 1992). Contracts implied less freedom vis-à-vis the public sector than before the arrangement. There seemed to be a tendency for the contracted organisations to narrow and specialise their programmes and activities. 'Odd' and unusual activities were abandoned so the organisations could focus on their contracted activities. Small voluntary organisations could not compete for contracts. The provider role increased efficiency but led to more bureaucracy. Contracted welfare provision presupposes specialisation and expertise, which, in turn, entails the need for employed professionals. The work can to a lesser extent build on volunteers and their involvement. Putnam (2000) found similar patterns in the US. Contracted relationships between the voluntary organisations and the public sector threaten the autonomy and particular distinctiveness of the voluntary sector, according to some research (Scott and Russell 2001). Studies in more recent years seem to confirm this trend internationally (Henriksen *et al.* 2012; Milbourne 2013). This would imply that what the voluntary organisations have to offer as contracted providers has increasingly come to resemble the services offered by the public sector or by for-profit providers. Milbourne (2013) wonders if is it possible at all to maintain autonomy, distinctive goals and values in welfare as a provider in a competitive welfare market. As for the Church, what would happen to its distinctive character that has so often been stressed in the Church discourse?

The question of whether the above-mentioned type of 'standardisation process' could become a problem if voluntary organisations become contracted providers, has to date hardly been studied in Sweden, according to Hammare (2013). Neither, he maintains, has systematic analysis been carried out, where welfare provision by voluntary organisations has been compared to the equivalent welfare provision by for-profit organisations or by the public sector. In his own study, focusing on the expertise and values in social work provision carried out by non-profit, for-profit and public provider organisations, Hammare found very small differences between the different types of organisations in terms of values, ideas and ideologies. These results hardly give support to the thesis of pluralism, nor do they point to value distinctiveness in voluntary organisations; in fact, they rather signal the contrary.

Conclusion

The Church of Sweden is at a crossroads, where important decisions must be made with an eye on the future. By tradition, it conducts extensive diaconal work, trusted by the Swedish public. Contrary to other religious bodies, as well as other voluntary organisations with social aims, the Church of Sweden is already highly professionalised in the welfare and care area. It is a modern service provider in various ways, with the capacity of a very large voluntary organisation. Viewed from this perspective, it might be argued that the Church of Sweden has a potential lead as a service provider compared to other voluntary organisations. For the Church, to take another step forward – into competing for contracts in the welfare market – would in one sense probably not be a very great change. However, what it could imply in terms of complications has been mentioned, i.e. narrowing of activities, specialisation and the mentioned risk of becoming too similar to public and for-profit providers. Some of these processes are probably inevitable. The dilemma of safeguarding the Church's own distinctive character and of providing welfare with a religious signature – actually the Church's main argument for its role in welfare provision – has to be addressed. Furthermore, it has been made clear by the Church centrally that contracted welfare provision would be the responsibility of each local parish. That such involvement could imply a loss of resources for everyday diaconal work and for 'odd' activities in the parish should not be overlooked.

The modern world has great need for organisations in civil society that can promote social integration, community and belonging, and where people can be involved. Here, the Church has a central, important mission, which in fact is rooted in a traditional theological tradition. In this area, the Church of Sweden actually has another privileged position: it has to do with its geographical 'lead' through its local parishes, which are, or could be, valuable spaces for local belonging, informal networks and the sort of care creation that is embedded in such a context. But involvement by the members in the Church of Sweden is decreasing and the Church is rather anonymous to many parishioners, who themselves are not known by the pastors and deacons. This undermines the possibility of providing the type of welfare and care that is motivated by a relational logic. It is hard to avoid suspecting that the present plans the Church is currently deliberating for a possible role as provider in the welfare market may be 'instead of' the kind of care and welfare that is formed through belonging and community, which the Church has difficulty creating. And, finally, if the Church takes on the role as contracted provider – what would happen to the religious part of it all, that which gives the Church its voice, its distinctive character and is, in fact, its raison d´être? So what should the Church of Sweden do? Should it work on developing its role as a welfare and care provider in civil society through increased community work and network creating within the parishes? Should it strengthen its religious voice and its distinctive, religious character? Or should the Church launch itself into the welfare market as one among many contracted welfare providers? Whatever road is taken, it will have consequences for the Church's future in Swedish society and for its role in welfare. Is it possible to have more than one welfare identity? It is probably possible but it remains a problematic issue for the Church of Sweden: there is perhaps the risk that the Church will end up not having any distinct identity at all.

Note

1 Parts of this chapter have been published in a longer version in Swedish: Jeppsson Grassman, E. (2014) 'Vilken väg? Svenska kyrkans omsorg i en tid av välfärdsförändringar', in A. Bäckström (ed) *Välfärdsinsatser på religiös grund: förväntningar och problem*, Skellefteå: Artos.

References

Engel, C. (2006) *Svenska kyrkans sociala arbete – för vem och varför? En religionssociologisk studie av ett diakonalt dilemma* [The Social Work in the Church of Sweden – for Whom and Why? a religion sociological study of a deaconry dilemma], Uppsala: Uppsala University.

Erlandsson, S., Storm, P., Stranz, A., Szebehely, M. and Trydegård, G-B. (2013) 'Marketising trends in Swedish eldercare: competition, choice and calls for stricter regulations', in G. Meagher and M. Szebehely (eds) *Marketisation in Nordic Eldercare: a research report on legislation, oversight, extent and consequences*, Stockholm: Stockholm University, Stockholm Studies in Social Work.

Halpern, D. (2005) *Social Capital*, Cambridge: Polity Press.

Hammare, U. (2013) *Mellan löften om särart och krav på evidens: en studies av kunskap och kunskapssyn i socialt inriktade ideella, privata och offentliga organisationer* [Between the Promise of Specificity and the Demand for Evidence: a study of knowledge and the approach to knowledge in socially oriented non-profit, private and public sector organizations], Stockholm: Stockholm University, Report 142 in Social Work.

Henriksen, L., Smith, S. and Zimmer, A. (2012) 'At the eve of convergence? Transformation of social service provision in Denmark, Germany and the United States', *Voluntas*, 23(2): 458–501.

Jegermalm, M. and Jeppsson Grassman, E. (2012) 'Helpful citizens and caring families: patterns of informal help and caregiving in Sweden in a 17-year perspective', *International Journal of Social Welfare*, 21(4): 422–32.

Jeppsson Grassman, E. (2001) *Socialt arbete i församlingens hägn* [Social Work in the Parish], Stockholm: Verbum.

Jeppsson Grassman, E. (2014) 'Vilken väg? Svenska kyrkans omsorg i en tid av välfärdsförändringar' [Which way? The Church of Sweden and its care at a time of welfare change], in A. Bäckström (ed) *Välfärdsinsatser på religiös grund: förväntningar och problem* [Welfare Achievements on Religious Grounds: expectations and problems], Skellefteå: Artos.

Jeppsson Grassman, E. and Svedberg, L. (2007) 'Civic participation in a Scandinavian welfare state: patterns in contemporary Sweden', in L. Trägårdh (ed) *State and Civil Society in Northern Europe: the Swedish model reconsidered*, New York: Berghahn Books.

Jeppsson Grassman, E. and Taghizadeh Larsson, A. (2013) 'Like coming home: the role of the Church of Sweden abroad for migrating senior Swedes', in A.L. Blaakilde and G. Nilsson (eds) *Nordic Seniors on the Move*, Lund: University of Lund, Lund Studies in Arts and Cultural Sciences 4.

Jeppsson Grassman, E. and Whitaker, A. (2009) 'Divergent logics of spiritual care: end of life and the role of the Church of Sweden', *Journal of Religion, Spirituality and Aging* 21(4): 344–60.

Johnson, N. (1992) 'The changing role of the voluntary sector in Britain from 1945 to the present day', in S. Kuhnle and P. Selle (eds) *Government and Voluntary Organisations*, Aldershot: Avebury.

Milbourne, L. (2013) *Voluntary Sector in Transition: hard times or new opportunities*, Bristol: Policy Press.

Nilsson, L. (2013) 'Välfärdspolitik och välfärdsopinionen 1986–2012: vinster i välfärden' ['Welfare Policies and Welfare Opinions 1986–2012: profits in welfare'], in L. Weibull, H. Oscarsson and A. Bergström (eds) *SOM-Undersökningen 2012* [The SOM-Study 2012], Gothenburg: University of Gothenburg, SOM-report 59.

Putnam, R. (2000) *Bowling Alone: the collapse and revival of American community*, New York: Simon & Schuster.

Sandberg, A. (2009) *Församlingen mot strömmen: befolkningsförändringar och verksamhetsutveckling på regional och lokal nivå inom Svenska kyrkan* [The Parish against the Stream: population changes and activity development at regional and local levels in the Church of Sweden], Uppsala: The Church of Sweden.

Scott, D. and Russell, L. (2001) 'Contracting: the experience of service delivery agencies', in M. Harris and C. Rochester (eds) *Voluntary Organisations and Social Policy in Britain: perspective on change and choice*, Basingstoke: Palgrave.

Sjödin, D. (2011) *Tryggare kan ingen vara: migration, religion och integration i en segregerad omgivning* [Nobody Can Be Safer: migration, religion and integration in a segregated environment], Lund: University of Lund, Lund Dissertations in Sociology, no. 98.

Swedish Government Official Report (1997) *Staten och trossamfunden* [The State and the Religious Communities], Stockholm: Fritzes, no. 55.

The Official Reports of the Church of Sweden (2013) *Att Färdas Väl: hur Svenska kyrkan kan navigera i välfärden* [To Fare Well: how the Church of Sweden can navigate in welfare], Uppsala: The Church of Sweden, no. 3.

Trägårdh, L. (ed) (2007) *State and Civil Society in Northern Europe: the Swedish model reconsidered*, New York and Oxford: Berghahn Books.

World Values Surveys (2011) *World Values Survey Wave 5 2005–2008*. Online. Available HTTP: www.worldvaluessurvey.org (accessed 28 October 2015).

Part V

Religion and spirituality across the lifespan

21

Spirituality

The missing component in trauma therapy across the lifespan

Heather Marie Boynton and Jo-Ann Vis

Introduction

Spirituality is a source of continual support, comfort and connectedness and a resource during difficult times for individuals of all ages. Trauma experienced in childhood or later in life, whether long term or short term, single incident or multiple events, has captured the attention of social workers and researchers for decades. Recently, the importance of spirituality in trauma, grief and loss has emerged. The ultimate goal for social workers and researchers is the desire to prevent or minimise posttraumatic effects that follow traumatic incidents (Raphael *et al.* 1996; van der Kolk *et al.* 1996).

Spirituality is one of the few phenomena that are integral across the lifespan, and it is related to physical and mental health, resilience, quality of life and overall wellbeing (Boynton 2011). Social workers will inevitably encounter individuals who are dealing with trauma and require spiritual support. While social workers are often trained in evidence-based trauma interventions and frameworks, spirituality is rarely discussed as part of these intervention frameworks.

Incorporating spirituality is a necessary approach to trauma treatment at all developmental stages of life. This incorporation has shown to promote improved outcomes and posttraumatic growth. It is imperative that social workers acquire a greater understanding of, and competence in, the area of trauma and spirituality. This chapter presents spirituality as integral to trauma in the salient areas of meaning making, coping and posttraumatic growth across the lifespan. It also discusses spirituality as a complement for common evidenced-based practices, such as Cognitive Behavioural Therapy [CBT] (Briere and Scott 2015), including Trauma Focused CBT (Cohen *et al.* 2012), Eye Movement Desensitisation and Reprocessing [EMDR] (Greyber *et al.* 2012) and Dialectical Behavioural Therapy [DBT] (Olenchek 2008).

Conceptualising trauma, grief and loss

There are a variety of traumas that can occur, including: the death of a significant other; abuse and violence; threats of injury or death to self or another; medical trauma; accidents; terrorism and war; natural and human-made disasters; and suicides. Traumatic events can be experienced directly or indirectly, and be linked to grief, loss, bereavement and mourning. These overlap with interrelated processes, creating complex responses, and making it difficult to distinguish between them (Cook *et al.* 2007). The terms are used interchangeably in the literature with overlap between the concepts, yet there are distinguishing definitions.

According to McCann and Pearlman (1990), a traumatic event is something that is sudden or beyond the norm, where an individual perceives an inability to meet the related demands of the trauma. The trauma may be physically or psychologically threatening, and affect one's sense of safety, security, survival or sense of self. A psychological trauma is described as a stress-related event involving intense feelings of distress, helplessness, anxiety, fear or disorientation, which challenge one's cognitive structures and perceptions regarding worldview, meanings and purpose in life (Vis and Boynton 2008).

Hooyman and Kramer (2006) convey that grief is a universal human response to the loss of an important person in one's life, or something of importance. It is a complex and individualised phenomenon encompassing a vast range of social and cultural responses and norms. They state that bereavement is the loss through death or separation, and that mourning is the social act or expression of grief. Complicated grief, also termed traumatic grief, can create intrusive, disturbing thoughts, images and memories that contribute to the pain, and to psychopathology. Given the complexity and interconnectedness of trauma, grief and loss, the word trauma will be used in this chapter with the understanding that grief and loss are incorporated.

Prevalence and symptoms of trauma

According to research, close to 70 per cent of individuals will experience one or more traumatic event(s) throughout their lifetime (Breslau *et al.* 1999; Calhoun and Tedeschi 1998; Saunders and Adams 2014). Significant problems can occur in the areas of affect, emotion regulation, behavioural responses, cognition, spirituality and dissociation. Janoff-Bulman (2006) professed that there is an experience of internal shock, with aspects of disintegration resulting from the psychological unpreparedness for the extremes of a new disrupted and altered reality. Various responses include confusion, preoccupation, rumination, dysphoria, pining, yearning and loneliness. Negative responses impinge on adaptation, disrupt daily functioning, restrain social activities and affect grieving responses.

Responses can differ in relation to development and individual context. Ogle *et al.* (2013) noted that in understanding the psychological impact of an event, it is vital to consider the developmental period in which it is experienced. Exposure to trauma in younger years may contribute to serious emotional and behavioural problems, and greater negative outcomes later in life (Goodman 2002; Ogle *et al.* 2013). Prior unresolved trauma influences stress reactions, and causes individuals to interpret future experiences as more traumatic and/or overwhelming. Difficulties in attachment, security, self-concept, self-esteem and spirituality can occur with developmental variances. Therefore, it is imperative to focus interventions on the mind, body and spirit across the developmental lifespan.

Spirituality: a missing component

Many of the models of trauma are pathology oriented, and previous frameworks are being challenged (Rothaupt and Becker 2007). The most researched models for various types of trauma treatment include CBT, DBT and EMDR, with CBT being the most researched therapy across the lifespan (Dinnen *et al.* 2015). All of these models incorporate skills and behaviours to manage distressing thoughts and impulses. Individuals are taught to utilise new skills in place of maladaptive responses induced by trauma. Cognitions that are deemed to be dysfunctional are identified and addressed.

Newer models of treatment are incorporating cultural and contextual factors; however, what is often missing in the theoretical conceptualisations, definitions and symptoms related to trauma exposure are spiritual aspects. Trauma is an existential injury that can wound the spirit (Thompson and Walsh 2010) and alter one's spiritual worldview and foundation of being. Trauma often creates a spiritual crisis or struggle, and affects one's sense of self and spiritual connections. A need for spiritual rumination, existential cogitation, spiritual meaning making, as well as spiritual rituals, ceremonies, practices and activities often emerge. Tapping into, accessing and nurturing one's authentic Self, spiritual passions, talents, skills and abilities contribute to overall wellbeing.

Spirituality is a multidimensional construct experienced by individuals in different ways, intersecting with religion and religiosity. It is shaped, formed and influenced through interactions with family, peers, community, sports, arts, cultural activities and the natural world. It is expressed through beliefs, narratives, rituals, activities and practices. Spiritual development is viewed to evolve like other developmental processes such as social, moral, emotional and cognitive aspects. Research has found that negative impacts from trauma occur in all of these developmental processes (Briere 2006; Ford 2002).

There are several definitions of spirituality in the social work literature that encompass the various dimensions and attributes, ranging from broad to succinct (Canda and Furman 1999; Crisp 2010; Sheridan 2004). Boynton (2016) described spirituality as a drive to find meaning in all life connections, purpose of life events, one's life's circumstances, existence in the universe and life purpose or destiny. It involves aspects of the mind including cognitions, beliefs, faith, hope, values, morals, identity formation, as well as the range of human emotions. Spirituality is associated with many virtues in life such as love, kindness, authenticity, integrity, fairness, compassion, honesty, loyalty and appreciation. It is experienced through the body via feelings and sensations, especially through the heart and core of the body.

Spirituality includes self-discovery, and an understanding of *Self* (the spiritual or divine aspect of oneself) (Burkhardt and Nagai-Jacobson 2002). Swinton (2001) characterises spirituality as a trifold experience. It is a quest for inner connectedness, which is intrapersonal, involving interpersonal social relationships reaching into the transcendent realms beyond self and others, making it transpersonal.

Spirituality is a domain of strength for individuals offering social, relational and psychological supports and resources (Koenig 2010; Rosmarin *et al.* 2011). It is an important factor in coping, resiliency, recovery and healing at all ages (Boynton 2016). It plays a critical role in how events are understood, experienced, managed and integrated into one's worldview (Pargament *et al.* 2006). It is also an important component in posttraumatic growth [PTG], where individuals are transformed by one's trauma experience. Individuals develop an awareness of personal strength while exploring and appreciating meaningful life possibilities, spiritual development and growth (Calhoun and Tedeschi 2006). Further positive post-trauma spiritual outcomes include a sense of closeness and nurturance in spiritual relationships, relaxation and peace from engaging in spiritual practices and rituals, as well as social support from congregations or spiritual groups.

Canda and Furman (2010) conceived spirituality to be at the heart of social work practice, empathy, compassion and care. Supporting this argument, social workers play an important role in assisting individuals to alleviate spiritual distress, struggles and crises. They are tasked with facilitating and supporting a positive spiritual outcome for clients. Therefore, spiritual competence to facilitate spiritual meaning making, nurture spiritual strengths and access the client's spiritual resources is required.

Bath (2008) outlined three pillars of trauma-informed treatment, which are feeling safe, self-regulation and connection in trusting relationships. The Child and Family Partnership (2010) also added agency and mastery, problem solving and executive functioning and meaning making including hope, faith and optimism. We propose that another necessary pillar of trauma treatment is spirituality.

Marrone (1999) identified four phases of trauma, consisting of cognitive restructuring, emotional expression, psychological reintegration and psycho-spiritual transformation. Spiritual transformation involves changes to central assumptions, attitudes and beliefs about death, life, compassion, love and a higher power. Spiritual relationships can be increased in number or strength; spiritual practices may evolve and increase; spiritual capacities may be heightened; and overall spiritual growth and development are possible.

Meaning making

Spirituality is a key component in the process of meaning making and interpreting one's life circumstances. The attributions one employs regarding the causes and reasons for a trauma often fall into the spiritual realm. Individuals are tasked with managing spiritual struggles and crises around meaning making. Trauma can create changes in a belief of a benevolent higher power, a loss of faith and struggles regarding sense of purpose, which can result in anger, distrust and a negative spiritual worldview. Meaning making involves the reconstruction of a spiritual worldview, and understandings in terms of spiritual relationships. Meaning is 'having a sense of direction, a sense of order, and a reason for existence, a clear sense of personal identity, and a greater social consciousness' (Reker 1997: 710).

The process of transcendent meaning making involves delving into deeper intuitive understandings regarding the event. It also comprises reflecting on ultimate values and belief systems, and on one's own existence in the world. Individuals who are able to construct positive spiritual or transcendent meanings experience less distress and fewer negative effects (Pargament *et al.* 2005).

In essence, meaning making is a natural evolutionary response following a traumatic experience that can damage or challenge confidence in one's spiritual worldview, sense of self and identity. This ever-evolving process incorporates a new reality or worldview. Meaning making is both a restorative and creative response to traumatic, life-altering experiences. The various interplays between physiological, physical, sensory, spiritual, social and behavioural factors significantly influence how one interprets or make sense of an event. Calhoun and Tedeschi (1999) argue that meaning connected to trauma includes two steps. One is to find meaning in the event and why it occurred, and the other involves retaining or creating a meaningful view of life despite the event. Meaning has a significant bearing on how individuals perceive the event in the present and future (LeDoux 1996; Schacter 1996; Schulz 1998; van der Kolk and Fisler 1995).

Coping and spirituality

Spirituality is an important aspect of coping in trauma as individuals rely on their spiritual beliefs, relationships, rituals, ceremonies, spiritual practices and activities. Many adults believe that spiritual aspects and concerns are not applicable for children, yet spiritual concerns, distress and struggles are quite salient for them. Many individuals find their spirituality is important to them, and assists in transcending adverse circumstances. Spiritual activities and engaging with a spiritual community can offer comfort and support. Individuals of all ages enjoy personal spiritual pursuits, such as writing, art, music, physical activity, various types of media, meditation, practicing mindfulness, focusing on the present or the positive and prayer. Spending time with pets and in nature, and/or collecting items from the natural world are other spiritual activities. It is evident that each person engages in practices that are suited to their own spiritual style. However, spiritual coping resources may be withheld or masked as spirituality is often deemed as socially weird and taboo (Boynton 2016).

Implications across the lifespan

Childhood

Children have robust spiritual lives and find spiritual coping practices, relationships and resources helpful in managing trauma (Boynton 2016). Youth with stronger spiritual resources and a sense of spirituality exhibit less delinquency, negative behaviours, emotional and psychological distress, school difficulties and psychopathology (Cheon and Canda 2010; Jackson *et al.* 2010; Mabe and Josephson 2004; Masten and Curtis 2000). Boynton (2016) revealed that traumatic events sparked and activated spiritual processes, behaviours and engagement in spiritual activities and in spiritual relationships for children. This was coupled with a catapulting of spiritual cogitations and a need for existential meaning making, resulting from spiritual rumination, questioning, reflection and analysis of the event, and on life itself. Children experiencing trauma are often viewed as growing up too fast, as they engage in mature spiritual reasoning. They are isolated as peers cannot relate, understand or even comprehend some of their spiritual cognitions experiences. This is even more of a concern when care givers are also impacted, or involved in their own traumatic meaning making struggles (Boynton 2016).

Many children believe in, seek out and communicate with an array of spiritual entities such as God, Creator, Mother Earth, Gaia, goddesses, guardian angels, spirit guides and animals (Boynton 2016). For the most part, children believe that spiritual entities are protective and caring, listen, watch over them and are ever present, guide them in their actions and communicate with them through the mind, heart and soul. Interestingly, Boynton (2016) found that children embrace and interact with spiritually symbolic objects, which provide children with a symbolic spiritual connection to a person or place, or a reminder of a spiritual relationship. Toys or personal objects representing nature or supportive relationships bring spiritual comfort, solace and reduce stress. During times of distress, children engage with these objects more frequently. Social workers can be cognisant of these aspects and nurture spiritual practices within traditional trauma interventions.

Adolescents

Cheon and Canda (2010: 123) stated that 'adolescence is a particularly intense period of ideological hunger, a striving for meaning and purpose, and a desire for relationships and connectedness'. Questioning, challenging and integrating alternate worldviews, societal structures, values and beliefs are part of adolescent identity development and belief formation. Engagement in complex thinking and global reasoning further develop during this phase of life.

Adolescents also employ a variety of spiritual coping practices that can easily complement trauma therapies. Jackson *et al.* (2010) found that adolescents felt that love and forgiveness helped them to heal. Spending time alone, or sharing problems with others, and listening to the advice and wisdom of elders were helpful. Engagement in these positive activities has been found to increase mental health and wellbeing, and life satisfaction for adolescents (Cotton *et al.*

2009; Jackson *et al.* 2010; Kelley and Miller 2007). Alternatively, adolescents engaging in negative spiritual coping or those that have impaired spiritual functioning experience higher levels of stress, depression, anxiety and PTSD symptoms (Bryant-Davis *et al.* 2012; Kim and Esquivel 2011; Van Dyke *et al.* 2009). These individuals tend to engage in substance use, sexual activity and delinquent behaviours, and have lower scores on psychological and existential wellbeing scales, poor academic performance and reduced self-esteem (Bryant-Davis *et al.* 2012; Cheon and Canda 2010; Kim and Esquivel 2011).

When trauma occurs, adolescents can encounter deep emotional pain that can result in them acting out, which Anglin (2003) describes as *pain behaviour*. Conversely, this behaviour may be a normal response to existential and spiritual injuries associated with soul or spiritual pain arising from disconnection or meaning making struggles. Attig (2004) describes soul pain as a loss of a sense of rootedness in normality, and spiritual pain as suffering due to a loss of sense of transcendence, and a loss of joy and hope. A critical task for adolescents in trauma is addressing the roots of their pain. Meaning making involved in self-identity and sense of self can be difficult during this stage, and it is even more confounded if a youth is separated from family and community through trauma (Carriere 2008). This would be a crucial spiritual component to augment evidence-based trauma interventions.

Adults

As individuals move into adulthood, greater complexity occurs in relation to meaning making, faith development and spirituality. McNamara Barry *et al.* (2010) discuss that the adult stage of development is one where an individual advances in terms of physical, cognitive and psychosocial development. These scholars believe that these advances support religious and spiritual exploration. During adulthood one may be more likely to manage post-trauma effects. Social workers ought to assess whether an individual is processing a single trauma event, or working through cumulative trauma experiences.

Ogle *et al.* (2014) elucidate that multiple traumatic events increase the likelihood of impact and severity of trauma. The issue regarding cumulative trauma is probably the most concerning for older adults. They may have experienced and managed trauma well in childhood or mid-life, but the decline in the later years in cognitive and physical functioning can create re-emerging trauma symptoms (Ogle *et al.* 2013; Petkus *et al.* 2009).

The biggest challenges for adults exposed to trauma are rumination and engaging in self-assessment and evaluation concerning one's full potential (Krause 2005). In Erikson's stage development (Erikson 1959), both younger and older adults focus on the important events of relationships, parenthood and work. Energy used to manage the trauma effects may impede success in other developmental tasks. Adults may become frustrated or feel a sense of disillusionment in their inability to meet these stage demands. Outcomes such as forming intimate and loving relationships, and nurturing others may become impossible tasks for some, as they are expelling their emotional energy on symptom management.

In his model of development, Erickson (1959) deemed that the last stage of maturity occurs at age 64 and older. In this stage, it is theorised that individuals reflect on life and evaluate whether one's life has brought fulfillment, and this is linked with meaning making. Older adults who can take meaning and weave the experience into their life review can create a reflective narrative that is more than loss and hopelessness, and is about growth and knowledge.

Within the last stage of development, seniors will both look back and have a sense of fulfilment, leading to wisdom, or a sense of despair, potentially leading to regret. Furthermore, a natural experience in aging is the increased likelihood of a loss of a loved one, as well as other transitional losses such as retirement, loss of family home and a sense of purpose (Ogle *et al.* 2013). Through positive meaning reflection, older adults can feel a sense of accomplishment, increased psychological benefits and physical improvements (Petkus *et al.* 2009). Krause (2005: 502) questions whether older adults 'will have greater difficulty finding a sense of meaning in life than older adults who have not encountered a traumatic event'. Trauma has the potential to create a negative view of one's life during self-reflection, and present 'undeniable evidence that things did not turn out as was hoped' (Krause 2005:504). The importance of positive spiritual meaning reflection is vital at this stage and should be a key element of trauma therapies.

Ogle *et al.* (2013) noted that adulthood may be the period in life stage development where one's experience of cognitive and social changes may be used to enhance psychological functioning following a traumatic incident. The authors postulated that emotion regulation skills improve in this stage, offering individuals new and adaptive skills to manage post-trauma exposure effects. Social supports were also seen as positive attributes to managing trauma effects, as well as relationship building and nurturing others. In this stage, resources in terms of developmental abilities and spiritual resources should be explored and utilised.

Summary

This chapter has argued the importance of incorporating spirituality within evidence-based trauma treatment across the lifespan. Spiritual meaning making and coping practices were presented as significant elements that should be part of evidence-based trauma therapies. It is believed that this would increase potential and capacity for post-traumatic growth. It is essential that social workers be trained and competent in the areas of stage development associated with trauma and spirituality across the lifespan in order to provide effective spiritually-sensitive trauma care.

References

Anglin, J. (2003) 'Staffed group homes for youth: toward a framework of understanding', in K. Kufeldt and B. McKenzie (eds) *Child Welfare: connecting research, policy and practice*, Waterloo: Wilfred Laurier University Press.

Attig, T. (2004) 'Disenfranchised grief revisited: discounting hope and love', *Omega*, 49(3): 197–215.

Bath, H. (2008) 'The three pillars of trauma-informed care', *Reclaiming Children and Youth*, 17(3): 17–21.

Boynton, H.M. (2011) 'Children's spirituality: epistemology and theory from various helping professions', *International Journal of Children's Spirituality*, 16(2): 109–27.

Boynton, H.M. (2016) 'Navigating in seclusion: the complicated terrain of children's spirituality', Unpublished doctoral dissertation, University of Calgary, Canada.

Breslau, N., Chilcoat, H.D., Kessler, R.C. and Davis, G.C. (1999) 'Previous exposure to trauma and PTSD effects of subsequent trauma: results from the Detroit area survey of trauma', *American Journal of Psychiatry*, 156(6): 902–7.

Briere, J. (2006) 'Dissociative symptoms and trauma exposure: specificity, affect dysregulation, and post-traumatic stress', *Journal of Nervous and Mental Disease*, 194(2): 78–82.

Briere, J.N. and Scott, C. (2015) *Principles of Trauma Therapy: a guide to symptoms, evaluation, and treatment (DSM-5 Update)*, Thousand Oaks, CA: Sage Publications.

Bryant-Davis, T., Ellis, M.U., Burke-Maynard, E., Moon, N., Counts, P.A. and Anderson, G. (2012) 'Religiosity, spirituality, and trauma recovery in the lives of children and adolescents', *Professional Psychology Research and Practice*, 43(4): 306–14.

Burkhardt, M.A. and Nagai-Jacobson, M.G. (2002) *Spirituality: living our connectedness*, Albany, NY: Delmar, Thomson Learning.

Calhoun, L. and Tedeschi, R.G. (1998) 'Beyond recovery from trauma: implications for clinical practice and research', *Journal of Social Issues*, 54(2): 357–71.

Calhoun, L.G. and Tedeschi, R.G. (1999) *Facilitating Posttraumatic Growth: a clinician's guide*, Mahwah, NJ: Lawrence Erlbaum Associates.

Calhoun, L.G. and Tedeschi, R.G. (2006) *Handbook of Posttraumatic Growth: research and practice*, Mahwah, NJ: Lawrence Erlbaum Associates.

Canda, E.R. and Furman, L.D. (1999) *Spiritual Diversity in Social Work Practice: the heart of helping*, New York: The Free Press.

Canda, E.R. and Furman, L.D. (2010) *Spiritual Diversity in Social Work Practice: the heart of helping,* 2nd edn, New York: The Free Press.

Carriere, J. (2008) 'Maintaining identities: the soul work of adoption and aboriginal children', *Pimatisiwin: a journal of Aboriginal and Indigenous community health*, 6(1): 61–79.

Cheon, J.W. and Canda, E.R. (2010) 'The meaning and engagement of spirituality for positive youth development in social work', *Families in Society*, 91(2): 121–6.

Cohen, J.A., Mannarino, A.P., Kliethermes, M. and Murray, L.A. (2012) 'Trauma-focused CBT for youth with complex trauma', *Child Abuse and Neglect*, 36(6): 528–41.

Cook, A., Spinazzola, J., Ford, J., Lanktree, C., Blaustein, M., Sprague, C., Cloitre, M., DeRosa, R., Hubbard, R., Kagan, R., Liautaud, J., Mallah, K., Olafson, E. and van der Kolk, B. (2007) 'Complex trauma in children and adolescents', *Focal Point,* 21(1): 4–8. Online. Available HTTP: www.pathway-srtc.pdx.edu/pdf/fpW0702.pdf (accessed 7 February 2016).

Cotton, S., Kudel, I., Roberts, Y.H., Pallerla, H., Tsevat, J., Succop, P. and Yi, M.S. (2009) 'Spiritual wellbeing and mental health outcomes in adolescents with or without inflammatory bowel disease', *Journal of Adolescent Health*, 44(5): 485–92.

Crisp, B.R. (2010) *Spirituality and Social Work*, Farnham: Ashgate.

Dinnen, S., Simiola, V. and Cook, J.M. (2015) 'Post-traumatic stress disorder in older adults: a systematic review of the psychotherapy treatment literature', *Aging and Mental Health*, 18(2): 144–50.

Erikson, E. (1959) *Identity and the Life Cycle*, New York: International University Press.

Ford, J.D. (2002) 'Traumatic victimization in childhood and persistent problems with oppositional-defiance', *Journal of Aggression, Maltreatment and Trauma*, 6(1): 25–58.

Goodman, R.F. (2002) *Caring for Kids After Trauma and Death: a guide for parents and professionals*, New York: The Institute for Trauma and Stress, NYU Child Study Center. Online. Available HTTP: www.nctsn.org/nctsn_assets/pdfs/Crisis%20Guide%20-%20NYU.pdf (accessed 7 February 2016).

Greyber, L.R., Dulmus, C.N. and Cristalli, M.E. (2012) 'Eye movement desensitization reprocessing, posttraumatic stress disorder, and trauma: a review of randomized controlled trials with children and adolescents', *Child Adolescent Social Work Journal*, 29(5): 409–25.

Hooyman, N.R. and Kramer, B.J. (2006) *Living through Loss: interventions across the life span*, New York: Columbia University Press.

Jackson, L.J., White, C.R., O'Brien, K., DiLorenzo, P., Cathcart, E., Wolf, M., Bruskas, D., Percora, P.J., Nix-Early, V. and Cabrera, J. (2010) 'Exploring spirituality among youth in foster care: findings from the Casey field office mental health study', *Child and Family Social Work*, 15(1): 107–17.

Janoff-Bulman, R. (2006) 'Schema-change perspectives on posttraumatic growth', in L.G. Calhoun and R.G. Tedeschi (eds) *Handbook of Posttraumatic Growth: research and practice*, Mahwah, NJ: Lawrence Erlbaum Associates.

Kelley, B.S. and Miller, L. (2007) 'Life satisfaction and spirituality in adolescents', *Research in the Social Scientific Study of Religion*, 18: 233–61.

Kim, S. and Esquivel, G.B. (2011) 'Adolescent spirituality and resilience: theory, research, and educational practices', *Psychology in the Schools*, 48(7): 755–63.

Koenig, H. G. (2010) 'Spirituality and mental health', *International Journal of Applied Psychoanalytic Studies*, 7(2): 116–22.

Krause, N. (2005) 'Traumatic events and meaning in life: exploring variations in three age cohorts', *Ageing and Society*, 25(4): 501–24.

LeDoux, J.E. (1996) *The Emotional Brain*, New York: Touchstone.

Mabe, P.A. and Josephson, A.M. (2004) 'Child and adolescent psychopathology: spiritual and religious perspectives', *Child and Adolescent Psychiatric Clinics of North America*, 13(1): 111–25.

Marrone, R. (1999) 'Dying, mourning, and spirituality: a psychological perspective', *Death Studies*, 23(6): 495–519.

Masten, A.S. and Curtis, J.W. (2000) 'Integrating competence and psychopathology: pathways toward a comprehensive science of adaptation in development', *Development and Psychopathology*, 12(3): 529–50.

McCann, L. and Pearlman, L. (1990) *Psychological Trauma and the Adult Survivor*, New York: Brunner/ Hazel.

McNamara Barry, C., Nelson, L., Davarya, S. and Urry, S. (2010) 'Religiosity and spirituality during the transition to adulthood', *International Journal of Behavioral Development*, 34(4): 311–24.

Ogle, C.M., Rubin, D.C. and Siegler, I.C. (2013) 'The impact of the developmental timing of trauma exposure on PTSD symptoms and psychosocial functioning among older adults', *Developmental Psychology*, 49(11): 2191–200.

Ogle, C.M., Rubin, D.C. and Siegler, I.C. (2014) 'Cumulative exposure to traumatic events in older adults', *Aging and Mental Health*, 18(3): 316–25.

Olenchek, C. (2008) 'Dialectical behavior therapy: treating borderline personality disorder', *Social Work Today*, 8(6): 22.

Pargament, K.I., Desai, K.M. and McConnell, K.M. (2006) 'Spirituality: a pathway to posttraumatic growth or decline?', in L.G. Calhoun and R.G. Tedeschi (eds) *Handbook of Posttraumatic Growth: research and practice*, Mahwah, NJ: Lawrence Erlbaum Associates.

Pargament, K.I., Magyar, G.M., Benore, E. and Mahoney, A. (2005) 'Sacrilege: a study of sacred loss and desecration and their implications for health and wellbeing in a community sample', *Journal for the Scientific Study of Religion*, 44(1): 59–78.

Petkus, A.J., Gum, A.M., King-Kallimanis, B. and Wetherell, J.L. (2009) 'Trauma history is associated with psychological distress and somatic symptoms in homebound older adults', *The American Journal of Geriatric Psychiatry*, 17(9): 810–18.

Raphael, B., Wilson, J., Meldrum, L. and McFarlane, A. (1996) 'Acute preventive interventions', in B. van der Kolk, A. McFarlane and L. Weisaeth (eds) *Traumatic Stress: the effects of overwhelming experience on mind, body, and society*, New York: Guilford Press.

Reker, G.T. (1997) 'Personal meaning, optimism, and choice: existential predictors of depression in community and institutional elderly', *The Gerontologist*, 37(6): 709–16.

Rosmarin, D.H., Wacholtz, A. and Ai, A. (2011) 'Beyond descriptive research: advancing the study of spirituality and health', *Journal of Behavioral Medicine*, 34(6): 409–13.

Rothaupt, J.W. and Becker, K. (2007) 'A literature review of western bereavement theory: from decathecting to continuing bonds', *The Family Journal: counseling and therapy for couples and families*, 15(1): 6–15.

Saunders, B.E. and Adams, Z.W. (2014) 'Epidemiology of traumatic experiences in childhood', *Child and Adolescent Psychiatric Clinics of North America*, 23(2): 167–84.

Schacter, D.L. (1996) *Searching for Memory: the brain, the mind and the past*, New York: BasicBooks.

Schulz, M.L. (1998) *Awakening Intuition*, New York: Three Rivers Press.

Sheridan, M.J. (2004) 'Predicting the use of spiritually-derived interventions in social work practice: a survey of practitioners', *Journal of Religion and Spirituality in Social Work*, 23(4): 5–25.

Swinton, J. (2001) *Spirituality and Mental Health Care: rediscovering a 'forgotten' dimension*, London: Jessica Kingsley Publishers.

The Child and Family Partnership (2010) *Resilience: successful navigation through significant threat*. Online. Available HTTP: www.reachinginreachingout.com/documents/MCYSResilienceReport11-16-10Dissemination.pdf (accessed 7 February 2016).

Thompson, N. and Walsh, M. (2010) 'The existential basis of trauma', *Journal of Social Work Practice*, 24(4): 377–89.

van der Kolk, B. and Fisler, R. (1995) 'Dissociation and the fragmentary nature of traumatic memories: overview and exploratory study', *Journal of Traumatic Stress*, 8(4): 505–25.

van der Kolk, B., McFarlane, A. and Weisaeth, L. (1996) 'Preface', in B. van der Kolk, A. McFarlane and L. Weisaeth (eds) *Traumatic Stress: the effects of overwhelming experience on mind, body, and society*, New York: Guilford Press.

Van Dyke, C., Glenwick, D., Cecero, J. and Kim, S. (2009) 'The relationship of religious coping and spirituality to adjustment and psychological distress in urban early adolescents', *Mental Health, Religion, and Culture*, 12(4): 369–83.

Vis, J. and Boynton, H.M. (2008) 'Spirituality and transcendent meaning making: possibilities for enhancing posttraumatic growth', *Journal of Religion and Spirituality in Social Work*, 27(1–2): 69–86.

22

Spirituality as a protective factor for children and adolescents

Linda Benavides

Introduction

The last 30 years have seen a shift in the social work profession from a dissociation of the religious/spiritual to an embracement of spirituality as an important human condition (Sheridan 2009; Weick *et al.* 1989). More recently, attention has turned to the spiritual lives of children and adolescents. Spiritual development from childhood to adolescence has been explored by several authors (Boyatzis *et al.* 2006; Coles 1990; Hart 2006; Hay 1994; Hay and Nye 2006; Hay *et al.* 2006; Rew *et al.* 2007; Schwartz *et al.* 2006; Smith and Denton 2005). Spirituality has been identified as a source of resiliency for at-risk children and adolescents (Crawford *et al.* 2006); as a source of decline in risk behaviours, such as substance use/abuse and early sexual experimentation (Blakeney and Blakeney 2006; Hodge *et al.* 2001; Rostosky *et al.* 2004), and as a factor in positive adolescent development (Benson *et al.* 2005; King and Benson 2006). The purpose of this chapter is to explore how spirituality can act as a protective factor for children and adolescents and consider the implications of this for social work practice.

Spirituality has been defined by Canda and Furman (2010: 5) as a 'universal and fundamental human quality involving the search for a sense of meaning, purpose, morality, wellbeing, and profundity in relationships with ourselves, others, and ultimate reality, however understood'. Hence, in this chapter, spirituality is understood as a search for meaning and purpose, for interconnectedness and transcendence, which can occur within and outside of religious practices (Canda and Furman 2010), as a source of strength (Benson *et al.* 2005; King and Benson 2006) and 'as an aspect of lived experience' (Crisp 2008: 367).

Spiritual lives of children and adolescents

The spiritual lives of children and adolescents have historically been neglected in the research literature. This is in part the result of the long-held belief that children and younger adolescents do not have the ability for abstract thought needed to contemplate spiritual issues. According to Hart (2006: 164), 'there is a prevalent presupposition that genuine spirituality requires adult abstract thinking and language ability', that reduces 'childhood spirituality into nothing more than a form of immaturity or inadequacy' (Hay and Nye 2006: 57). As a result, earlier explorations and understandings of spirituality in children and adolescents were tied with religious beliefs and practices.

Research with children over the last three decades has pointed to the innate nature of spirituality. In his book *The Spiritual Life of Children*, Robert Coles (1990) presents his findings from extensive interviews with over 500 children and adolescents from different countries and of various religions and nonreligious backgrounds. Coles, who met with over 100 of these children at least 25 times over the course of a few years, found that what he had originally thought were expressions of religiosity, upon further reflection were expressions of participants' spirituality. Coles (1990: 37) concluded that 'Where do we come from? What are we? Where are we going? are the eternal questions children ask more intensely, unremittingly, and subtly than we sometimes imagine'.

Similarly, other researchers (Hay and Nye 2006) have explored spirituality from a biological and evolutionary viewpoint, which 'asserts the existence of an embodied spiritual awareness or "relational consciousness" that is antecedent to both religious and ethical beliefs' (Hay *et al.* 2006: 51). Spirituality is understood as a trait that has survived in humans for its usefulness to human growth and development. If spirituality was not essential it would not have survived within the species (Hay 1998).

Consequently, there is growing support for the idea that spirituality is an innate process whereby individuals are born spiritual, and this spiritual self is either supported or stifled through the individual's environment, including family and friends (Boyatzis *et al.* 2006; Rew *et al.* 2007; Schwartz *et al.* 2006). King has claimed:

> This potential or capacity for spirituality is present in every human being, but it needs to be activated and realised. Its awakening and development during childhood is of great importance, but it requires that parents and teachers will recognize this hidden potential.
>
> (King 2013: 6)

Similarly, Hay asserts that children and adolescents need guidance from family and friends to 'become "aware of their awareness" and to reflect on this experience in the light of the culture within which it emerges' (1998: 13). It is important to note that for many, this spiritual growth occurs within traditional religious contexts. As such, an appreciation of the innateness of spirituality that thrives within different cultures, within or outside of religious contexts, is important.

The conceptual and empirical research into the spiritual life of children and adolescents has opened the door to the exploration of spirituality as a protective factor for this population. The literature on resiliency and protective factors will be reviewed before exploring spirituality as a protective factor for children and adolescents.

Protective factors

Research on resiliency and protective factors began in the 1970s with the work of Werner and Smith (1977). Through their longitudinal study with a group of children born in the 1950s in Hawaii, Werner and Smith brought attention to the fact that despite adverse circumstances (poverty, homelessness, exposure to violence, etc.) many individuals are able to overcome challenges and have positive developmental trajectories. Resilience is understood as 'a variable quality that derives from a process of repeated interactions between a person and favourable features of the surrounding context in a person's life' (Gilligan 2004: 94). These favourable strengths are known in the research literature as protective factors (Howard *et al.* 1999). Protective factors are defined as those strengths, internal and external, which enable individuals to successfully adapt to stressful life events (Alvord and Grados 2005; Howard *et al.* 1999). Protective factors are 'hypothesized to interact with sources of risk such that they reduce the probability of negative outcomes under conditions of high risk' (Compas *et al.* 1995: 273). As such, protective factors can be seen as the 'building blocks' (Minnard 2002: 235) of resilience. Protective factors have been identified as both internal and external strengths of children and adolescents. Internal protective factors identified in the literature include hope, internal locus of control, self-esteem, self-regulation, intelligence and positive interpersonal relationships (Carbonell *et al.* 2002; Kliewer *et al.* 2004; Luthar 1991). Three primary systems in a child's life (family, school and community) have been identified as categories of external protective factors (Howard *et al.* 1999). Recently, spirituality as an internal protective factor has begun to receive attention in the literature.

Spirituality as protective factor for children and adolescents

Spirituality has been identified as a source of strength for children and adolescents exposed to stressful life events, such as homelessness (Bender *et al.* 2007; Williams 2004), exposure to domestic violence – including intimate partner violence and child abuse (Benavides 2012), and community violence – including wars and armed conflicts (Betancourt and Khan 2008; Bryant-Davis and Wong 2013). In his qualitative study on homeless youth, Kidd (2003: 250) found that for these participants, 'when they were feeling very down, this sense of spirituality gave some meaning to their suffering, and that there was a "reason" why they had survived up to that point'.

Spirituality has also been found to moderate the development of mental health problems (Cotton *et al.* 2005; Davis *et al.* 2003). In their study on the impact of spirituality on depression, Cotton *et al.* (2005: 529e12) found that adolescents with 'higher levels of spiritual wellbeing, in particular existential wellbeing, had fewer depressive symptoms and fewer risk-taking behavior'. Spirituality has also been identified as a protective factor for substance use/abuse (Hodge *et al.* 2001; Knight *et al.* 2007; Ritt-Olson *et al.* 2004; Sussman *et al.* 2006), early sexual behaviours (Rostosky *et al.* 2004) and as a strong predictor of happiness in children (Holder *et al.* 2010). Hodge *et al.* (2001: 159) elaborate, stating 'because spirituality may enhance self-esteem and perceptions of personal efficacy, youths may develop the internal resources to be able to make choices that are consistent with their own values and beliefs'.

These studies indicate that spirituality is a fundamental form of resilience that enhances positive development and can protect children and adolescents from the development of at-risk behaviours. Spirituality, however, is not experienced and expressed the same by all. In the following section, we will explore diverse ways in which children and adolescents express their spirituality and how those expressions serve as a protective mechanism.

Children and adolescents of distinct cultures and/or faiths express their spirituality in diverse ways. For some, spirituality is tied to traditional religious experiences, while for others expressions of spirituality are non-traditional, such as art and music. For some it is both. Through the act of participating in religious activities and/or creative pursuits, these expressions of spirituality protect the child or adolescent from the development of adverse developmental outcomes.

Traditional religious expressions

For children and adolescents who express their spirituality through traditional religious expressions, attending services, participating in youth activities, praying/meditating and/or celebrating religious holidays can provide the means by which they are able to continue to grow and express their spiritual selves. It is through this process by which spirituality serves as a protective factor. For example, in a study of young African members of a Pentecostal church in South Africa, the researchers found that for the participants, involvement in 'praise and worship activities allowed them to "cope and escape" while the music participation was linked with upliftment, transformation, and feelings of wellbeing' (Tshabalala and Patel 2010: 80). Similarly, in their study of Muslim adolescents in India, Annalakshmi and Abeer (2011) found that those adolescents with a religious personality were more likely to be resilient.

For many children and adolescents, religious rituals celebrating milestones or transitions serve as protective factors. In the Latino Catholic community, Quinceneras are an important part of a young Catholic female's life. Quinceneras, which celebrate a female's fifteenth birthday, marks the transition from a young girl to a young woman accepting responsibility for her faith in God and the responsibilities that this entails. As part of the religious ceremony, Quinceneras renew their baptismal promises and recite a special prayer to the Virgen de Guadalupe asking for guidance in following the footsteps of Jesus and being faithful to her baptismal promises (Cantu 2002). Similarly, in the Jewish tradition, adolescent males and females celebrate coming of age rituals. At the age of 13, males celebrate their Bar Mitzvah in which they are considered as having the same rights and responsibilities as grown men. Jewish females celebrate their Bat Mitzvah at the age of 12, which signifies the transition from a young girl to a woman with the responsibility to carry forth her own faith and traditions (Patai and Bar-Itzhak 2013). For these adolescents, their sense of responsibility towards their faith and the promises made during the Quincenera and Bar/Bat Mitzvah celebrations, serve to deter risk behaviours and serve as a protective mechanism. This could be, as expressed by Bhagwan (2009: 229), because 'rituals awaken the mysterious and stir up emotions of wonder, reverence, awe, and openness to new possibilities'.

Rituals are also important protective factors in other cultures. In their study of Muslim adolescents, Annalakshmi and Abeer (2011) found that Islamic rituals served as a source of strength for the participants. The authors elaborated, stating:

> the highly resilient were higher on Islamic rituals (religious practice and ritual behaviour indicative of the manifestation of one's religious worldview) and on Mu'amalat (religiously guided behaviours towards one's family, fellow human beings and the rest of creation including animals and the natural environment).
>
> (Annalakshmi and Abeer 2011: 731)

For Native American and First Nation children and adolescents, participation in tribal ceremonies such as sweat lodges, pow wows and talking circles, serve as traditional healing practices (Portman and Garrett 2006) and leads to a sense of 'belonging and communal meaningfulness' (Garrett et al. 2014: 485).

Non-traditional expressions

Children and adolescents express their spirituality in diverse ways, both within and outside of traditional religious practices. For some children and adolescents, creative expressions, such as writing, drawing, playing musical instruments, etc. are a means by which they connect to their spiritual selves.

For many children and adolescents, music – either through the act of playing a musical instrument or through the process of listening to music – helps transcend the individual to a space where they are able to process and make sense of their world. This may be, as expressed by Gellel (2013: 217–8), a result of spirituality being 'tied with the search for meaning and for the self, as well as with the aesthetic and with emotions and concepts that are difficult to express in words'.

Similarly, writing (e.g. journaling, storytelling, etc.) and art are powerful tools that provide opportunities for children and adolescents to connect to their spiritual selves. It also provides 'the means and opportunity by which they can rediscover a positive self-image in order to struggle against the development of a self-destructive and negative sense of self' (Kollontai 2010: 269–70).

Spirituality can also be expressed through other means, such as playing sports (Smith and Denton 2005) and dancing (Broadbent 2004). As expressed by Snowber (2007: 1453), 'dance is the garden where we can let our soul take both roots and wings, connecting to ourselves, others, and most importantly, to that which is mystery'.

Implications and conclusion

Social work practitioners who work with children and adolescents should be encouraged by the literature supporting spirituality as a protective factor. Practitioners should strive to provide opportunities for children and adolescents to explore their spirituality from the beginning of their work together. It is important, however, that social work practitioners do not bias their work with children and adolescents with their own spiritual beliefs and/or practices. In particular, the idea that children and younger adolescents are not spiritual should be avoided. Practitioners must continuously engage in a process of self-assessment to prevent bias from entering their work with children and adolescents.

As spirituality is experienced and understood in diverse ways, practitioners would do well to consider conducting spiritual assessments to best meet the spiritual needs of the children and adolescents they work with. David Hodge's (2015) book, *Spiritual Assessment in Social Work and Mental Health Practice*, might be useful towards this aim. It is also important for practitioners to realise that for some children and adolescents their spirituality may be experienced through both traditional and non-traditional expressions.

Social work practitioners can, through their knowledge of the spiritual lives of children and adolescents, provide a safe space for children and adolescents to express, process and practice their spirituality. Social work practitioners can incorporate interventions such as music therapy, sacred play, sand–tray therapy, art therapy, writing and poetry therapy, and dance therapy, to name a few interventions in their work with children and adolescents (Bhagwan 2009; Derezotes 2006; Land 2015). These interventions can also be incorporated into group work with children and adolescents. Through interventions such as these, practitioners can create a space for spiritual expressions and growth. Derezotes (2006: 155) addresses the importance of a safe space for interventions, such as sacred play, to be successful, stating, 'sacred play both requires and creates more spiritual freedom. When a child is allowed to freely follow his or her own natural interests, play can be an expression of soul and Creative Spirit'.

As such, it is imperative that social workers advocate for the inclusion of creative expressions in schools, especially in lower socioeconomic school districts where the arts are typically the first programmes cut. Social work practitioners can advocate for the development of programmes within existing social service agencies that foster creative expressions. Social workers can also provide needed resources, such as art supplies, for their clients to use at home.

For children and adolescents whose spirituality is experienced through religious expressions, social workers can incorporate into their interventions elements of the faith community their clients identify with. For example, Bhagwan (2009) suggests the use of spiritual stories found in different faiths and/or cultures as a way to engage the client in dialogue about their spirituality and how their spirituality can be a source of strength. Similarly, Land (2015) suggests that expressive therapies, such as music therapy and sand-tray therapy, can be modified to include important religious practices and beliefs that clients can relate to. In addition, practitioners can assist their clients with connecting to the faith communities they belong to. Sometimes it is as simple as setting up transportation to church, synagogue, temple, parish, mosque, etc.

In order to be competent, ethical social workers, it is important that practitioners make an effort to meet the spiritual needs of the children and adolescents they work with. Unfortunately, spirituality is not taught consistently in social work programmes nor is it addressed in practice consistently (Oxhandler *et al.* 2015; Sheridan 2009). It is imperative that as social workers we work to change this.

In conclusion, spirituality is a strength inherent in children and adolescents that can moderate the effects of negative life experiences and contributes to overall positive development. The current chapter provided an understanding of spirituality as a protective factor and addressed the process by which spirituality serves as a protective mechanism. Implications and recommendations for social work practice were addressed.

References

Alvord, M.K. and Grados, J.J. (2005) 'Enhancing resilience in children: a proactive approach', *Professional Psychology: Research and Practice*, 36(3): 238–45.

Annalakshmi, N. and Abeer, M. (2011) 'Islamic worldview, religious personality and resilience among Muslim adolescent students in India', *Europe's Journal of Psychology*, 7(4): 716–38.

Benavides, L.E. (2012) 'A phenomenological study of spirituality as a protective factor for adolescents exposed to domestic violence', *Journal of Social Service Research*, 38(2): 165–74.

Bender, K., Thompson, S.J., McManus, H., Lantry, J. and Flynn, P.M. (2007) 'Capacity for survival: exploring strengths of homeless street youth', *Child and Youth Care Forum*, 36(1): 25–42.

Benson, P.L., Scales, P., Sesma, A. and Roehlkepartain, E.C. (2005) 'Adolescent spirituality', in K. Moore and L. Lippman (eds) *What Do Children Need to Flourish? Conceptualizing and measuring indicators of positive development*, New York: Kluwer Academic/Plenum.

Betancourt, T.S. and Khan, K.T. (2008) 'The mental health of children affected by armed conflict: protective processes and pathways to resilience', *International Review of Psychiatry*, 20(3): 317–28.

Bhagwan, R. (2009) 'Creating sacred experiences for children as pathways to healing, growth, and transformation', *International Journal of Children's Spirituality*, 14(3): 225–34.

Blakeney, R.F and Blakeney, C.D. (2006) 'Delinquency: a quest for moral and spiritual integrity?', in E.C. Roehlkepartain, P.E. King, L. Wagener and P.L. Benson (eds) *The Handbook of Spiritual Development in Childhood and Adolescence*, Thousand Oaks: Sage Publications.

Boyatzis, C.J., Dollahite, D.C. and Marks, L.D. (2006) 'The family as a context for religious and spiritual development in children and youth', in E.C. Roehlkepartain, P.E. King, L. Wagener and P.L. Benson (eds) *The Handbook of Spiritual Development in Childhood and Adolescence*, Thousand Oaks: Sage Publications.

Broadbent, J. (2004) 'Embodying the abstract: enhancing children's spirituality through creative dance', *International Journal of Children's Spirituality*, 9(1): 97–104.

Bryant-Davis, T. and Wong, E.C. (2013) 'Faith to move mountains: religious coping, spirituality, interpersonal trauma recovery', *American Psychologist*, 68(8): 675–84.

Canda, E.R. and Furman, L.D. (2010) *Spiritual Diversity in Social Work Practice: the heart of helping*, 2nd edn, New York: Oxford University Press.

Cantu, N.E. (2002) 'Chicana life-cycle rituals', in N.E. Cantu and O. Najera-Ramirez (eds) *Chicana Traditions: continuity and change*, Urbana & Chicago: University of Illinois Press.

Carbonell, D.M., Reinherz, H.Z., Giaconia, R.M., Stashwick, C.K., Paradis, A.D. and Beardslee, W.R. (2002) 'Adolescent protective factors promoting resilience in young adults at risk for depression', *Child and Adolescent Social Work Journal*, 19(5): 393–412.

Coles, R. (1990) *The Spiritual Life of Children*, Boston: Houghton Mifflin.

Compas, B.E., Hinden, B.R. and Gerhardt, C.A. (1995) 'Adolescent development: pathways and processes of risk and resilience', *Annual Review of Psychology*, 46: 265–93.

Cotton, S., Larkin, E., Hoopes, A., Cromer, B.A., and Rosenthal, S.L. (2005) 'The impact of adolescent spirituality on depressive symptoms and health risk behaviors', *Journal of Adolescent Health*, 36(6): 529e7–14.

Crawford, E., Wright, M.O. and Masten, A.S. (2006) 'Resilience and spirituality in youth', in E.C. Roehlkepartain, P.E. King, L. Wagener and P.L. Benson (eds) *The Handbook of Spiritual Development in Childhood and Adolescence*, Thousand Oaks: Sage Publications.

Crisp, B.R. (2008) 'Social work and spirituality in a secular society', *Journal of Social Work*, 8(4): 363–75.

Davis, T.L., Kerr, B.A. and Kurpius, S.E. (2003) 'Meaning, purpose, and religiosity in at-risk youth: the relationship between anxiety and spirituality', *Journal of Psychology and Theology*, 31(4): 356–65.

Derezotes, D.S. (2006) *Spiritually Oriented Social Work Practice*, Boston: Pearson Education, Inc.

Garrett, M.T., Parrish, M., Williams, C., Grayshield, L., Portman, T.A.A., Rivera, E.T. and Maynard, E. (2014) 'Fostering resilience among Native American youth through therapeutic intervention', *Journal of Youth Adolescence*, 43(3): 470–90.

Gellel, A.M. (2013) 'Traces of spirituality in the Lady Gaga phenomenon', *International Journal of Children's Spirituality*, 18(2): 214–26.

Gilligan, R. (2004) 'Promoting resilience in child and family social work: issues for social work practice, education, and policy', *Social Work Education*, 23(1): 93–104.

Hart, T. (2006) 'Spiritual experiences and capacities of children and youth', in E.C. Roehlkepartain, P.E. King, L. Wagener and P.L. Benson (eds) *The Handbook of Spiritual Development in Childhood and Adolescence*, Thousand Oaks: Sage Publications.

Hay, D. (1994) 'The biology of God: what is the current status of Hardy's hypotheses?' *The International Journal for the Psychology of Religion*, 4(1): 1–23.

Hay, D. (1998) 'Why should we care about children's spirituality?', *Pastoral Care in Education*, 16(1): 11–16.

Hay, D. and Nye, R. (2006) *The Spirit of the Child*, revised edn, London: Jessica Kingsley Publishers.

Hay, D., Reich, K.H. and Utsch, M. (2006) 'Spiritual development: intersections and divergence with religious development', in E.C. Roehlkepartain, P.E. King, L. Wagener and P.L. Benson (eds) *The Handbook of Spiritual Development in Childhood and Adolescence*, Thousand Oaks: Sage Publications.

Hodge, D.R., Cardenas, P. and Montoya, H. (2001) 'Substance use: spirituality and religious participation as protective factors among rural youths', *Social Work Research*, 25(3): 153–61.

Hodge, D.R. (2015) *Spiritual Assessment in Social Work and Mental Health Practice*, New York: Columbia University Press.

Holder, M.D., Coleman, B. and Wallace, J.M. (2010) 'Spirituality, religiousness, and happiness in children aged 8–12 years', *Journal of Happiness Studies*, 11(2): 131–50.

Howard, S., Dryden, J. and Johnson, B. (1999) 'Childhood resilience: review and critique of literature', *Oxford Review of Education*, 25(3): 307–23.

Kidd, S.A. (2003) 'Street youth: coping and interventions', *Child and Adolescent Social Work Journal*, 20(4): 235–61.

King, P.E. and Benson, P.L. (2006) 'Spiritual development and adolescent wellbeing and thriving', in E.C. Roehlkepartain, P.E. King, L. Wagener and P.L. Benson (eds) *The Handbook of Spiritual Development in Childhood and Adolescence*, Thousand Oaks: Sage Publications.

King, U. (2013) 'The spiritual potential of childhood: awakening to the fullness of life', *International Journal of Children's Spirituality*, 18(1): 4–17.

Kliewer, W., Cunningham, J.N., Diehl, R., Parrish, K.A., Walker, J.M., Atiyeh, C., Neace, B., Duncan, L., Taylor, K. and Mejia, R. (2004) 'Violence exposure and adjustment in inner city youth: child and caregiver emotion regulation skill, caregiver–child relationship quality, and neighborhood cohesion as protective factors', *Journal of Clinical Child and Adolescent Psychology*, 33(3): 477–87.

Knight, J.R., Sherritt, L., Harris, S.K., Holder, D.W., Kulig, J., Shrier, L.A. and Chang, G. (2007) 'Alcohol use and religiousness/spirituality among adolescents', *Southern Medical Journal*, 100(4): 349–55.

Kollontai, P. (2010) 'Healing the heart in Bosnia-Herzegovina: art, children, and peacemaking', *International Journal of Children's Spirituality*, 15(3): 261–71.

Land, H. (2015) *Spirituality, Religion, and Faith in Psychotherapy: evidence-based expressive methods for mind, brain, and body*, Chicago: Lyceum Books, Inc.

Luthar, S.S. (1991) 'Vulnerability and resilience: a study of high-risk adolescents', *Child Development*, 62(3): 600–16.

Minnard, C.V. (2002) 'A strong building: foundation of protective factors in schools', *Children and Schools*, 24(4): 233–46.

Oxhandler, H.K., Parrish, D.E., Torres, L.R. and Achenbaum, W.A. (2015) 'The integration of clients' religion and spirituality in social work practice: a national survey', *Social Work*, 60(3): 228–37.

Patai, R. and Bar-Itzhak, H. (eds) (2013) *Encyclopaedia of Jewish Folklore and Traditions*, New York: Routledge.

Portman, T.A.A. and Garrett, M.T. (2006) 'Native American healing traditions', *International Journal of Disability, Development, and Education*, 53(4): 453–69.

Rew, L., Wong, J., Torres, R. and Howell, E. (2007) 'Older adolescents' perceptions of the social context, impact, and development of their spiritual/religious beliefs and practices', *Issues in Comprehensive Pediatric Nursing*, 30(1–2): 55–68.

Ritt-Olson, A., Milam, J., Unger, J.B., Trinidad, D., Teran, L., Dent, C.W. and Sussman, S. (2004) 'The protective influence of spirituality and "health-as-a-value" against monthly substance use among adolescents varying in risk', *Journal of Adolescent Health*, 34(3): 192–9.

Rostosky, S.S., Wilcox, B.L., Wright, M.L.C. and Randall, B.A. (2004)' 'The impact of religiosity on adolescent sexual behavior: a review of the evidence', *Journal of Adolescent Research*, 19(6): 677–97.

Schwartz, K.D., Bukowski, W.M. and Aoki, W.T. (2006) 'Mentors, friends, and gurus: peer and nonparent influences on spiritual development', in E. Roehlkepartan, P. King, L. Wagner and P. Benson (eds) *The Handbook of Spiritual Development in Childhood and Adolescence*, Thousand Oaks: Sage Publications.

Sheridan, M.J. (2009) 'Ethical issues in the use of spiritually based interventions in social work practice: what we are doing and why', *Journal of Religion and Spirituality in Social Work*, 28(1): 99–126.

Smith, C. and Denton, M.L. (2005) *Soul Searching: the religious and spiritual lives of American teenagers*, Oxford: Oxford University Press.

Snowber, C.N. (2007) 'The soul moves: dance and spirituality in educative practice', L. Bresler (ed) *International Handbook of Research in Arts Education*, New York: Springer.

Sussman, S., Skara, S., Rodriguez, Y. and Pokhrel, P. (2006) 'Non drug use-and drug use-specific spirituality as one-year predictors of drug use among high-risk youth', *Substance Use and Misuse*, 41(13): 1801–16.

Tshabalala, B.G. and Patel, C.J. (2010) 'The role of praise and worship activities in spiritual wellbeing: perceptions of a Pentecostal youth ministry group', *International Journal of Children's Spirituality*, 15(1): 73–82.

Weick, A., Rapp, C., Sullivan, W.P. and Kisthardt, W. (1989) 'A strengths perspective for social work practice, *Social Work*, 34(4): 350–4.

Werner, E.E. and Smith, R. S. (1977) *Kauai's Children Come of Age*, Honolulu: The University Press of Hawaii.

Williams, N.R. (2004) 'Spirituality and religion in the lives of runaway and homeless youth: coping with adversity', *Journal of Religion and Spirituality in Social Work*, 23(4): 47–66.

23

Responding to child abuse in religious contexts

Philip Gilligan

Contexts, complexities and challenges

Abuse of children is perpetrated in a wide variety of contexts. It occurs in all cultures and countries (UNICEF 2014). Measuring its breadth and impact is challenging and its occurrence in different contexts is unevenly documented. Astbury (2013) stresses the importance of understanding each situational context, but concludes that cultural and religious contexts have been researched inadequately. Even when data are available, their scope may also be very limited. As in other situations, abuse in religious contexts may be physical, sexual or emotional; occur in multiple settings and may be perpetrated by individuals or groups or both. Both perpetrators and victims/survivors adhere to religious beliefs to varying degrees.

Awareness of abuse in religious contexts has increased over the past 25 years, notably since the explosion of disclosures about abuse perpetrated by Roman Catholic clergy in the USA, Ireland, England and Wales, Australia and elsewhere, and revelations about inappropriate responses by church authorities (John Jay College 2004; Keenan 2011; Pilgrim 2011; Scorer 2014; Terry 2014). However, both the quality and quantity of information regarding the many different phenomena that can be categorised as child abuse in a religious context remain extremely variable.

Reports of child abuse in religious contexts involve the full spectrum of faith groups, sects and denominations. Examples can be cited from Islam (Abrams 2011; Singleton 2010), Hinduism (Cahill 2012), Judaism (Borchelas-dan 2015; Otterman and Rivera 2012) and Buddhism (Pathirana 2012), but much more information is available regarding abuse in Christian churches, especially in industrialised and Anglophone countries, and this provides the bulk of current knowledge.

At the same time, the responses of many religious institutions to revelations by and demands from survivors and other campaigners for justice, openness and acknowledgement has often been one of defensiveness. This results in public controversy. Minister and Clergy Child Sexual Abuse Survivors [MACSAS], for example, suggest that 'the failure of institutions such as the Catholic Church to hear, to respond and to accept responsibility is a scandal to the Christianity (sic)' (MACSAS 2011), while the McLellan Commission (2015: 12) reports admissions by some church leaders that they 'feel total shame with regard to past cover-up'.

The definition of 'child abuse in religious contexts' is not straightforward. Some actions are widely recognised as abusive (e.g. contact sexual abuse or physical assaults on children resulting in injury or death), but other behaviours, considered abusive by many professionals, remain both lawful and tolerated by society and are presented as essential to children's spiritual wellbeing or membership of a faith community. They include physically non-violent exorcism of children accused of being possessed by evil spirits (Briggs *et al.* 2011; Stobart 2006) and medically unnecessary circumcision of male infants (Hinchley 2007; Patrick 2007). Questions such as the appropriate limits to parents' rights to withhold recommended medical treatment from children on religious grounds remain contended and inadequately conceptualised in law (Humphrey 2008), while some would continue to argue that all religious indoctrination of children should be viewed as 'child abuse' (Hitchens 2007).

There are also questions about whether particular categories of abuse should be seen as occurring in a religious context. Genital mutilation or cutting of young women (FGM/C) provides one example of such questions. Programmes designed to eradicate FGM/C often place emphasis on the idea that those involved are being asked to abandon 'cultural', rather than 'religious' traditions (e.g. Innocenti Research Centre 2010), but this perhaps serves to demonstrate the need for practitioners to remember that, in the worldview of the individuals involved, their 'abusive' behaviour often results from a belief that they are fulfilling religious obligations. FGM/C is sanctioned by no sacred text and by no major religious authority, but pronouncements by religious authorities do not necessarily determine what individuals or communities believe to be their religious obligation. However, it is often associated with 'religion' because religion, tradition and culture are, in practice, intertwined (Innocenti 2010).

Impact of abuse in religious contexts

At the extreme, children die or suffer irreversible life-changing physical injuries, as the direct result of phenomena such as their carers' or a faith community's belief in spirit possession or in the need to trust to God alone for recovery from illness. Such children have been subjected to physically violent exorcisms or 'deliverance' (Laming 2003; Stobart 2006) or deprived of recommended medical treatment (Asser and Swan 1998).

In more mainstream contexts, reports, particularly into abuse perpetrated by religious authority figures, reveal that victims/survivors experience profound suffering (Department of Justice and Law Reform 2009; Government of Ireland 2009; John Jay College 2004; McLellan Commission 2015; Philadelphia Grand Jury 2011; Tentler 2007). Indeed, Astbury (2013) notes that research suggests '(c)lergy-perpetrated sexual abuse of children can catastrophically alter the trajectory of victims' psychosocial, sexual, and spiritual development' and notes arguments that there are many similarities between incest and clergy abuse, especially where the families of victims are closely allied with their church.

There is also considerable evidence to suggest that abuse in religious contexts has additional and specific impact on victims/survivors. The John Jay Research Team reports that some psychological effects of clergy-perpetrated child sexual abuse occur repeatedly in testimonies. These include major symptoms of post-traumatic stress disorder, substance abuse, emotional changeability, relational conflicts and a profound alteration in individual spirituality and religious practices associated with a deep sense of betrayal by the individual perpetrator and the church (John Jay College 2004, 2006; McMackin *et al.* 2008). Farrell and Taylor (2000) report symptoms such as self-blame, guilt, psychosexual disturbances, self-destructive behaviours, substance abuse and re-victimization. In a study of Mormon women survivors of church childhood sexual abuse, Gerdes *et al.* (2002) found that women's healing journeys were especially difficult because the church pervaded so much of their social lives.

Farrell *et al.* (2010: 124) argue that sexual abuse perpetrated by clergy should be seen as a distinct form of trauma, generating 'unique posttraumatic symptoms not accounted for within the existing Posttraumatic Stress Disorder conceptual frameworks'. These include 'significant anxiety and distress in areas such as theological belief, crisis of faith, and fears surrounding the participant's own mortality'. For some, the experience of abuse, especially by clergy, is experienced not only as betrayal by trusted authority figures, but as abuse within which God is perceived as 'integral' (Farell 2009: 39). On the basis of work with mainly female Christian survivors, Kennedy concludes:

> Victims of abuse find it incredibly difficult to understand why it is that God/Jesus did not protect them. They blame God/Jesus for their abuse. It's quite something to feel betrayed by your human family, but really huge to feel betrayed by an all-powerful deity.
>
> (Kennedy 2003: 4)

Ryan (1998: 47) found that, while some writers argue that ongoing spiritual practice offers survivors a variety of benefits including 'providing meaning for life and the traumatic experience, feeling less alone in the world and maintaining hope', others find impediments to recovery in some spiritual belief systems. Impediments include fatalism, patriarchal hierarchies, stoicism, emphasis on forgiveness, self-blame and over-reliance on spiritual systems to the exclusion of other resources. At the same time, Doyle (2001, 2006) emphasises that religion can provide reassurance to victims of abuse and identifies 'religiosity' as a positive factor in children's resilience.

Social work, religion and child abuse

Given the complexities involved, it is unsurprising that studies suggest social workers and others are often reluctant to engage with issues arising from religion and religious beliefs (Furness and Gilligan 2010) and that such reluctance impacts on their responses to survivors/victims of child abuse in religious contexts (Gilligan 2009). The nature of their responses may also be complicated further by the idea that social work and all forms of spirituality are in 'opposition' (Crisp 2010) and by individual experiences and beliefs that, in the absence of adequate reflection, may significantly influence practice. As a result, there seem to be great variations in practitioners' willingness to consider the potential for service users' religious beliefs to enhance their emotional wellbeing, to heighten their distress or to do both at the same time.

Religion is, however, significant in determining the ways in which some people interpret events, resolve dilemmas, make decisions and view themselves, their own and others' actions and how they respond to these (Beit-Hallahmi and Argyle 1997; Hunt 2005). This is likely to be especially so in situations such as child abuse in religious contexts. Practitioners may not, therefore, be able to engage or to facilitate appropriate interventions if they take too little account of these aspects of people's lives or consider them on the basis of inaccurate, ill-informed or stereotyped 'knowledge' (Hodge *et al.* 2006). At the same time, whatever the context, social workers need to adopt an approach that recognises that individual constructions of religion reflect the nature of individual experience (Hunt 2005). Thus, without more detailed information and dialogue, the fact that someone is known to be 'Roman Catholic', 'Sikh', 'agnostic' or whatever will, in itself, tell a social worker very little about that person's specific attitudes, needs, strengths, beliefs or potential support networks. In the UK and other parts of Europe, an increasing majority of those who report that they are 'Christian' do so without any formal or regular participation in the activities of any particular church or sect. Their approach to religion is individual and privatised (Hunt 2005). Practitioners, therefore, need to understand what, if anything, religion means to a particular individual.

In practice, social workers need to respond to actual and immediate situations, to recognise the potential significance of individuals' religious beliefs and practices, and to assess the extent to which they are potentially beneficial, harmful or both in particular situations. On occasions, they may be involved with carers who believe they have a 'religious' duty to do something the wider society views as unacceptable. They may be involved with individuals who draw positive benefit from 'religious' practices that fall outside conventional categorisations. They also need to recognise that some victims/survivors will find contexts beyond their original faith community in which to express and benefit from their religious beliefs, including informal and formal religious services organised by survivors' groups both independently and in cooperation with religious authorities.

The response of religious institutions

Moules (2006: 23) reminds us that 'Children can be abused in any environment' and that 'It would be naïve to assume that child abuse could not happen within our faith'. Few would now argue that membership of any faith community provides protection from child abuse and in recent decades many religious institutions have established child protection policies and procedures (e.g. Archbishop's Council 2011). In the UK, these can often be accessed online (e.g. Catholic Safeguarding Advisory Service 2015; The Methodist Church in England 2015). There have also been notable collaborations between safeguarding boards and Muslim organisations in relation to safeguarding in mosque schools and other Islamic study centres (e.g. Ahmed and Riasat 2013) and between majority black churches, safeguarding boards and organisations such as the Churches' Child Protection Advisory Service and Africans Unite Against Child Abuse (Briggs et al. 2011).

Religious institutions have developed policies at very different speeds and implementation of them has not always been consistent. All members of Churches Together in Britain and Ireland agreed to implement the recommendations of *Time for Action* (Galloway and Gamble 2002), including those regarding the development of support services for survivors of sexual abuse in their churches. Some did so, but in its submission to the Cumberlege Commission, MACSAS (2006) claims, for example, that the Catholic Church did not. Subsequently, in 2015, writing of the year ahead, the chair of the National Catholic Safeguarding Commission [NCSC] admitted that 'the one area where we will be most challenged is in listening to and meeting with survivors which is not an area of consistently good practice' (NCSC 2015: 5). However, he also reported that 'The working party on pastoral support for survivors has made real progress and … we believe we have a model that can be implemented gradually across all our Dioceses and Religious Communities' (NCSC 2015: 4).

The model referred to by the NSCS is that developed by the *Hurt by Abuse* pilot in Sheffield, England in the Diocese of Hallam (2015), which makes explicit use of *A Vision of a Catholic Church which Supports and Cares for Those Who Have Been Harmed* (Markham 2010). This document emphasises the need to convey messages that child protection reflects core Gospel imperatives.

Among many other things, Markham (2010) promotes the idea of children's advocates, for the church to communicate in its actions that allegations are taken seriously and for no-one to be deterred from reporting concerns. Markham also encourages victims/survivors to be used as expert witnesses and advisers, for the church to properly resource healing centres and demonstrate that it understands that victims/survivors have different needs, for holistic services to families, for dedicated spiritual support and recognition of victim experiences in liturgical material. He sees a need for church leaders to recognise the complexity of gospel exhortations to forgive and the pressure these may place on victims, and for the church to ensure that it has the mechanisms to provide practical support and appropriate restitution for victims.

It is clear from their testimonies that for some victims and survivors, continuing religious practice, attendance at services and active involvement in their faith community is important to their ongoing ability to cope with having been abused, even when the perpetrator is a member of the clergy. Indeed, some writers suggest that ongoing participation in religion can provide reassurance to victims of abuse, who report that they gain strength from their belief that God loves them unconditionally (Crompton 1998; Doyle 2001, 2006). They suggest that spirituality benefits survivors by assisting them to transcend the violent experience as it is happening, providing meaning for both life and specific experiences and helping them to feel less alone in the world. Kennedy (1995: 34) emphasises that 'for a great many Christian children who have been abused, if they see God as loving, then the continuation of a Christian practice is essential for healing'. At the same time, many of the same writers recognise impediments to recovery from the trauma of child abuse in certain spiritual belief systems. Kennedy (2003), for example, argues that Christian beliefs may shape victims' acceptance of abuse and cause them to see their suffering as redemptive.

There are also some notable examples of churches and religious institutions exploring systems for restorative justice and compensation. These aim at restoring harm by including affected parties in user-led processes and encounters (direct and indirect) that promote understanding through honest dialogue, in which offenders take full responsibility for what they have done and institutions accept that they are accountable to the victims for helping them restore or be compensated for what they have lost (Gavrielides 2007, 2013; McKay 2014).

Criticisms of the responses of religious institutions

Many survivors' groups and other observers remain extremely dissatisfied with the responses of religious institutions and hierarchies both in general and in specific cases, while others express concern that some religious communities remain unaware of the abuse occurring among them. Specific examples illustrate the types of difficulties that may arise across all faiths and religious institutions to varying degrees. Neustein and Lesher (2008) discuss the ways in which, in Orthodox Jewish communities, religious judicial processes may prevent individuals abused by rabbis from obtaining justice through secular legal processes; Gerdes *et al.* (2002) found that victims/survivors report that the typical reaction of the Mormon church was to tell them to forgive the perpetrator or to deny the facts. I have highlighted elsewhere (Gilligan 2012b) the apparent failure of the Roman Catholic church in England and Wales, a decade after acceptance of the Nolan Report (Nolan 2001), to implement its declared policies regarding the laicisation of clergy convicted of child sexual abuse offences by criminal courts. In 2006, Siddiqui (2006: 1) suggested that 'The Muslim community is at present in a state of denial—denial of the fact that child abuse takes place in places of worship including in mosques, *madrasas* (mosque schools) and families' while the Methodist Church in Britain (2015: 20) found that 'ministers not only have difficulty recognising and accepting that abuse has taken place when the perpetrator is a colleague but also struggle to recognise it when it is a lay person abusing'.

In relation to the Roman Catholic church in England and Wales, the Cumberlege Commission (Cumberlege 2007: 22) stated concerns that five years after Lord Nolan reported, 'Bishops and Congregational Leaders may be minimising the distressing consequences, the harmful impact and the anguish that follows in the wake of child abuse', while, in Scotland, the McLellan

Commission (2015: 10) reported that 'No point was made more consistently to the Commission by survivors than their sense that they had not been listened to and not believed'.

I have previously argued that, where institutions seek to serve conflicting legitimacy communities, they risk alienating victims/survivors, especially where survivors' experiences have left them feeling that the institution has prioritised financial interests and reputation over what they had come to expect in the context of rhetoric promising openness, honesty and sensitivity (Gilligan 2012a). In considering such a mismatch it is relevant to recall what we know from attachment theory: that is, a child who has the experience that 'things did not turn out as he was led to believe' learns that cognition 'is not to be trusted' (Crittenden 1999: 54) and that those who have had such experiences 'always feel in danger of being manipulated by those who make promises' (Howe 2005: 128).

At the same time, recognition that institutional hierarchies, formal authorities and faith leaders do not necessarily understand or represent the views or needs of individual members of their faith communities is of crucial importance in responding appropriately to the needs of those abused in religious contexts. Religion and religious activities may provide contexts where they can find recovery and build their resilience (Crompton 1998; Doyle 2001, 2006; Kennedy 1995). However, it is equally clear that especially for those for whom religious beliefs are of ongoing importance, failure by religious institutions to respond sensitively and adequately has heightened their distress (Lawrence 2011; MACSAS 2006).

Meeting the needs of victims/survivors of child abuse in religious contexts

The needs, strengths and responses of each victim/survivor are a unique result of the interaction of many factors. In this context, these factors are likely to include the impact of individuals' religious beliefs on their experience of being abused and the impact of being abused on their religious beliefs (Farrell 2009). Some victims/survivors remain active members of their original faith community or join another, while others cease all involvement with religion or may become active critics of religion *per se*.

Meanwhile, survivors groups and individual victims/survivors have made clear statements regarding their needs. While some are satisfied with the response of religious institutions or express no further interest in relevant issues, many campaign actively for improved responses. They increasingly advocate the use of restorative justice, which, in addition to meeting the particular needs of individuals, also emphasises the need for victims/survivors to know that they have been believed, their pain is acknowledged both by perpetrators and religious institutions, they will be appropriately compensated and the faith community will maximise the protection of others and respond appropriately and sensitively to victims/survivors in the future. In 2014, Stop Church Child Abuse, an alliance of survivor support groups in England and Wales, advocated for a complaints system that is independent of churches, tailor-made support and therapy, and an improved system of redress and mandatory reporting of abuse (Stop Church Child Abuse 2015). Survivors NI (2011), meanwhile, called for reparation that will 'redress all the consequences of the abuse suffered ... be based on the needs, views and circumstances of the individual and ... proportionate to the gravity of the violation and the resulting harm'. Survivors NI (2011) also suggest that such packages 'should include restitution, compensation, rehabilitation, satisfaction and guarantees of non-repetition', that institutions should contribute to costs to the extent to which they are accountable and that any individual or entity found liable should either provide that reparation or compensate the state for doing so.

Acknowledgement and validation are essential components of healing (Salter 1995) and, for at least some, experience of an adequate response from their religious institution or faith

215

community is crucial to recovery. Those involved in survivors' groups are also likely to benefit from the sense of solidarity, empathy and understanding inherent in knowing they are not alone, but such emotionally secure bases may not be available to or accessed by all victims/survivors. Those who are not in contact with survivors' organisations will remain particularly dependent on other sources of support. They will ultimately benefit indirectly from the work of survivors' groups in pressing for more appropriate and consistent responses from religious institutions and others, including social workers in secular organisations, but much work remains to be done to establish both their needs and the most effective and sensitive ways of meeting these.

Professionals seeking to respond appropriately to individuals need to recognise that they are likely to have needs particular to them and their situation, as well as needs that appear to be shared by most victims/survivors of child abuse in religious contexts. Policy makers and law givers would, in turn, do well to note the conclusion of Bottoms *et al.* (1995: 109), who emphasise that 'in the long run, society should find ways to protect children from religion-related abuse and to help religions evolve in the direction of better treatment of children'. Freedom to choose and to practice a religion should not include freedom to abuse children.

References

Abrams, F. (2011) *Child Abuse Claims at UK Madrassas 'Tip of Iceberg'*. Online. Available HTTP: www.bbc.co.uk/news/education-15256764 (accessed 25 October 2015).

Ahmed, I. and Riasat, A. (2013) *Children Do Matter,* Bradford: Council of Mosques. Online. Available HTTP: www.bradford-scb.org.uk/mosques.htm (accessed 25 October 2015).

Archbishop's Council (2011) *Responding Well to Those Who Have Been Sexually Abused*, London: Church House Publishing. Online. Available HTTP: www.churchofengland.org/media-centre/news/2011/07/responding-well-to-those-who-have-been-sexually-abused-new-policy-and-guidance.aspx (accessed 30 October 2015).

Asser, S.M. and Swan, R. (1998) 'Child fatalities from religion-motivated medical neglect', *Pediatrics,* 101(4): 625–9.

Astbury, J. (2013) *Child Sexual Abuse in the General Community and Clergy-Perpetrated Child Sexual Abuse: a review paper prepared for the Australian Psychological Society to inform an APS response to the Royal Commission into Institutional Responses to Child Sexual Abuse,* Melbourne: The Australian Psychological Society. Online. Available HTTP: www.psychology.org.au/inpsych/2013/october/astbury/ (accessed 15 November 2015).

Beit-Hallahmi, B. and Argyle, M. (1997) *The Psychology of Religious Behaviour, Belief and Experience*, London: Routledge.

Borchelas-dan, A. (2015) 'Advocate calls for global Jewish child-abuse commission', *The Times of Israel,* 16 February 2015. Online. Available HTTP: www.timesofisrael.com/advocate-calls-for-global-jewish-child-abuse-commission/ (accessed 25 October 2015).

Bottoms, B., Shaver, P., Goodman, G. and Qin, J. (1995) 'In the name of God: a profile of religion-related child abuse', *Journal of Social Issues*, 51(2): 85–111.

Briggs, S., Whittaker, A., Linford, H., Bryan, A., Ryan, E. and Ludick, D. (2011) *Safeguarding Children's Rights: exploring issues of witchcraft and spirit possession in London's African communities*, London: Trust for London.

Cahill, D. (2012) *A Holy and Unholy Mess: child sexual abuse and the world's major religious traditions in the Australian context*. Online. Available HTTP: http://religionsforpeaceaustralia.org.au/news/royal-commission/411-sexual-abuse-in-religions.html (accessed 25 October 2015).

Catholic Safeguarding Advisory Service (2015) *Catholic Safeguarding Resource Area*. Online. Available HTTP: www.csas.uk.net/resource-area/ (accessed 15 November 2015).

Crisp, B.R. (2010) *Spirituality and Social Work*, Farnham: Ashgate.

Crittenden, P. (1999) 'Child neglect: causes and contributors', in H. Dubowitz (ed) *Neglected Children: research, practice and policy*, Thousand Oaks: Sage.

Crompton, M. (1998) *Children, Spirituality, Religion and Social Work*, Aldershot: Ashgate.

Cumberlege, J. (2007) *Safeguarding with Confidence: keeping children and vulnerable adults safe in the Catholic Church. The Cumberlege Commission Report*, London: Catholic Truth Society.

Department of Justice and Law Reform (2009) *Report by Commission of Investigation in the Catholic Archdiocese of Dublin (The Murphy Report)*. Dublin: Department of Justice and Law Reform.

Diocese of Hallam (2015) *Hurt by Abuse*. Online. Available HTTP: http://hallam-diocese.com/safeguard-ing/hurt-by-abuse/ (accessed 15 November 2015).

Doyle, C. (2001) 'Surviving and coping with emotional abuse in childhood', *Clinical Psychology and Psychiatry*, 6(3): 387–402.

Doyle, C. (2006) *Working with Abused Children: from theory to practice*, 3rd edn, Basingstoke: Palgrave Macmillan.

Farrell, D. (2009) 'Sexual abuse perpetrated by Roman Catholic priests and religious', *Mental Health, Religion and Culture*, 12(1): 39–53.

Farrell, D., Dworkin, M., Keenan, P. and Spierings, J. (2010) 'Using EMDR with survivors of sexual abuse perpetrated by Roman Catholic priests', *Journal of EMDR Practice and Research*, 4(3): 125–33.

Farrell, D.P. and Taylor, M. (2000) 'Silenced by God: an examination of unique characteristics within sexual abuse by clergy', *Counselling Psychology Review*, 15(1): 22–31.

Furness, S. and Gilligan, P. (2010) *Religion, Belief and Social Work: making a difference*, Bristol: Policy Press.

Galloway, K. and Gamble, D. (2002) *Time for Change: sexual abuse, the churches and a new dawn for survivors*, London: Churches Together in Britain and Ireland.

Gavrielides, T. (2007) *Restorative Justice Theory and Practice: addressing the discrepancy*, Helsinki: European Institute for Crime Prevention and Control, affiliated with the United Nations (HEUNI).

Gavrielides, T. (2013) 'Clergy child sexual abuse and the restorative justice dialogue', *Journal of Church and State*, 55(4): 617–39.

Gerdes, K.E., Beck, M.N. and Miller, H. (2002) 'Betrayal of a sacred trust: "Sanctuary trauma" in sexual abuse survivors', *Social Work Today*, 2(7): 6–11.

Gilligan, P. (2009) 'Considering religion and beliefs in child protection and safeguarding work: is any consensus emerging?' *Child Abuse Review*, 18(2): 94–110.

Gilligan, P. (2012a) 'Contrasting narratives on responses to victims and survivors of clerical abuse in England and Wales: challenges to Catholic Church discourse', *Child Abuse Review*, 21(6): 414–26.

Gilligan, P. (2012b) 'Clerical abuse and laicisation: rhetoric and reality in the Catholic Church in England and Wales', *Child Abuse Review*, 21(6): 427–39.

Government of Ireland (2009) *The Commission to Inquire into Child Abuse (The Ryan Report)*, Dublin: The Stationery Office.

Hinchley, G. (2007) 'Is infant male circumcision an abuse of the rights of the child? Yes', *British Medical Journal*, 335(7631): 1180.

Hitchens, C. (2007) *God Is Not Great: how religion poisons everything*, New York: Twelve.

Hodge, D., Baughman, L. and Cummings, J. (2006) 'Moving toward spiritual competency: deconstructing religious stereotypes and spiritual prejudices in social work literature', *Journal of Social Service Research*, 32(4): 211–32.

Howe, D. (2005) *Child Abuse and Neglect: attachment, development and intervention*, Basingstoke: Palgrave MacMillan.

Humphrey, T. (2008) 'Children, medical treatment and religion: defining the limits of parental responsibil-ity', *Australian Journal of Human Rights*, 14(1): 141–69.

Hunt, S. (2005) *Religion and Everyday Life*, London: Routledge.

Innocenti Research Centre (2010) *The Dynamics of Social Change: towards the abandonment of female genital mutilation/cutting in five African countries*, Florence: The UNICEF Innocenti Research Centre. Online. Available HTTP: www.unicef-irc.org/publications/618 (accessed 5 November 2015).

John Jay College (2004) *The Nature and Scope of Sexual Abuse of Minors by Catholic Priests and Deacons in the United States 1950–2002*, Washington, DC: United States Conference of Bishops. Online. Available HTTP: www.usccb.org/search.cfm?q=The+Nature+and+Scope+of+Sexual+Abuse+of+Minors+b y+Catholic+Priests+and+Deacons+in+the+United+States+1950-2002 (accessed 25 October 2015).

John Jay College (2006) *The Nature and Scope of Sexual Abuse of Minors by Catholic Priests and Deacons in the United States: supplementary data analysis*, Washington, DC: United States Conference of Bishops.

Keenan, M. (2011) *Child Sexual Abuse and the Catholic Church: gender, power, and organizational culture*, Oxford: Oxford University Press.

Kennedy, M. (1995) *Submission to the National Commission of Inquiry into the Prevention of Child Abuse*, London: Christian Survivors of Sexual Abuse.

Kennedy, M. (2003) *Christianity and Child Sexual Abuse: survivors informing the care of children following abuse*. Online. Available HTTP: www.rcpsych.ac.uk/pdf/Margaret%20Kennedy%201.11.03%20Christ

ianity%20and%20Child%20Sexual%20Abuse%20-%20Survivors%20informing%20the%20care%20 of%20children%20following%20abuse.pdf (accessed 5 November 2015).

Laming, Lord (2003) *The Victoria Climbié Inquiry: report of an inquiry*, London: HMSO.

Lawrence A. (2011) *The Stones Cry Out: report on the MACSAS survey 2010*, Brentford: MACSAS.

Markham, L. (2010) *A Vision of a Catholic Church which Supports and Cares for Those Who Have Been Harmed*. Online. Available HTTP: http://hallam-diocese.com/milanesa/uploads/2015/08/Vision-of-a-Catholic-Church.pdf (accessed 5 November 2015).

McKay, R. (2014) (Revised 24 November 2014) *Redress Schemes: submission to the Royal Commission into institutional responses to child sexual abuse*, Sydney: Centre for Peace and Conflict Studies.

McLellan Commission (2015) *A review of the current safeguarding policies, procedures and practice within the Catholic Church in Scotland*. Online. Available HTTP: https://www.mclellancommission.co.uk/report (accessed 5 November 2015).

McMackin, R.A., Keane, T M. and Kline, P.M. (2008) 'Introduction to special issue on betrayal and recovery: understanding the trauma of child sexual abuse', *Journal of Child Sexual Abuse*, 17(3–4): 197–200.

Minister and Clergy Sexual Abuse Survivors [MACAS] (2006) *Time to Hear: submission to Cumberlege Commission*. Online. Available HTTP: www.macsas.org.uk/MACSAS%20Resources.html (accessed 24 October 2015).

Minister and Clergy Sexual Abuse Survivors [MACAS] (2011) *MACSAS end 'Exploratory Talks' with the Catholic Church*. Press release, 11 October 2011.

Moules S. (2006) 'The Catholic churches' response to allegations of child abuse', in *Child Protection in Faith-based Environments: a guideline report*, London: Muslim Parliament of Great Britain.

National Catholic Safeguarding Commission [NSCS] (2015) *Annual Report*, London: NCSC. Online. Available HTTP: www.catholicsafeguarding.org.uk/documents.htm (accessed 30 October 2015).

Neustein, A. and Lesher, M. (2008) 'A single-case study of rabbinic sexual abuse in the Orthodox Jewish community', *Journal of Child Sexual Abuse*, 17(3–4): 270–89.

Nolan, Lord (2001) *A Programme for Action: final report of the independent review on child protection in the Catholic Church in England and Wales*, London: Catholic Bishops' Conference of England and Wales.

Otterman, S. and Rivera, R. (2012) 'Ultra-Orthodox shun their own for reporting child sexual abuse', *New York Times*, 9 May 2012. Online. Available HTTP: www.nytimes.com/2012/05/10/nyregion/ultra-orthodox-jews-shun-their-own-for-reporting-child-sexual-abuse.html?pagewanted=all&_r=0 (accessed 25 October 2015).

Pathirana, S. (2012) *Sri Lanka's Hidden Scourge of Religious Child Abuse*. Online. Available HTTP: www.bbc.co.uk/news/world-south-asia-15507304 (accessed 25 October 2015).

Patrick, K. (2007) 'Is infant male circumcision an abuse of the rights of the child? No', *British Medical Journal*, 335(7631): 1181.

Philadelphia Grand Jury (2011) *Investigation of Sexual Abuse by Clergy II*, Philadelphia: Office of the District Attorney.

Pilgrim, D. (2011) 'The child abuse crisis in the Catholic Church: international, national and policy perspectives', *Policy and Politics*, 39(3): 309–24.

Ryan, P. (1998) 'Spirituality among adult survivors of childhood violence: a literature review, *The Journal of Transpersonal Psychology*, 30(1): 39–51.

Salter, A.C. (1995) *A Guide to Understanding and Treating Adult Survivors of Child Sexual Abuse: transforming trauma*, London: Sage.

Scorer, R. (2014) *Betrayed: the English Catholic Church and the child sex abuse crisis*, London: Biteback Books.

Siddiqui, G. (2006) 'Breaking the taboo of child abuse', in *Child Protection in Faith-based Environments: a guideline report*, London: Muslim Parliament of Great Britain.

Singleton, R. (2010) *Physical Punishment: improving consistency and protection*, London: Department for Education.

Stobart, E. (2006) *Child Abuse Linked to Accusations of 'Possession' and 'Witchcraft'*, London: Department for Education and Skills.

Stop Church Child Abuse (2015) *Stop Church Child Abuse*. Online. Available HTTP: http://stopchurch-childabuse.co.uk/ (accessed 15 November 2015).

Survivors NI (2011) *Submission to the Historical Institutional Abuse Taskforce of the Northern Ireland Executive*, Belfast: Survivors and Victims of Institutional Abuse in Northern Ireland. Online. Available HTTP: www.survivorsni.org/ (accessed 2 November 2015).

Tentler, L. (ed) (2007) *The Church Confronts Modernity: Catholicism since 1950 in the United States, Ireland and Quebec*, Washington, DC: Catholic University of America Press.

Terry, K.J. (2014) 'Child sexual abuse within the Catholic Church: a review of global perspectives', *International Journal of Comparative and Applied Criminal Justice*, 39(2): 139–54.

The Methodist Church in Britain (2015) *Methodist Safeguarding Policy*. Online. Available HTTP: www. methodist.org.uk/ministers-and-office-holders/safeguarding/methodist-safeguarding-policy (accessed 15 November 2015).

UNICEF (2014) *Hidden in Plain Sight: a statistical analysis of violence against children*, New York: United Nations Children's Fund, Data and Analytics Section. Online. Available HTTP: www.unicef.org/publications/index_74865.html (accessed 25 October 2015).

24

Queer meaning

Mark Henrickson

Introduction

It is may be both surprising and challenging to encounter a chapter on queer people in a volume on religion, spirituality and social work. For many people, both queer and non-queer, the very notion that we might talk about religion and spirituality at the same time we consider sexual and gender minorities is epistemologically dissonant. These seem to be exclusive categories that simply do not fit together in either historical or contemporary discourse. Yet a major task of a minoritised identity or experience of difference is to make sense of that identity or difference (Park and Folkman 1997; Plattner and Meiring 2006; Solomon 2012). If we understand spirituality as a kind of meaning making activity (Lips-Wiersma 2002), then there is something quite spiritual about a minoritised or marginalised individual's search for meaning. On the other hand, religions, which are formalised institutions with specific codes of beliefs, practices and boundaries that usually reflect dominant social norms, often have difficulties managing differences of the sexual kind (Boellstorff 2005; Buchanan *et al.* 2001; Congregation for the Doctrine of the Faith 1986; Fone 2000; Siraj 2012). The challenge to social work, with its core principles of social justice and human rights, and its mandate to respect diversities (International Federation of Social Workers [IFSW] and the International Association of Schools of Social Work [IASSW] 2014), is to support clients, and the families, institutions and policymakers with which they engage, to manage these differences and challenges. Providing a perspective from which to do that is the goal of this chapter.

This chapter will not address the profound spiritual crisis caused by HIV disease particularly in gay male communities since the 1980s. This is not to ignore the importance of this pandemic in any way; rather, this spiritual crisis merits specific attention, and has already been addressed by a rich literature (see for instance, Cotton *et al.* 2006; Fortunato 1987; Jacobson *et al.* 2006; Miller 2005; Simoni *et al.* 2002).

A note on language

The taxonomy of sexual identity is complex, and there is little agreement even (or perhaps especially) among people who write and talk frequently about sexual and gender identities. Western notions of identity are reflected in English language labels such as 'gay', 'lesbian', 'bisexual', 'trans★', and so forth, but in many cultures such essentialised and individuated categories have no meaning, and there are cultures and languages with more than two gender signifiers. Binary identities such as 'gay' and 'straight', and even 'male' and 'female', have been replaced by contemporary understandings of sexualities and genders as multidimensional continua (Teich 2012). Current academic writing often uses the inclusive language 'sexual and gender minorities' as an attempt to reflect the broad scope of these concepts, and that is the language that will be used here. In this chapter the word 'queer' is also used deliberately, to underscore and reclaim a term of bullying and hate, to align with the contemporary scholarships of queer theory and queer theology (e.g. Cheng 2011; Cornwall 2010), and to highlight the multifarious meanings of queer – which synonyms can include surprising, astonishing, funny, perplexing, odd, curious and unexpected. Sexual and gender minorities are all of those things. Words (such as 'heterosexual', which did not appear in print until the 1930s) are used anachronistically for the sake of brevity and clarity.

Heteronormativity

Much of social work theory and education has used the heuristic of the cultural 'other' about sexual and gender minorities in order to learn *about* them as separate phenomena or cultural variants (Mallon 2008). Enlightened introductory social work textbooks now include sections on how important it is to learn to work with sexual and gender minorities because of high rates of depression and other mental health disorders, substance misuse, suicidality and other social problems in these communities. Such approaches can label sexual and gender minorities as broken – as sad, mad and bad. *Coming out* is constructed as a kind of ontological crisis, which the young (or mature) person must undergo as though it were an unavoidable rite of passage to an essential sexual or gender minority identity. Coming out is understood as a coming to terms with the 'real' (essentialised) self, and rejecting the norms, conventions and ways of validating knowledge with which the individual has been brought up. Thus constructed, coming out is not an isolated event, but is a process that the gender or sexual minority person undertakes throughout their entire lifespan, often beginning with a family of origin, and continuing through teachers, coaches, health care providers, national censuses, workplaces, social gatherings, banks, insurance documents, religious institutions, hotel clerks, lawyers and funeral directors.

However, this taken-for-granted step fails to recognise that the need to come out is necessitated by a socio-political context that constructs minoritised sexual and gender identities as unusual or variant. This socio-political context is called *heteronormativity*, the assumption that heterosexuality, and its accompanying rights, institutions and privileges (including reproduction) is natural, inevitable or desirable (Kitzinger 2005; Montgomery and Stewart 2012). Heteronormativity assumes heterosexuality implicitly, and explicitly writes it into the laws of many nations and states: the assumptions, for instance, that opposite-sex marriage was somehow divinely instituted, and remained intact and consistent for all classes throughout human history; normal families require both a mother and father; and/or certain kinds of sexual behaviour are criminal. The management of sexual and gender minorities with arrest, incarceration, shock treatment, physical and chemical castration and (in some nations) torture, stoning and death, are examples of how the state has managed and continues to manage sexual and gender minorities (Fone 2000). Although she was speaking of women, Adrienne Rich, the late American poet, could have been speaking of all sexual and gender minorities when she wrote 'Heterosexuality has had to be imposed, managed, organized propagandized and maintained by force' (1980/1986: 50). It is these realities that make coming out as a sexual minoritised person hardly a taken-for-granted step, but an act of great courage and integrity. Acknowledgement of one's sexual or gender minority status also requires resituating oneself in the context of one's cultural norms; this, in turn, creates the need to rediscover or redefine the meaning of one's identity.

Religious institutions are inheritors, and even guardians, of cisgendered heteronormativity. Religious scriptures are (often selectively) interpreted as condemning anything other than heterosexuality as aberrant, sinful or disgraceful. Heterosexual milestones such as marriage and birth are celebrated with public ceremony. Since about 1000 CE (Fone 2000), church leaders have often been at the forefront of ensuring that heterosexual values are retained and promoted; and these messages of exclusion and stigma have been widely circulated in popular and social media. It is these messages that sexual and gender minority persons read, mark, learn and inwardly digest; they know that they are not welcome.

While the gaze of social work on sexual and gender minorities as cultural variants is perhaps an inevitable and positive first step in breaking away from the power of the state and religion, contemporary queer discourse challenges this heuristic because such an approach constructs sexual and gender minorities as objects of knowledge (Hicks 2008). Such approaches problematise sexual and gender minorities, and fail to critique the dominant paradigm of cisgendered heteronormativity, which creates the experience of alienation in the first instance. It is not the minoritised sexual or gender identity, then, that creates the crisis of meaning: it is the larger social-political and religious context of heteronormativity that creates the spiritual crisis.

To complicate matters further, there is a growing challenge within sexual and gender minority communities in developed Western nations to an emerging phenomenon called *homonormativity*. Homonormativity is a late-twentieth and twenty-first century notion that equality with middle class, cisgendered heterosexuals – the rights to marry, to birth or adopt children, etc. – is a desirable goal (Cocker and Hafford-Letchfield 2010). A complex challenge has emerged for sexual and gender minorities: on the one hand, legal and social inequalities remain battles (like marriage equality) that once engaged cannot be lost; on the other, sexual and gender minorities increasingly insist that only they have the right to establish ontological and epistemic meaning for themselves (why reproduce the meaning of heterosexual marriage in same-sex relationships?). This challenge could easily be misconstrued as mere political discourse, and to non-queer people something akin to perseverating at trivia. Yet striving for autonomy – the right to define oneself, to establish where one belongs and to create a meaningful way of living – is a meaning-making activity, and thus a spiritual one.

Meaning-making is not simply an activity that asks relatively simple questions about whether a queer person is acceptable to their god. The awareness that one is not as one thought, that one is ontologically different from one's family, one's peers, one's culture and society, is a shattering one. The self is fractured. The known reality is forever and completely changed; all the 'truths' that the queer person has learned about themselves either implicitly or explicitly must be reassessed, and reinterpreted into the new identity, or rejected. The meaning-making process for a sexual or gender minority person is a multidimensional one, which seeks to locate the person horizontally in family, society and culture, vertically in one's beliefs about the universe, and historically both in the life course of a person and in their sociopolitical context.

Heteronormativity, then, creates a crisis of identity in queer people, which perplexes non-queer people – Why do they always have to talk about it? – and which queer people must resolve in some way. As we shall see, for people who understand themselves as religious, both queer and non-queer, it is not surprising that a primary resource to addressing this crisis is a faith community.

Spirituality and religion as meaning-making

One of the essential challenges of a sexual or gender minority identity is the experience of alienation, or not belonging. The early and ontological experience of (usually) being different from one's birth family and one's peer group is at the core of the experience of self (Solomon 2012) as the sexual or gender minority person attempts to find meaning in the experience of difference. A queer identity is an individuated identity – it is not something that is shared with a family, tribe or kin collective, and so the process of finding meaning in the identity is, inevitably, an individual one. Much of the contemporary literature in the field of sexuality and spirituality comes from the counselling discipline. The literature is almost universal in demonstrating the importance for individual mental health of reconciling one's identity with one's religious and spiritual values. While it is admirable that counsellors are researching and publishing in this area, the predominant paradigm in counselling is a reflexive-therapeutic one, which locates problems in individuals, and helps individuals to adjust to an unchanging or unchangeable environment. A core challenge to the helping professionals who work with sexual and gender minorities is not to replicate the oppression of problematising those individuals by *a priori* locating the problem in them rather than the social context. In other words, simply because the meaning-making process is individuated does not mean that the problem is in the individual. Social work, on the other hand, accesses a variety of paradigms when working with clients, and recognises that sometimes problems are in environments. We shall return to this later in the chapter.

Searching for meaning by sexual and gender minority persons not infrequently begins in the context of a formal religious organisation (Buchanan *et al.* 2001; Figueroa and Tasker 2014; Gold and Stewart 2011; Hattie and Beagan 2013; Yip 2002). However, as we have seen, many, if not most, formal religious organisations have had at best an antipathetic relationship with sexual and gender minorities; many of these religions, while outwardly expressing love and charity, struggle to navigate from outright condemnation to tolerance (Hamblin and Gross 2014; Melendez and LaSala 2006). A major developmental task of sexual and gender minority individuals is to reconcile their personal experiences of identity with the discourse of exclusion by their faith communities (Guttiérrez 2012; Kocet *et al.* 2011; Levy and Reeves 2011; Murr 2013; Siraj 2012; Walker and Longmire-Avital 2013). Screeds of text, some of it useful, have been written about what religions and religious texts, particularly the monotheistic Abrahamic religions, have claimed about sexual and gender minorities (Hunt 2003; Irby 2014; Rosik *et al.* 2007), and Hunt's (2015) extensive anthology contains an array of articles on managing the queer self in Christianity, Judaism and Islam. The experience for most sexual and gender minority persons is that what religions have to say about them is often unhelpful, and at worst hateful. Reviewing and responding to that literature and those theologies is beyond the scope of this chapter. Contemporary scholarship and queer theologies propose alternative hermeneutics and ways of approaching problematic texts.

The negotiation of sexuality in the context of formal religions can be a major life task in the lives of emerging sexual and gender minorities, and for some remains contended throughout the life course (Boellstorff 2005; Cheng 2011) as they struggle to maintain a relationship with formal religions (Dollahite and Lambert 2007; Eliason *et al.* 2011; Henrickson and Staniforth 2012). The resolution for many is to leave their faith communities. A New Zealand study, for instance, found that lesbian, gay and bisexual respondents to a national survey were leaving Christianity at 2.37 times the rate of the general population (which was also increasingly unchurched). Sexual minority respondents who claimed 'no religion' experienced significantly more support from their families of origin, and reported that their families were significantly more likely to include a same-sex partner in family occasions, than those who reported that they were currently

Christian (Henrickson 2007). Tan (2005) found that lesbian and gay respondents who had high existential wellbeing, or spiritual lives, had higher self-esteem, lower internalised homophobia and a lower sense of alienation than those who expressed a sense of religious wellbeing. He suggests that this may be because his respondents had to look beyond organised religion to seek more comprehensive answers to the meaning of existence and faith. Indeed, there is evidence to support that the longer a gay or lesbian person has lived that identity, the more satisfied they are with their lives, even when compared with life satisfaction in heterosexual persons (Henrickson and Neville 2012). Apparently it really does get better, but as queer youth now ask, why should they have to wait?

There are some mainstream religious organisations that welcome sexual and gender minorities (e.g. see chapter on 'LGBTQ affirming environments' in Hunt 2015), and recent polls, such as the May 2015 vote on marriage equality in traditionally Roman Catholic Ireland, and the evolving position of mainstream churches on marriage equality (e.g. the Anglican Church of Canada), suggest that some established religions may be becoming more flexible in respect of full and open inclusion of sexual and gender minorities. There are queer-affirming groups in many mainstream religions today, including the Latter Day Saints and Islam. The dissolution of the 'ex-gay' Christian organisation Exodus International in 2013, and their public apology for the pain and hurt their so-called 'reparative therapies' (which seek to 'repair' homosexuals by claiming to convert them to heterosexuality) had caused (Sundby 2013) seems a step towards recognising how fraught relationships have been between some faith communities and sexual and gender minorities. It is also a public recognition of the futility of attempting to change something as fundamental as sexuality. Additionally, there are established parallel religious organisations catering specifically for sexual and gender minorities. However, Maher (2006) has suggested that such parallel organisations are on the fringes of both religious life and gay and lesbian life.

The role of social work

Social workers are often motivated by their own religious and spiritual beliefs to altruism and to help others. Social workers and gender and sexual minorities who encounter one another in these complex processes and contexts therefore face significant challenges. Social work in this practice area has, I suggest, four tasks:

1   Social workers must understand themselves, and their personal values and motivations around sexuality and gender. Social work values are clearly set out in international ethics documentation (International Federation of Social Work 2012): principles such as human rights, human dignity and social justice set a framework for self-determination, the right to participation, treating each person as a whole, and identifying and developing strengths are a part of our natural discourse; we oppose negative discrimination, recognise diversity and challenge unjust policies and practices. At the same time many social workers come to their work with their own religious and spiritual backgrounds and beliefs about an alphabet of social issues from abortion through to young girls and the Human Papillomavirus (HPV) vaccine. Some workers may be members of faith communities that are hostile or antipathetic to sexual and gender minorities. If a social worker approaches a sexual or gender minority client with an attitude of 'I'm going to save you', or even 'I don't believe in your lifestyle but I can work with you anyway', then the work is doomed from the start. Such attitudes are unprofessional, uninformed and arrogant. The client will sense such attitudes immediately, and will react by closing down or not engaging. Claims have been

made – and addressed – that ignoring the heteronormative values of a practitioner is a kind of oppression, but such claims ignore the tremendous position of privilege and power that heterosexuals enjoy. The social worker with such attitudes has more work to do on him/ herself before they can work in this area.

2   Social workers must have a clear understanding of their personal beliefs about sexual and gender identities, and understand how those beliefs are informed by science. Social workers must be very careful not to replicate gender and sexual binaries. Social workers need to understand that we encounter individuals at moments in time, and that identities, behaviours and relationships evolve over time – and sometimes very brief amounts of time. A young woman who identified herself as lesbian last week may well describe an intimate romantic relationship she is having with a man today. A client who self-identified as male a month ago may identify as genderqueer today. We need to set aside our own expectations and simply encounter the client where they are. Healthy and respectful curiosity is useful in a social worker, because when we engage respectfully with clients we can help them to articulate the questions they have about themselves and their beliefs.

3   Social workers must understand the importance of meaning-making for queer clients, and how important it is to reconcile individual identities with spiritual and religious beliefs. This means that social workers must understand the underlying experience of alienation that gender and sexual minority communities feel from cisgendered, heteronormative institutions such as marriage, families and religions. It requires empathy for the confusion and often deep longing that accompanies this experience of alienation, particularly when these institutions are important to the client. Such empathy may mean respectfully challenging, and perhaps helping someone to exit from, faith systems or institutions that oppress or exclude them, or insist that they change or conform in order to be re-accepted. But social workers who treat sexual and gender minority persons as broken, or in need of help or guidance solely because of their sexuality, do so at their peril, for in doing so they may fail to recognise and critique their own complicity in promoting heteronormative values.

4   Social workers must have a clear understanding of the pervasiveness of cisgendered heteronormativity, and the effect heteronormativity has on themselves, on sexual and gender minorities and on religious institutions. They must work beyond a reflexive therapeutic paradigm that locates problems in individuals, and recognise that sometimes environments must also change. If a religious institution in a community is still touting 'reparative therapy', for instance, then social workers must use their advocacy skills to shut it down as both dangerous and unethical. Good social workers will know the supportive individuals and resources in their communities, and be able to link sexual and gender minority individuals with those resources. It is not the role of social work specifically to address matters of faith or belief, of course. But it is part of our responsibility to point out where those beliefs become self-oppressive, and how maintaining negative beliefs can affect the entire ecology of an individual. Meaning-making can occur in healthy, life- and identity-affirming ways, and the social worker can accompany the client and their families on that important journey.

This chapter promised a perspective to support social workers in helping clients, families, institutions and policymakers to manage differences associated with being a sexual or gender minority. That perspective is quite simply to be an informed, self-aware social worker, who does not replicate heteronormative oppression and stigma. The praxis is to work with clients from a vantage of respect for both person and process. This is both easy and difficult. Readers will know how to be good social work practitioners, but somehow when it comes to something as fundamental as gender, sexuality and identity, professional values can become lost in personal values, opinions and experiences. Our task is to be aware of those personal values, opinions and experiences, to learn from them, and as always allow our clients to teach us so that we will find richer meaning in our own lives.

References

Boellstorff, T. (2005) 'Between religion and desire: being Muslim and gay in Indonesia', *American Anthropologist*, 107(4): 575–85.

Buchanan, M., Dzelme, K., Harris, D. and Hecker, L. (2001) 'Challenges of being simultaneously gay or lesbian and spiritual and/or religious: a narrative perspective', *American Journal of Family Therapy*, 29(5): 435–49.

Cheng, P.S. (2011) *Radical Love: an introduction to queer theology*, New York: Seabury.

Cocker, C. and Hafford-Letchfield, T. (2010) 'Out and proud? Social work's relationship with lesbian and gay equality', *The British Journal of Social Work*, 40(6): 1996–2008.

Congregation for the Doctrine of the Faith. (1986) *Letter to the Bishops of the Catholic Church on the Pastoral Care of Homosexual Persons*. Online. Available HTTP: www.vatican.va/roman_curia/congregations/cfaith/documents/rc_con_cfaith_doc_19861001_homosexual-persons_en.html (accessed 20 February 2008).

Cornwall, S. (2010) *Sex and Uncertainty in the Body of Christ: intersex conditions and Christian theology*, London: Equinox.

Cotton, S., Puchalski, C.M., Sherman, S.N., Mrus, J M., Peterman, A.H., Feinberg, J., Pargament, K.I., Justice, A.C., Leonard, A.C. and Tsevat, J. (2006) 'Spirituality and religion in patients with HIV/AIDS', *Journal of General Internal Medicine*, 21(Supplement 5): S5–13.

Dollahite, D.C. and Lambert, N.M. (2007) 'Forsaking all others: how religious involvement promotes marital fidelity in Christian, Jewish and Muslim couples', *Review of Religious Research*, 48(3): 290–307.

Eliason, M.J., Burke, A., Van Olphen, J. and Howell, R. (2011) 'Complex interactions of sexual identity, sex/gender, and religious/spiritual identity on substance use among college students', *Sexuality Research and Social Policy*, 8(2): 117–25.

Figueroa, V. and Tasker, F. (2014) '"I always have the idea of sin in my mind….": family of origin, religion, and Chilean young gay men', *Journal of GLBT Family Studies*, 10(3): 269–97.

Fone, B. (2000) *Homophobia: a history*, New York: Metropolitan Books.

Fortunato, J.E. (1987) *AIDS, The Spiritual Dilemma*, San Francisco: Harper & Row.

Gold, S.P. and Stewart, D.L. (2011) 'Lesbian, gay, and bisexual students coming out at the intersection of spirituality and sexual identity', *Journal of LGBT Issues in Counseling*, 5(3–4): 237–58.

Guttiérrez, R. (2012) 'Islam and sexuality', *Social Identities: Journal for the Study of Race, Nation and Culture*, 18(2): 15–59.

Hamblin, R.J. and Gross, A.M. (2014) 'Religious faith, homosexuality, and psychological wellbeing: a theoretical and empirical review', *Journal of Gay and Lesbian Mental Health*, 18(1): 67–82.

Hattie, B. and Beagan, B.L. (2013) 'Reconfiguring spirituality and sexual/gender identity: "It's a feeling of connection to something bigger, it's part of a wholeness"', *Journal of Religion and Spirituality in Social Work*, 32(3): 244–68.

Henrickson, M. (2007) 'A queer kind of faith: religion and spirituality and lesbian, gay and bisexual New Zealanders', *Aotearoa Ethnic Network Journal*. Online. Available HTTP: www.aen.org.nz/journal/2/2index.html (accessed 12 February 2008).

Henrickson, M. and Neville, S. (2012) 'Identity satisfaction over the life course in sexual minorities', *Journal of Gay and Lesbian Social Services*, 24(1): 80–95.

Henrickson, M., and Staniforth, B. (2012) 'Living the dream: religion in the construction of sexual identities', *Fieldwork in Religion*, 7(2): 117–33.

Hicks, S. (2008) 'Thinking through sexuality', *Journal of Social Work*, 8(1): 65–82.

Hunt, S. (2003) 'Saints and sinners: the role of conservative Christian pressure groups in the Christian gay debate in the UK', *Sociological Research Online*, 8(4). Online. Available HTTP: www.socresonline.org.uk/8/4/hunt.html (accessed 14 August 2016).

Hunt, S. (2015) *Religion and LGBTQ Sexualities: critcal essays*, Farnham: Ashgate.

International Federation of Social Work (2012) *Statement of Ethical Principles*. Online. Available HTTP: http://ifsw.org/policies/statement-of-ethical-principles/ (accessed 12 June 2015).

International Federation of Social Workers [IFSW] and International Association of Schools of Social Work [IAASW] (2014) *Global Definition of Social Work*. Online. Available HTTP: http://ifsw.org/get-involved/global-definition-of-social-work/ (accessed 3 August 2016).

Irby, C.A. (2014) 'Moving beyond agency: a review of gender and intimate relationships in conservative religions', *Sociology Compass*, 8(11): 1269–80.

Jacobson, C.J., Luckhaput, S.E., Delaney, S. and Tsevat, J. (2006) 'Religio-biography, coping, and meaning-making among persons with HIV/AIDS', *Journal for the Scientific Study of Religion*, 45(1): 39–56.

Kitzinger, C. (2005) 'Heteronormativity in action: reproducing the heterosexual nuclear family in after-hours medical calls', *Social Problems*, 52(4): 477–98.

Kocet, M.M., Sanabria, S. and Smith, M.R. (2011) 'Finding the spirit within: religion, spirituality, and faith development in lesbian, gay, and bisexual individuals', *Journal of LGBT Issues in Counseling*, 5(3-4): 163–79.

Levy, D.L. and Reeves, P. (2011) 'Resolving identity conflict: gay, lesbian, and queer individuals with a Christian upbringing', *Journal of Gay and Lesbian Social Services*, 23(1): 53–68.

Lips-Wiersma, M. (2002) 'The influence of spiritual "meaning-making" on career behavior', *Journal of Management Development*, 21(7): 497–520.

Maher, M.J. (2006) 'A voice in the wilderness: gay and lesbian religious groups in the western United States', *Journal of Homosexuality*, 51(4): 91–117.

Mallon, G.P. (ed) (2008) *Social Work Practice with Lesbian, Gay, Bisexual and Transgender People*, 2nd edn, New York: Routledge.

Melendez, M.P. and LaSala, M.C. (2006) 'Who's oppressing whom? Homosexuality, Christianity and social work', *Social Work*, 51(4): 371–7.

Miller, R.L. (2005) 'An appointment with God: AIDS, place and spirituality', *Journal of Sex Research*, 42(1): 35–45.

Montgomery, S.A. and Stewart, A.J. (2012) 'Privileged allies in lesbian and gay rights activism: gender, generation and resistance to heteronormativity', *Journal of Social Issues*, 68(1): 162–77.

Murr, R. (2013) '"I became proud of being gay and proud of being Christian": the spiritual journeys of queer Christian women', *Journal of Religion and Spirituality in Social Work*, 32(4): 349–72.

Park, C.L. and Folkman, S. (1997) 'Meaning in the context of stress and coping', *Review of General Psychology*, 1(2): 115–44.

Plattner, I.E. and Meiring, N. (2006) 'Living with HIV: the psychological relevance of meaning making', *AIDS Care*, 18(3): 241–5.

Rich, A. (1980/1986) 'Compulsory heterosexuality and lesbian existence', in A. Rich (ed) *Blood, Bread and Poetry*, London: Virago.

Rosik, C.H., Griffith, L.K. and Cruz, Z. (2007) 'Homophobia and conservative religion: toward a more nuanced understanding', *American Journal of Orthopsychiatry*, 77(1): 10–19.

Simoni, J.M., Martone, M.G. and Kerwin, J.F. (2002) 'Spirituality and psychological adaptation among women with HIV/AIDS: implications for counseling', *Journal of Counseling Psychology*, 49(2): 139–47.

Siraj, A. (2012) '"I don't want to taint the name of Islam": the influence of religion on the lives of Muslim Lesbians', *Journal of Lesbian Studies*, 16(4): 449–67.

Solomon, A. (2012) *Far from the Tree: parents, children and the search for identity*, New York: Scribner.

Sundby, A. (2013) *Exodus International, Controversial Ministry Offering 'Alternative to Homosexuality,' to Shut Doors*. Online. Available HTTP: www.cbsnews.com/news/exodus-international-controversial-minis try-offering-alternative-to-homosexuality-to-shut-doors/ (accessed 12 June 2015).

Tan, P.P. (2005) 'The importance of spirituality among gay and lesbian individuals', *Journal of Homosexuality*, 49(2): 135–44.

Teich, N.M. (2012) *Transgender 101: a simple guide to a complex issue*, New York: Columbia University Press.

Walker, J.J. and Longmire-Avital, B. (2013) 'The impact of religious faith and internalized homonegativity on resiliency for black lesbian, gay, and bisexual emerging adults', *Developmental Psychology*, 49(9): 1723–31.

Yip, A.K.T. (2002) 'The persistence of faith among nonheterosexual Christians: evidence for the neosecularization thesis of religious transformation', *Journal for the Scientific Study of Religion*, 41(2): 199–212.

25

From entanglement to equanimity

An application of a holistic healing approach into social work practice with infertile couples

Yao Hong and Celia Hoi Yan Chan

Introduction

Infertility is a 'disease of the reproductive system defined by the failure to achieve a clinical pregnancy after 12 months or more of regular unprotected sexual intercourse' (Zegers-Hochschild *et al.* 2009: 1522). According to a global estimate of infertility prevalence, it was reckoned that approximately 50 million couples were affected by infertility in 2010 (Mascarenhas *et al.* 2012). Many of these infertile couples live with infertility as an unresolved event and suffer the biographical disruption it causes for a lengthy period of time. A growing body of literature is identifying the psychosocial consequences and demands associated with infertility and its relevant treatments (Berger and Henshaw 2013; Boivin and Gameiro 2015).

Given the prevalence of infertility, this chapter argues that social workers need to understand the needs of infertile couples. In this chapter, we will:

1   identify the entanglement state experienced by individuals and couples in the context of infertility;
2   conceptualise the equanimity with the presence of infertility with reference to Eastern philosophy and Traditional Chinese Medicine beliefs;
3   explain the components of spirituality bridging between infertility-associated entanglement and equanimity; and
4   introduce principles and techniques fostering the transformation from entangled state to equanimous state.

Entanglement in relation to infertility

In a pronatalist world, the experience of infertility is a stressful life event among infertile couples, which negatively affects their personal, marital, familial, cultural and social integrity (Greil *et al.* 2010). Across many cultures, couples experience a state of entanglement with a mixture of emotional responses when they are diagnosed as infertile, such as grief, depression, anger, guilt, shock, denial and anxiety (Joja *et al.* 2015; Petok 2006; Sternke and Abrahamson 2014). Loss of identity, self-esteem and social roles tend to cause high levels of depression and anxiety for infertile couples. For women especially, infertility experiences often lead to feelings of being 'inadequate', 'flawed as a woman' and 'embarrassed' (Domar *et al.* 2012).

Theoretically, entanglement refers to a mental state in which the emotive and cognitive mind is preoccupied with a conceptualised idea, hindering one's capacity to experience calmness, inner peace, freedom of choice, which as a result generates pain and suffering. Entanglement could be understood as a sense of affliction rooted in Chinese culture, denoting 'holding on, rigid attachments, and fixation on desirable attributes, values, and behaviours as determined by the individual' (Lee *et al.* 2009: 35). The state of entanglement with regards to infertility could be considered from four aspects: affective responses, inflexible thoughts, maladaptive behaviours and spiritual struggles. For both dyads within infertile couples, anticipatory loss of the child caused by infertility is emotionally abominable, cognitively unacceptable, behaviourally dysfunctional and existentially meaningless.

In the Chinese context, entanglement in relation to infertility happens for good reason. For couples, having children after marriage has not only been viewed as the next developmental task, but also an action essential in order to fulfill their obligations to their family and society at large. Chinese traditional childbearing attitudes are based on Confucianism, in which family values are highly emphasised. Children have been regarded as gifts from nature and family expansion, stability and relationship harmony as being achieved through reproduction (Chin 2005). These beliefs reinforce the importance of childbearing within Chinese families, requiring that the couples responsibly complete their reproductive mission after marriage. Therefore, failure to produce children is seen by Chinese couples as the biggest violation of filial piety and a disgraceful affront to family and ancestors. When childbearing carries symbolic meanings, failure to achieve this mission might bring stress and potential havoc into the lives of individuals, couples and their families.

Within the context of infertility, entanglement may mainly originate from the unresolved perplexing ambiguity regarding the living status of the desired child. Unlike losses resulting from death, infertility retains a physical or psychological presence with child 'in an ongoing manner' (Harris 2011: 2), which results in reoccurring ambiguity and uncertainty. This ambiguity allows infertile couples, and their extended families, to continue hoping for pregnancy success and family building; grief is frozen, relationships stagnate and the uncertainty is ongoing (Boss *et al.* 2011). For infertile couples, their yearnings for a child may not only be ongoing but also co-exist with a state of anticipatory loss due to the physical absence of a child, which may represent their long-term reality.

What is equanimity?

The concept of equanimity comes from the Latin word aequus meaning balanced, and animus meaning spirit or internal state. Aequanimitas is a mental equilibrium that requires clinical thinking and effort in emotional regulation. Major religions, including Buddhism, Hinduism, Judaism, Christianity and Islam, all support the notion of an ideal mentality in which people are able to detach from thoughts, and some even extol the virtue and value of equanimity as one of the sublime states. Equanimity is the ground for developing wisdom and freedom and the nurturing soil of compassion and love. Humanity filled with equanimity is characterised as 'abundant, exalted, immeasurable, and without hostility and without ill will' (from MN 99: Subha Sutta; II 206–8, in Bodhi 2005).

Equanimity is a fundamental technique for emotional regulation and self-exploration for the infertile population. It is difficult for infertile individuals or couples to maintain a balanced mind given exposure to strong internal and external stressors. Looking into infertility experiences, the pain point is right in the middle of extreme emotional contrasts.

Table 25.1 Symbolic manifestations of opposite extremes within infertility context

Infertility-relevant	Fertility-relevant
Loss	Gain
Failure	Success
Incompleteness	Wholeness
Inadequacy	Competence
Despair	Hope
Disappointment	Satisfaction
Sorrow	Happiness
Blame	Honour
Dark	Light
Weakness	Strength
Sickness	Health

When confronted with infertility, individuals and couples might oscillate between the opposite extremes of emotions, presented in Table 25.1. These waves of emotion carry them up and fling them down when efforts to conceive have once again failed. Similar to falling off balance in a physical sense, infertile people who lose emotional sense of balance can end up enduring physical, psychological, spiritual, cultural and social consequences if they become stuck at the infertility-relevant end of the emotional spectrum.

Equanimity is equilibrium of mind, rooted in spiritual insights. Colloquially, equanimity could be considered as an ideal state of wellbeing, in which authentic happiness occurs despite an absence of pleasure. Emotional states associated with equanimity include inner peace, being in love and experiencing joy and pleasure. Infertile individuals who are able to enter into a state of equanimity are not unaware of their infertile status but actively engaged in spiritual healing, and finding internal peace while acutely sensitive to the external desire not to be childless. Therefore, equanimity is not only absence of emotional disturbance, but an active process of building meaningful life alongside the presence of infertility or other stressful events (Chan *et al.* 2014).

Spirituality bridging between entanglement and equanimity

Infertile people frequently mention their religious or spiritual struggles relating to involuntary childlessness. In many cultures, the significance of childbearing is so overwhelming that infertility is accompanied with loss of meaning in their profane and sacred lives. Infertility sometimes discredits individuals' beliefs in faith and is interpreted as punishment for their past mistakes, such as engaging in premarital sex or moral wrong doing (Berger and Henshaw 2013; Dyer *et al.* 2002).

Religious coping has been proven effective in improving health and mental health in nursing practices; for instance, seeking spiritual support, redefining any stressors through religion and engaging in religious activities are associated with health enhancement (Pargament *et al.* 1998, 2004; Weaver *et al.* 2003). Higher levels of religious coping or spiritual wellbeing in infertile women are significantly associated with fewer pathological symptoms and less infertility distress (Domar *et al.* 2001).

Spirituality is increasingly differentiated from religiosity, and understood as embodying fundamental values, beliefs and life meanings. Religiosity refers to a particular doctrinal system that guides sacred beliefs and practices about a higher power (e.g. God), while spirituality refers to 'beliefs and practices that connect people with sacred and meaningful entities beyond themselves' (Roudsari *et al.* 2007: 142).

As spirituality is a broader and more personal overarching construct than religion, spiritual healing for the infertile should entail more general humanistic meanings (e.g. self-compassion, altruism, familyism, nature), rather than narrowly defined as religious coping. Spirituality is supposed to be 'an active investment in internalised beliefs that bring a sense of meaning, wholeness and connection with others' (Walsh 2006: 73). Although infertility is such an overwhelming adversity, it might potentially jeopardise all available experiences of positively-nurtured spirituality, it can also reveal one's values and sense of life meanings in terms of personal identity, family beliefs and life attitudes.

Given to the infertility context, Chan *et al.* (2012) have identified tranquility, letting go of control over pregnancy outcomes and making meanings of children and family as crucial components of spirituality for women undergoing assisted reproductive treatments. Table 25.2 identifies the key spiritual concerns in the context of infertility as life meanings, transcendence and relationship wellbeing. All these proximal variables attached to infertility experiences can be regarded as spirituality, helping the infertile population to survive and transform. In clinical

Table 25.2 Proximal variables of spirituality with infertility

Concepts	Definitions	In the context of infertility
Meaning of life	Significances of living or human existence in general	Infertility is an unexpected threat to one's self values, family beliefs, religious faith, and meanings in work and family life. Infertile people may become disoriented with uncertainty pertaining to childbearing and future life. Infertility is accompanied by a series of losses, such as loss of reproductive rights and ability, family line continuum, self and identity, hope and future, control and so forth. These senses of loss resulted in negative meanings and interpretations towards life. Infertile people will experience a sense of injustice, perplexity and confusion towards life meanings
Transcendence	A sense of being that goes beyond time and space	For many individuals and couples, infertility is ambiguous, nonfinite and unresolved loss. Infertile people often felt stagnant in a transition period, which is characterised by uncertainty and powerlessness. People in liminal stage may feel frustrated and hopeless in developing their identity through fertility. Practicing transcendence focuses on developing self-awareness and self-empowerment, which could help the infertile to go through and grow in infertility experiences. Ultimately, a transcendent person is capable of identifying himself/herself with the reality of infertility throughout time and space
Relationship wellbeing	Connection with self, family, social networks, the world or sacred power	Infertility is both a personal stressor and a relationship crisis. Although marital disruption and marital benefits have been found among couples with fertility problems, it is common for infertile couples to experience uncertainty and instability of the marital relationship and reduced marital satisfaction. Others in the social network may be incapable of providing proper help, resulting in unhelpable behaviours or social isolation. To avoid embarrassment and traumatisation, infertile partners may choose to isolate themselves from familial and social activities

practices, spirituality could be considered as a working focus to help infertile clients transform from entanglement to equanimity

From an Eastern perspective, spiritual wellbeing encompasses one's capacity to endure, and even to accept and value suffering or misfortune; it also includes the capacity to construct and reconstruct meanings in terms of adversities, as well as to maintain peace of mind, spirit and sense of direction in the face of harsh external circumstances (Ng *et al.* 2005). Nurturing this kind of spirituality might equip individuals and couples with the skills needed to accept their infertility, work on readjusting life goals and in turn develop a fulfilling, meaningful life.

Ways to achieve equanimity in response to infertility

In clinical work with infertility, one of the primary goals and obligations of professionals is to facilitate individuals, couples and families to achieve transition from an entangled state to an equanimous balance of life. Spirituality as a domain of human existence is a critical dimension in the interconnectedness of body, mind, spirit and environment. Spiritual healing reaches beyond symptom reduction with the aim of attaining intrapersonal and interpersonal growth. In the specific case of infertility, acknowledging entanglement, creating new meanings from infertility, reconnecting body, mind and spirituality, inviting compassion from social networks and encouraging interdependence within couples are found to be helpful to the healing process.

Acknowledging entanglement

One of the main aims of counselling is to help infertile individuals or couples learn how to tolerate, manage and resolve the difficult experience of infertility (Covington and Burns 2006). For infertile individuals, failure to give birth often leads to a variety of negative emotional responses, such as guilt, shame and inadequacy (Greil *et al.* 2010). Entanglement is also normal for the infertile, irrespective of whether their infertility is temporary or prolonged, treatable or untreatable. Professionals may need to help clients to acknowledge their state of entanglement in an effort to normalise their feelings and thoughts. Expressing their complicated emotions is an important first step for clients to being understood both by themselves and others (e.g. spouse, doctors, therapists, social workers, etc.). In turn, this facilitates further possibilities for meaning exploration and positive self-awareness. Acknowledging their entanglement may be essential if infertile people are to develop an equanimity in which they achieve an acceptance of their infertility.

Reworking meanings attached to infertility

Loss in relation to infertility often undermines spiritual integrity. Unreliability in religiosity and spirituality can bring tremendous pain and despair. Hence, it has been proposed that coming to terms with loss requires a spiritual transformation rather than relinquishment of emotional bonds. In other words, acknowledging and reworking the existing working models of self and the world in the wake of loss may be necessary for meaning reconstruction (Attig 2001). For infertile couples, it is not just meanings directly associated with infertility, but also the implications of this for them as a couple that require validation. Once identified, meanings that are more adaptive, healthy and future-oriented can be fostered, while others that are destructive and detrimental can be challenged.

In terms of practice, the first step for professionals is to learn how to appreciate meanings they find in infertility experiences, even if those are destructive meanings. As there is a possibility that those destructive meanings are coping strategies for other detrimental, life-threating behaviours (e.g. suicide or self-harm), the second step is to understand how these meanings influence the healing process. This process emphasises eliciting, discussing and expressing emotions and thoughts, which could be very healing and transforming. In this step, the professionals should help the clients to confront with meanings they made for infertility. By conceptualising and operationalising alternative meanings, professionals can help infertile people to make sense of their infertility and their lives. The ultimate step is to create new meanings that help the infertile couple to successfully live with the ambiguity of involuntary childlessness.

Reconnecting body, mind and spirituality

Viewing body and mind as two distinct and independent entities may have benefited humanity as the foundation for advances in surgery, trauma care, pharmaceuticals and many other forms of health treatment, but has also inhibited scientific inquiries into humans' emotional and spiritual life, and greatly underestimated the innate ability to heal in many situations. However, since the late twentieth century, there have been considerable efforts to explore the relationship between mind, body and spirit, and this has established the positive impact on physical and mental health of meditation, mindfulness, yoga and other activities that explicitly connect mind, body and spirit (James and Spiegel 2007). Thus, physical health, psychosocial wellbeing and spiritual integrity are interconnected.

Infertility has been historically treated as a physiological disease with a variety of psychological consequences (Greil *et al.* 2010). Entangled emotions, thoughts, beliefs, attitudes and expectations are characterised as complicated mental experiences, which could in turn affect physical health and spiritual wellbeing (Domar *et al.* 2005). The integrative approach has been gradually adopted to help infertile individuals to regain connection of body–mind–spirit and perform self-healing through practicing equanimity (Chan *et al.* 2006).

Accumulating evidence supports that physical and psychological health are associated with spiritual wellbeing. One study interviewed women 20 years after their unsuccessful IVF treatments, and found that adaptive psychosocial functioning could be achieved when the infertile women were capable of developing meaningful interpretations of their infertility experiences (Wirtberg *et al.* 2007). Meaningful interpretation towards infertility experiences provided possibilities for the infertile to find release from preoccupation with childbearing, rebalance the body–mind–spirit connection and achieve feelings of equanimity. One of the most useful skills in order to foster spirituality is to be mindful of when equanimity is absent. For the infertile couples, honest awareness of what makes them imbalanced internally helps them to learn how to regain the balance of body–mind–spirit.

Inviting compassion from social networks

Given that pronatalism is widespread, infertile couples are often severely stressed by pressures from parents, relatives, colleagues, friends, casual acquaintances, religious teachings and society at large (Sternke and Abrahamson 2014). Social disengagement, withdrawal or even isolation are strategies commonly used by couples to escape from the embarrassing moments when asked about childbearing plans. However, not engaging with familial and social networks also makes positive social support unavailable for some couples (Mousavi *et al.* 2015).

Under many circumstances, people from social networks are willing to offer assistance to infertile couples, but may be lacking the capacity and proper methods to provide appropriate help. For instance, maternal or paternal parents might have difficulty in progressing to the role and developmental stage of 'grandparent' if their own offspring remain childless. Although they might share the sadness of the infertile couples, parents' unrealistic expectations and excessive concerns about fertility can turn into pressure, emotional entanglement and psychological distress for the infertile couples, which cause them to withdraw from familial and social engagements.

To maintain social integrity after a diagnosis of infertility, infertile individuals may need to learn how to invite compassion from their social networks. Compassion is different from sympathy or moral judgment. Compassion could be considered as an affective state that is aroused by witnessing another's suffering and that motivates a subsequent desire to help (Goetz *et al.* 2010). When disclosure is made, infertile couples reluctant to express, communicate and negotiate their expectations of support from family and friends will need to overcome their reluctance if support is to be forthcoming.

Encouraging interdependence within dyads

In the process of transition from infertility to involuntary childlessness, one characteristic of childless acceptance is the possible presence of new and meaningful dyadic relationships. This relational transformation requires re-examinations of choices, life goals and future dreams that couples made jointly. It is very likely that husbands and wives differed from each other in terms of childbearing attitudes, treatment decisions, lifestyle choices and so forth. Marital conflicts might be encountered when one partner decides to invest more to continue treatments, while the other partner might be ready to accept the childless lifestyle. Within the infertility context, dyadic incongruence might serve as one primary challenge for counselling. Clinical experiences suggest that infertile couples staying together have the capacity to recommit to each other and reorganise the chaotic situation, though tension and conflicts were inevitable during infertility experiences.

Conclusion

Entanglement and equanimity are both commonly experienced by the infertile as emotional responses to infertility. Spiritual, religious or meaning-oriented reorganisation could be considered as a working focus in promoting holistic wellbeing for infertile people in psychosocial interventions. To realise the therapeutic goals, acknowledging entanglement, reworking meanings attached to infertility, reconnecting links among body, mind and spirit, inviting compassion from social networks and encouraging interdependence within dyads are useful in helping infertile individuals and couples to survive and transform from infertility.

References

Attig, T. (2001) 'Relearning the world: making and finding meanings', in R.A. Niemeyer (ed) *Meaning Reconstruction and the Experience of Loss*, Washington DC: American Psychological Association.

Berger, R., Paul, M.S. and Henshaw, L.S. (2013) 'Women's experience of infertility: a multi-systemic perspective', *Journal of International Women's Studies*, 14(1): 54–70.

Bodhi, B. (2005) *In the Buddha's Words: an anthology of discourses from the Pali Canon*, Somerville, MA: Wisdom Publications.

Boivin, J. and Gameiro, S. (2015) 'Evolution of psychology and counseling in infertility', *Fertility and Sterility*, 104(2): 251–9.

Boss, P., Roos, S. and Harris, D.L. (2011) *Grief in the Midst of Ambiguity and Uncertainty: an exploration of ambiguous loss and chronic sorrow*, New York, London: Routledge.

Chan, C.H., Chan, C.L., Ng, E.H., Ho, P.C., Chan, T.H., Lee, G.L. and Hui, W.H. (2012) 'Incorporating spirituality in psychosocial group intervention for women undergoing in vitro fertilization: a prospective randomized controlled study', *Psychology and Psychotherapy*, 85(4): 356–73.

Chan, C.H., Ng, E.H., Chan, C.L., Ho, P.C. and Chan, T.H. (2006) 'Effectiveness of psychosocial group intervention for reducing anxiety in women undergoing in vitro fertilization: a randomized controlled study', *Fertility and Sterility*, 85(2): 339–46.

Chan, C.H.Y., Chan, T.H.Y., Leung, P.P.Y., Brenner, M.J., Wong, V.P.Y., Leung, E.K.T., Wang, X., Lee, M.Y., Chan, J.S.M. and Chan, C.L.W. (2014) 'Rethinking wellbeing in terms of affliction and equanimity: development of a Holistic Wellbeing Scale', *Journal of Ethnic and Cultural Diversity in Social Work*, 23(3–4): 289–308.

Chin, P. (2005) *Chinese*, San Francisco: UCSF Nursing Press.

Covington, S.N. and Burns, L.H. (2006) *Infertility Counseling: a comprehensive handbook for clinicians*, Cambridge: Cambridge University Press.

Domar, A., Gordon, K., Garcia-Velasco, J., La Marca, A., Barriere, P. and Beligotti, F. (2012) 'Understanding the perceptions of and emotional barriers to infertility treatment: a survey in four European countries', *Human Reproduction*, 27(4): 1073–9.

Domar, A.D., Nielsen, B., Dusek, J., Paul, D., Penzias, A.S. and Merari, D. (2001) 'The impact of spirituality/religiosity on distress in infertile women', *Fertility and Sterility*, 76(3): S198.

Domar, A.D., Penzias, A., Dusek, J.A., Magna, A., Merarim, D., Nielsen, B. and Paul, D. (2005) 'The stress and distress of infertility: does religion help women cope?', *Sexuality, Reproduction and Menopause*, 3(2): 45–51.

Dyer, S.J., Abrahams, N., Hoffman, M. and van der Spuy, Z.M. (2002) '"Men leave me as I cannot have children": women's experiences with involuntary childlessness', *Human Reproduction*, 17(6): 1663–8.

Goetz, J. L., Keltner, D. and Simon-Thomas, E. (2010) 'Compassion: an evolutionary analysis and empirical review', *Psychological Bulletin*, 136(3): 351–74.

Greil, A.L., Slauson-Blevins, K. and McQuillan, J. (2010) 'The experience of infertility: a review of recent literature', *Sociology of Health and Illness*, 32(1): 140–62.

Harris, D.L. (2011) 'Infertility and reproductive loss', in D.L. Harris (ed) *Counting Our Losses: reflecting on change, loss, and transition in everyday life*, New York: Routledge.

James, L. and Spiegel, D. (2007) 'Overview and significant trends', in J.H. Lake and D. Spiegel (eds) *Complementary and Alternative Treatments in Mental Health Care*, Washington DC: American Psychiatric Publishing.

Joja, O.D., Dinu, D. and Paun, D. (2015) 'Psychological aspects of male infertility: an overview', *Procedia: Social and Behavioral Sciences*, 187: 359–63.

Lee, M.Y., Ng, S-M., Leung, P.P.Y. and Chan, C.L.W. (2009) *Integrative Body-Mind-Spirit Social Work: an empirically based approach to assessment and treatment*, Oxford: Oxford University Press.

Mascarenhas, M.N., Flaxman, S.R., Boerma, T., Vanderpoel, S. and Stevens, G.A. (2012) 'National, regional, and global trends in infertility prevalence since 1990: a systematic analysis of 277 health surveys', *PLoS Medicine*, 9(12): e1001356. doi: 10.1371/journal.pmed.1001356.

Mousavi, S.S., Kalyani, M.N., Karimi, S., Kokabi, R. and Piriaee, S. (2015) 'The relationship between social support and mental health in infertile women: the mediating role of problem-focused coping', *Scholars Journal of Applied Medical Sciences*, 3(1D): 244–8.

Ng, S.M., Yau, J.K.Y., Chan, C.L.W., Chan, C.H.Y. and Ho, D.Y.F. (2005) 'The measurement of body-mind-spirit wellbeing: toward multidimensionality and transcultural applicability', *Social Work in Health Care*, 41(1): 33–52.

Pargament, K.L., Koenig, H.G., Tarakeshvar, N. and Hahn, J. (2004) 'Religious coping methods as predictors of psychological, physical and spiritual outcomes among medically ill elderly patients: a two year longitudinal study', *Journal of Health Psychology*, 9(6): 713–30.

Pargament, K.L., Smith, B.W., Koenig, H.G. and Perez, L. (1998) 'Patterns of positive and negative religious coping with major life stressors', *Journal for the Scientific Study of Religion*, 37(4): 710–24.

Petok, W.D. (2006) 'The psychology of gender-specific infertility diagnoses', in S.N.L. Covington and L.H. Burns (eds) *Infertility Counseling: a comprehensive handbook for clinicians*, Cambridge: Cambridge University Press.

Roudsari, R.L., Allan, H.T. and Smith, P.A. (2007) 'Looking at infertility through the lens of religion and spirituality: a review of the literature', *Human Fertility*, 10(3): 141–9.

Sternke, E.A. and Abrahamson, K. (2014) 'Perceptions of women with infertility on stigma and disability', *Sexuality and Disability*, 33(1): 3–17.

Walsh, F. (2006) *Strengthening Family Resilience,* 2nd edn, New York: Guilford.

Weaver, A.J., Flannelly, L.T., Garbarino, J., Figley, C.R. and Flannelly, K.J. (2003) 'A systematic review of research on religion and spirituality in the "Journal of Traumatic Stress" 1990–1999', *Mental Health, Religion and Culture,* 6(3): 215–28.

Wirtberg, I., Moller, A., Hogstrom, L., Tronstad, S.E. and Lalos, A. (2007) 'Life 20 years after unsuccessful infertility treatment', *Human Reproduction,* 22(2): 598–604.

Zegers-Hochschild, F., Adamson, G.D., de Mouzon, J., Ishihara, O., Mansour, R., Nygren, K., Sullivan, E. and Vanderpoel, S. (2009) 'International Committee for Monitoring Assisted Reproductive Technology (ICMART) and the World Health Organization (WHO) revised glossary of ART terminology, 2009', *Fertility and Sterility,* 92(5): 1520–4.

26

Life's end journey

Social workers in palliative care

Martha Wiebe

Introduction

The profession of social work has its historic roots in religion. Much of the early work done by social workers was initiated and funded by churches caring for the poor, the disabled, the orphaned and other marginalised people in society (Cnaan *et al.* 2004; Crisp 2010; Graham *et al.* 2006; Schmidt 2008). As social work became more prominent and strived to become a respected, scientifically-based profession it moved away from religion. Things of the spirit defy scientific measurement and explanation. Evidence-based practice could not incorporate the immeasurable spiritual and religious dimensions and thus they were seen as incompatible with professionalism. Indeed social work made efforts to distance itself from its beginnings and particularly from religion (Gilligan and Furness 2006; Henery 2003; Sheridan and Amato-von Hemert 1999; Streets 2009). In part it was also the case that governments started taking a more active role in delivering many social services and churches thus had a less prominent role to play.

Over the past 20 years, however, there has been renewed interest in spirituality and its interface with social work (Callahan 2009; Canda 1998; Coates *et al.* 2007; Crisp 2010; Furman *et al.* 2004; Graham *et al.* 2006). In this chapter I will explore both the role and importance of spirituality and religion in end of life care. I will also make a case for the inclusion in social work curricula of topics that deal with spirituality and religious thought. In particular, I will point to the significance of religion particularly at the end of life and will draw on my experience as a volunteer working in a hospice setting. The case examples in this chapter do not represent any person, alive or dead but are composites of people I have encountered at the hospice. Names have been changed and no other identifying information is used.

This chapter is based on my experiences of working in Canada. Religion continues to play a significant role in the lives of many Canadians. A recent survey found that 'a solid core of Canadians continue to embrace the Christian faith and other religious traditions' (Angus Reid Institute 2015). Thirty per cent of Canadians surveyed embrace religion, and for people over the age of 55 this was slightly higher. Another 44 per cent indicated some ambivalence to religion but did not reject it. Of the people who indicated that they embraced religion, eight out of ten indicated that their faith strengthened them. Another finding in this survey was that 'more than 70 per cent of Canadians today express belief in a "Supreme Being"' and 66 per cent expressed a belief in life after death. These are important findings when considering work in palliative care. To dismiss religion as irrelevant is problematic and perilous.

Definitions

While spirituality has saliency in recent social work literature, religion continues to be viewed with some suspicion and scepticism in many quarters of the profession (Cnaan *et al.* 2004). The literature on spirituality has dissociated itself from religion (Henery 2003). The concern about proselytising has discouraged social work from paying attention to the religious dimension as a part of many people's lives. Proselytising would be in violation of the code of ethics and any attempt to evangelise is unethical; however, taking into account the role of religion in some people's lives should be an important piece of an assessment (Furman *et al.* 2004). Of course, spirituality and religion are not two distinctive entities exclusive of one another; indeed, there is a great deal of overlap. A person who is religious adheres to a set of beliefs and doctrines generally shared in a community of other like-minded believers. Spirituality on the other hand is seen as a personal experience that does not necessarily subscribe to a community's shared beliefs or rituals (Callahan 2009; Jacobs 2004; Streets 2009). In this chapter I will refer to both spirituality and religion.

Hospice care and palliative care will be used interchangeably. Palliative care is defined by the World Health Organization [WHO] as care of people when a cure is no longer available for their illness. The focus in palliative care is on physical comfort and in addressing spiritual and emotional needs (Sepulveda *et al.* 2002; WHO 2002). The objective is to provide comfort measures so that people can have the best quality of life possible in their remaining days or months. Hospice care is a subset of palliative care that tends to take place outside of a hospital, either in the home or in a community hospice facility.

End of life issues

When patients and their families receive the news that all treatment options have been exhausted and that palliative care is recommended, it can be devastating. Disbelief, hopelessness and anger are emotions that frequently surface. Staring into the abyss, the unknown, is daunting. The dying process is enveloped in mystery. Questions emerge: What will happen to me? How and when will the end come? What happens after that? Is there life after death? What is the meaning of my death? And what is the meaning of my life? Can there be meaning to my suffering and if so what is it? These existential questions raise profound issues that can be deeply spiritual whether or not people are religious. Callahan (2009: 169–70) has noted that 'even when patients denied having religious beliefs, they expressed spiritual needs that included a desire for meaning, purpose and transcendence'.

People working in palliative care must be skilled in responding to existential questions and issues. The directive in palliative care is to consider the physical, emotional, social and spiritual needs of the person. The holistic approach of social work parallels that of palliative care. The emphasis is on caring for the person regardless of their social class, ethnicity, race, sexual orientation, gender or religion (Berzoff and Silverman 2004; Csikai 2004; Gilligan and Furness 2006).

While social work purports to view the whole person, most social workers have limited or no training in addressing religious and spiritual questions and frequently lack confidence in dealing with these issues when they arise (Hegarty *et al.* 2010). Canadian social workers in a recent study indicated that they felt unprepared for working with dying people and their families (Bosma *et al.* 2010). Similarly an American study found that workers were trained and competent in preparing advanced health directives but felt inadequate in addressing cultural differences and religious and spiritual issues (Csikai and Raymer 2005). Many expressed discomfort in dealing with questions related to God, the soul and life after death. These were seen as the purview of the chaplain. While the chaplain may be at ease in addressing these concerns, in many facilities chaplains are present only periodically. When these issues arise it is important that the helper in the room, whether it is a nurse, doctor or social worker, be able to respond in a caring and appropriate manner.

In many respects social workers should be well positioned to work in the area of terminal/palliative care in that they have a family focus and are familiar with helping people deal with loss (Clausen *et al.* 2005; Gwyther *et al.* 2005). Lloyd (1997: 175) identified that 'working with loss and grief has long been identified as integral to core social work skills, social workers recognizing the pervasive and cumulative effects of loss on so many of their clients'. Social workers are familiar with supporting people when they experience the loss of employment, the apprehension of children, the loss of their health or of their home. The distinguishing characteristic of working with the dying and the bereaved is the spiritual or religious dimension of the work. Lloyd found that:

> when focusing on the experiences of dying or bereaved persons, a total of 82 per cent of the social workers thought that *spiritual pain* was always, most times or sometimes present; 77 per cent also felt that *philosophical questioning* was always, most time or sometimes present.
>
> (Lloyd 1997: 184)

Skills for working in palliative care

The requisite social work skills of listening, supporting and empowering are fundamental to working in palliative care. However, when people are dying, many of them will seek religious and spiritual support to help them cope with their terminal illness (Callahan 2009). The skills already incorporated into the social worker's tool kit require additional honing to take into account the importance of faith.

A social worker's childhood and personal experience with religious institutions may have left them feeling disenchanted and possibly hostile toward religion. To work in palliative care it is important that workers critically analyse how their view of religion may be shaping and distorting their practice with people who are struggling with existential questions as they near the end of their life (Todd 2007). Consequently, 'by not re-examining personal biases social workers may overlook the importance of religion and thus forego the opportunity to connect in a deep and meaningful way with the people they are serving' (Wiebe 2014: 343).

Open communications

Workers need to be open to hearing people's stories and listening to their feelings of doubt, anxiety and fear, and accompanying them in their attempts to find meaning in their suffering.

> It is the ability to hear people talk about their faith and their religious beliefs and to recognize how these may be an anchor for them in their end of life journey. This might include being present in meditation and prayer with the patient. The role of the helper is to try to understand fully the person who is dying. While we will never be able to understand fully what that person is experiencing, the importance is in listening, and attempting to understand.
>
> (Wiebe 2014: 344)

It is imperative that workers are not dismissive of the spiritual dimension and recognise in a respectful way the importance of religious beliefs and personal faith. When the worker has a level of comfort with and an understanding and appreciation of the patient's religion, it can form the basis of a trusting, genuine relationship between them.

Empathy

Empathy is the ability to feel along with a person, trying to step into the other person's shoes and hear where that person is coming from. It is the ability to have a compassionate presence. A recent study of cancer patients in Toronto found that the ability of the therapist to respond in a caring and empathical manner was the most helpful attribute (Nissim *et al.* 2012). While I was at the hospice one evening I heard a woman calling out from her bed: 'I can see the headline in the newspaper now; "woman dies and no one cares".' I walked into the room, sat with her and held her hand, reassuring her that I cared. She was feeling very anxious and fearful that she might die in the middle of the night when no one was in the room. I understood her anxiety and reassured her that the staff at the hospice were available 24 hours a day and that we tried very hard to ensure that no one died alone. Holding her hand seemed to calm her and she started verbalising her fear of dying. She mentioned that she used to believe in God but had stopped going to church some years ago and now felt abandoned by God. We spoke at some length about her family who had visited her earlier that evening and with whom she appeared to have a good relationship. I listened to her and reassured her that God's love shone through other people and going to church was not God's prerequisite. She smiled as I left the room and soon fell asleep.

It is important that workers are vigilant to recognise spiritual distress and be open to hearing people's fears and anxieties. Plantive (2015) suggests that we be bold in the questions we ask and the discussion we invite with people in palliative care. Giving patients permission to have the difficult discussions also means allowing them to control the conversation (Gawande 2014).

Reviewing the past

Our daily lives are frequently marked by planning for the future – what we need to accomplish today or this week or in the coming months, where we plan to travel, what our short- and long-term career goals are and so on. Our view tends toward what lies ahead. At the end journey a somewhat different pattern emerges, that of looking back. This is a time when people look in the rear view mirror of what their lives have been. It can be a time to contemplate significant relationships and one's accomplishments but also to consider the unfinished business in one's personal life. Engaging with people in reviewing their lives is a therapeutic role the social worker can play.

A recent experience I had at the hospice was with a 65-year-old woman. When Matilda was admitted she expressed disappointment and anger at being referred to the hospice. She resisted the idea of palliative care but all treatment options had been exhausted. Her chart indicated that staff and volunteers should avoid using the term hospice or palliative care with Matilda – she did not want to face the fact that a cure was no longer an option for her. Matilda was a single woman with no family nearby. During her time at the hospice she had few visitors and indeed requested that a note be taped on her door asking visitors who came to restrict their visit to 15 minutes. Matilda appeared to be depressed. Nolan (2011) reminds us that when patients lose hope that recovery is possible they can fall into profound despair.

One evening after I had assisted her in eating her dinner I asked her about her work and learned that she had held a high level professional job in government. She spoke about the challenges in her work but also how rewarding it was. I asked her about the things she was proudest of and she mentioned the many accolades she had received when she retired a year previously. She noted that when she looked back she felt privileged to have had such a full professional life. She was raised Catholic and although she didn't attend church she indicated that she still had a belief in God. When I was ready to leave her bedside she took my hand and with a smile on her face said, 'Thank you for this. It was so good to have a meaningful conversation'. When I returned a few days later I learned that Matilda had died peacefully the previous evening.

Providing opportunities for reconciliation

In looking back at one's life, people sometimes focus on unresolved issues. There are regrets about disrupted relationships. When someone is admitted into the hospice we periodically receive information from the patient or the family that one or another of the family members is estranged from the dying person. Sometimes the patient does not wish to discuss this, but at other times they struggle with the estrangement and want to find ways of mending the relationship. Releasing a burden the dying person is carrying may happen through the simple act of listening without judgment and encouraging the patient to talk. Social workers can also try to facilitate reconciliation. If both parties to the estrangement are open to talking, a bridge can be built; however, this is not always an option. When Philip was admitted into the hospice, he had not had contact with his son for over 15 years and had no information about where he might be and no way to reach him. Indeed he did not even know whether his son was still alive. It was clear that there was a great deal of residual psychic pain around this fractured relationship. Although a reunion was not possible, I encouraged Philip to speak about the relationship. He spoke about what went wrong and how he wished he had reacted differently to his son. He mentioned that his son had a serious drug problem and how this caused Philip a great deal of worry, anger and pain. Then at some point he looked up from his pillow and said, 'I forgive him and hope that he can forgive me'.

At the hospice a common refrain in the dying chapters of someone's life is dealing with regrets. 'Social workers can help give expression to these regrets, encouraging patients not only to review their lives but also to gently help them find forgiveness, both of others, and of themselves' (Wiebe 2014: 347). Dealing with unfinished business has particular urgency in a palliative care setting for both patients and their loved ones. It is important to validate the pain but also to point out and recognise that failure is human and we have all made mistakes. Trying to work through regrets and unfinished business to forgiveness will help the person find peace. Spiritual comfort and guidance can help people come to terms with past conflicts, feelings of guilt and regret and to see the divine hand in forgiveness.

Importance of rituals

Jacobs (2004: 192) suggests that 'the use of rituals, prayer, meditation, or scripture may elicit feelings of joy, comfort and peace'. Rituals can be one of the significant comfort measures at the end of life. Prayer and meditation are commonly-used methods that hospice patients rely on (Callahan 2013; Jacobs 2004). Workers who are uncomfortable with this miss an opportunity for a profound encounter with the patient at a critical time in life. Social workers need to recognise and be at ease with prayer and with talking about God.

I have frequently observed the importance of religious rituals for the dying person as well as for those sitting at their bedside. Religious symbols are often in evidence; a crucifix hung over the doorway or the Torah on the bedside table. Some Muslims request that we position the hospice bed so that the dying person faces toward the Holy Mosque in Mecca. For Catholics there is the request for the last rites and many find comfort in praying the rosary. Michel had lost much of his sight so he asked his family to tape a picture of Jesus on the railing of his bed so that when he woke up he could see it. Susan had a rosary on her bedside table and would pray the rosary when she woke up at night and felt fearful. She would also ask me to read to her from the Bible, particularly from the Psalms. All these measures can provide some degree of support and comfort to dying people and their loved ones.

Social work education for end of life care

Schools of social work for the most part do not have spirituality or religion as part of the core curricula (Canda and Furman 2010; Csikai and Raymer 2005; Oxhandler and Pargament 2014). This lack of training is particularly critical for those who will work with the dying and the bereaved. A recent US survey of clinical social workers reported a low level of integrating clients' religion and spirituality in their clinical practice (Oxhandler et al. 2015). Yet in palliative care an appreciation and understanding of religion and spirituality is an important professional asset. Furness and Gilligan (2010: 2186) have argued that 'those affected by ill health and life crisis may turn to religious or other belief systems as ways to support and comfort them in times of need, especially when conventional health treatment has failed to cure or aid recovery'. While some workers might feel uncomfortable with religious talk, they must be vigilant in recognising spiritual distress and be open to engaging sensitively with patients' spiritual concerns.

In our highly secularised society, many students may have had very limited exposure to religious thought and faith. Curriculum content should include 'models of spiritual development and religious traditions, content on understanding and accepting diversity in religious and spiritual values, and assessment and intervention skills related to religious and spiritually sensitive practice' (Sheridan and Amato-von Hemert 1999: 127). Although they may not be religious, students need to develop an awareness of their own values and beliefs particularly regarding their own mortality and learn about the importance of faith. An exploration of this in the classroom could offer an opportunity for them to reflect on their own concepts regarding death. Thinking about their own spirituality can help workers guide patients in an exploration of their spiritual beliefs and needs. Students also need to broaden the frame and learn about religious values, beliefs and practices across different cultures and faiths. Inviting this discussion in the classroom must be done in such a way as not to imply a certain kind of answer or to evangelise. In the same way inviting this discussion at the bedside must be done sensitively:

> the prohibition on proselytizing should not be construed as a prohibition on asking patients about their spiritual or religious beliefs and practices. Skillful spiritual screening, history-taking, and assessments should not be threatening to patients or specific to one denomination, faith, tradition or philosophical orientation.
>
> (Puchalski et al. 2009: 901)

Conclusion

Many Canadians in the twenty-first century believe in a God or Supreme Being. Faith can be an anchor in people's lives and tends to have particular significance and poignancy toward the end of life's journey. This dimension of people's lives however has been ignored to a large extent in the training of social workers. While social work education provides students with the essential skills of helping people deal with pain and loss, the religious element has not been given prominence. Recognising and undergirding the religious beliefs and faith that support people as they face death is an area in social work curricula that requires more attention. An appreciation of spirituality and religion can contribute to rich and meaningful relationships as people enter the final chapter of their lives.

References

Angus Reid Institute (2015) *Religion and Faith in Canada Today: strong belief, ambivalence and rejection define our views*. Online. Available HTTP: http://angusreid.org/faith-in-canada/ (accessed 25 November 2015).

Berzoff, J. and Silverman, P.R. (eds) (2004) *Living with Dying: a handbook for end-of-life healthcare practitioners*, New York: Columbia University Press.

Bosma, H., Johnston, M., Cadell, S., Wainwright, W., Abernethy, N., Feron, A. and Nelson, F. (2010) 'Creating social work competencies for practice in hospice palliative care', *Palliative Medicine*, 24(1): 79–87.

Callahan, A.M. (2009) 'Spiritually-sensitive care in hospice social work', *Journal of Social Work in End-of-Life and Palliative Care*, 5(3–4): 169–85.

Callahan, A. (2013) 'A relational model for spiritually-sensitive hospice care', *Journal of Social Work in End-of-Life and Palliative Care,* 9(2–3): 158–79.

Canda, E.R. (ed) (1998) *Spirituality in Social Work: new directions*, Binghamton, NY: The Haworth Press.

Canda, E.R. and Furman, L.D. (2010) *Spiritual Diversity in Social Work Practice: the heart of helping*, 2nd edn, New York: Oxford University Press.

Clausen, H., Kendall, M., Murray, S., Worth, A., Boyd, K. and Benton, F. (2005) 'Would palliative care patients benefit from social workers' retaining the traditional "casework" role rather than working as care managers? A prospective serial qualitative interview study', *The British Journal of Social Work*, 35(2): 277–85.

Cnaan, R A., Broddie, S.C. and Danzig, R.A. (2004) 'Teaching about organized religion in social work: lessons and challenges', *Journal of Religion and Spirituality in Social Work*, 23(3): 67–84.

Coates, J., Graham, J.R., Swartzentruber, B. and Quellette B. (eds) (2007) *Spirituality and Social Work: select Canadian readings*, Toronto: Canadian Scholars' Press.

Crisp, B.R. (2010) *Spirituality and Social Work*, Farnham: Ashgate.

Csikai, E.L. (2004) 'Social workers' participation in the resolution of ethical dilemmas in hospice care', *Health and Social Work*, 29(1): 67–76.

Csikai, E.L. and Raymer, M. (2005) 'Social workers' educational needs in end-of-life care', *Social Work in Health Care*, 41(1): 53–72.

Furman, L.D., Benson, P.W., Grimwood, C. and Canda, E. (2004) 'Religion and spirituality in social work education and direct practice at the millennium: a survey of U.K. social workers', *The British Journal of Social Work*, 34(6): 767–92.

Furness, S. and Gilligan, P. (2010) 'Social work, religion and belief: developing a framework for practice', *The British Journal of Social Work*, 40(7): 2185–202.

Gawande, A. (2014) *Being Mortal: medicine and what matters in the end*, Toronto: Random House.

Gilligan, P. and Furness, S. (2006) 'The role of religion and spirituality in social work practice: views and experiences of social workers and students', *The British Journal of Social Work,* 36(4): 617–37.

Graham, J., Coholic, D. and Coates, J. (2006) 'Spirituality as a guiding construct in the development of Canadian social work: past and present considerations', *Critical Social Work*, 7(1). Online. Available HTTP: www1.uwindsor.ca/criticalsocialwork/spirituality-as-a-guiding-construct-in-the-development-of-canadian-social-work-past-and-present-cons (accessed 25 November 2015).

Gwyther, L.P., Altilio, T., Blacker, S., Christ, G., Csikai, E. L., Hooyman, N., Kramer, B., Linton, J. M., Raymer, M. and Howe, J. (2005) 'Social work competencies in palliative and end-of-life care', *Journal of Social Work in End-of-Life and Palliative Care*, 1(1): 88–120.

Hegarty M.M., Abernethy, A.P., Olver, I. and Currow, D.C. (2010) 'Former palliative caregivers who identify that additional spiritual support would have been helpful in a population survey', *Palliative Medicine*, 25(3): 266–77.

Henery, N. (2003) 'The reality of visions: contemporary theories of spirituality in social work', *The British Journal of Social Work*, 33(8): 1105–13.

Jacobs, C. (2004) 'Spirituality and end-of-life care practice for social workers', in J. Berzoff and P.R. Silverman (eds) *Living with Dying: a handbook for end-of-life healthcare practitioners*, New York: Columbia University Press.

Lloyd, M. (1997) 'Dying and bereavement, spirituality and social work in a market economy of welfare', *The British Journal of Social Work*, 27(2): 175–90.

Nissim, R., Freeman, E., Lo, C., Zimmerman, C., Gagliese, L., Rydall, A., Hales, S. and Rodin, G. (2012) 'Managing cancer and living meaningfully (CALM): a qualitative study of a brief individual psychotherapy for individuals with advanced cancer', *Palliative Medicine*, 26(5): 713–21.

Nolan, S. (2011) 'Hope beyond (redundant) hope: how chaplains work with dying patients', *Palliative Medicine*, 25(1): 21–5.

Oxhandler, H.K. and Pargament, K.I. (2014) 'Social work practitioners' integration of clients' religion and spirituality in practice: a literature review', *Social Work*, 59(3): 271–9.

Oxhandler, H.K., Parrish, D.E., Torres, L.R. and Aschenbaum, W.A. (2015) 'The integration of clients' religion and spirituality in social work practice: a national survey', *Social Work*, 60(3): 228–37.

Plantive, R. (2015) *Suffering in Palliative Care: an overview of methods to alleviate suffering*, Maycourt Hospice, Ottawa: Canada.

Puchalski, C., Ferrell, B., Virani, R., Otis-Green, S. and Baird, D. (2009) 'Improving the quality of spiritual care as a dimension of palliative care: the report of the consensus conference', *Journal of Palliative Medicine*, 12(10): 885–904.

Schmidt, G. (2008) 'Social work and the social gospel in Canada: historical overview and implications for future practice', *Social Work and Christianity*, 35(2): 167–78.

Sepulveda, C., Marlin, A., Yoshida, T. and Ullrich, A. (2002) 'Palliative care: the World Health Organization's global perspective', *Journal of Pain and Symptom Management*, 24(2): 91–6.

Sheridan, M.J. and Amato-von Hemert, K. (1999) 'The role of religion and spirituality in social work education and practice: a survey of student views and experiences', *Journal of Social Work Education*, 35(1): 125–41.

Streets, F. (2009) 'Overcoming a fear of religion in social work education and practice', *Journal of Religion and Spirituality in Social Work*, 28(1–2): 185–99.

Todd, S. (2007) 'Feminist community organizing: the spectre of the sacred and the secular', in J. Coates, J.R. Graham, B. Swartzentruber and B. Quellette (eds) *Spirituality and Social Work: select Canadian readings*, Toronto: Canadian Scholars' Press.

Wiebe, M. (2014) 'Social work, religion, and palliative care', *Journal of Religion and Spirituality in Social Work*, 33(3–4): 339–52.

World Health Organization [WHO] (2002) *WHO Definition of Palliative Care*. Online. Available HTTP: www.who.int/cancer/palliative/definition/en/ (accessed 22 November 2013).

27

Social work and suffering in end-of-life care

An arts-based approach

Irene Renzenbrink

Introduction

Social workers encounter profound human suffering in many fields of service and are called upon to help and support people at critical points in their lives. There are times when the suffering can be alleviated and other times when solutions will be extremely difficult to find. End-of-life care and bereavement are areas of social work practice that call for a response to suffering that goes beyond the usual repertoire of psychosocial interventions. This chapter will explore some of the challenges that social workers face in end-of-life care and bereavement support and, in particular, how the expressive and creative arts can provide resources that enhance coping and resilience for patients, families and for the workers themselves. Case vignettes drawn from my work as an art therapist and social worker in palliative care will be used to illustrate these themes. Arts-based research is a relatively new field of qualitative research and its methods of inquiry are increasingly being used to further understanding of this very complex area of human service and engagement with people who are vulnerable as they prepare for death. The potential of using collage as a particular example of an arts-informed method for research and practice will be discussed in relation to dying and bereavement.

Facing death: a spiritual challenge

As Kearney (1996) reminds us, death remains the ultimate separation and no matter how skilled and humane our care, there is nothing that can make it all better. For some people, he says, 'dying has become a time of terrified struggle or meaninglessness despite the best efforts of family and caregivers to comfort and palliate their distress' (Kearney 1996: 23). Social workers may themselves be engaged in 'terrified struggle' from time to time as they explore some of the biggest questions about life, death, suffering and fairness – the questions to which Rabbi Harold Kushner (2004) refers in his book, *When Bad Things Happen to Good People*. Struggling to find meaning in his son's death from a rare disease at the age of 14, Kushner decided that although life is not always fair, and 'the wrong people get sick and the wrong people get robbed and the wrong people get killed in wars and in accidents' (2004: 52), it is the compassionate response to tragedy and the sharing of others' pain and vulnerability that ultimately helps us to make sense of suffering. When we respond to pain and vulnerability in others, it could be said that we enter the spiritual domain, defined in the broadest sense by Holloway (2005: ix–x) as 'the inner life of human beings, all that is left when you have fed or sheltered them, and that's just about everything that's important to them'. A more succinct and focused definition of spirituality, arrived at by a group of palliative care practitioners led by Puchalski, is as follows:

> Spirituality is the aspect of humanity that refers to the way individuals seek and express meaning and purpose and the way they experience their connectedness to the moment, to self, to others, to nature, and to the significant or sacred.
>
> (Puchalski *et al.* 2009: 887)

This is echoed by Eckersley (2007: 54) when he describes spirituality as 'a deeply intuitive, but not always consciously expressed, sense of connectedness to the world in which we live'. When I think about the patients I have met in palliative care over the years it is this connectedness that stands out. They live the remainder of their life in precious moments with family, friends and their professional caregivers, often surrounded by special objects and mementoes, acutely aware of the beauty of nature. While this might sound idealised and not easily achieved in a hospital environment unless the rooms are specially designed and oriented towards gardens and sky, it is important to try to create an environment in which the patient feels at home and at peace. For some people home is the best place to die but for others it can be the worst. It will depend on the resources and support that is available to them. Although relief of pain and other distressing symptoms is vitally important if there are to be healing conversations and leave taking, many encounters in end-of-life care and expressions of love and devotion go beyond words. The creative and expressive arts can play an important role. Self-awareness, willingness to face one's own mortality and give expression to grief that is experienced both personal and professionally is a vital prerequisite for working effectively in end-of-life care. The reward for this effort, apart from enriching encounters with patients and their families, is the development of a deeper spiritual awareness and appreciation of life for the practitioner.

Spiritual pain

The suffering experienced by people facing their own death has been referred to as 'spiritual pain'. Dame Cicely Saunders, a nurse, social worker and physician who founded St. Christopher's Hospice in London in 1967, is recognised as the 'outstanding innovator' in the field of hospice and palliative care (Clark 2002: 905). It was Saunders who established a new kind of scientifically-based tender loving care for dying people and their families. In contrast to previous medical neglect, there was a new openness about the terminal condition that recognised the importance of fostering dignity, meaning and the patient's humanity. Although suffering was no longer seen as a symptom or a problem to be solved, there was a need for some kind of acknowledgement and conceptualisation of the complexity of the dying experience. Saunders developed the concept of 'total pain', which included physical, emotional, social, financial and spiritual pain. She understood the interplay of practical and emotional struggles but also the pain that comes 'from the depths of a person's being' (Kearney 1996: 14). Saunders (1988) also acknowledged the needs of staff in this work when she said, 'It is hard to remain near pain, least of all an anguish for which we feel we can do nothing. We are wounded healers and we need the support of our whole group in this work.'

Michael Kearney, an Irish palliative care physician, uses the term *soul pain* to describe a particular form of suffering for the dying person. He has written that 'We may fear anticipated physical pain and distress, the emotional pain of separation from those we love and the dependency and loss of control, which, we imagine, lie ahead' (Kearney 1996: 15). However, soul pain refers to a deeper layer of fear, an 'existential and primal fear of the unknown that is more like our fear of the dark' (Kearney 1996: 15), and Kearney goes on to describe soul pain as a 'wasteland of meaninglessness and hopelessness' (1996: 1).

Eckhart Tolle (2003) says that it is a great privilege and a sacred act to be present at a person's death as a witness and companion. Yet, social workers are not always comfortable with this aspect of their helping role and may wish to call on the chaplain or another professional team member to engage with patients and families at such a time. However, the ability to respond to a dying patient is a rare opportunity and Tolle urges us to surrender to every aspect of that experience. He says, 'do not deny what is happening and do not deny your feelings. The recognition that there is nothing you can do may make you feel helpless, sad or angry ... you are not in control' (Tolle 2003: 111).

As social workers that also offer bereavement counselling and support to individuals and families after someone dies, we need to recognise this helplessness, especially when the death is unexpected or particularly complicated. As Parkes (1972: 175) explains, 'The helper cannot bring back the person who's dead and the bereaved cannot gratify the helper by seeming helped'.

Sharing in brokenness

Social workers in end-of-life care are asked to enter into places of pain and to respond with compassion and wisdom based on their professional and personal life experiences. In his exploration of compassion in end-of-life care, Larkin (2016: 4) refers to Henri Nouwen's belief that compassion asks us to go 'where it hurts, to enter into places of pain, to share in brokenness, fear, confusion and anguish'. Larkin (2016: 7) argues that compassion requires 'resilience, fortitude, and sometimes risk taking, but always tenacity and determination'. It is not enough to feel compassion. A compassionate response is an active one.

The extent to which compassionate involvement can be sustained will depend on many things, including the resources available to us in the workplace as we struggle to make sense of tragedy. Skilled supervision and support from our superiors and colleagues can help us to set realistic goals and acknowledge our achievements. We will need a balanced workload with opportunities for creativity or 'something for the soul' as a wise senior social worker once suggested. Sometimes there will be a need for personal therapy and healing activities such as meditation or other spiritual practices. At other times, 'time out', physical exercise and laughter with family and friends will alleviate stress and cast away thoughts of difficult work encounters. Most importantly and often neglected is the grieving that we need to do ourselves, not only for the actual or fantasised deaths of people close to us but also for the little deaths or dyings we experience in life. The poet Kenneth Patchen (1957: 3) captures this idea perfectly with the words, 'There are so many little dyings it doesn't matter which one of them is death'.

David Browning (2004: 22) believes that when we accompany others through tragic life events, 'our own experiences with suffering and the sense we make of those experiences, constitute both the starting and ending points of these explorations'. Using his mother's death when he was 13 as a starting point for an exploration of what he has learned as an oncology social worker and in his work with dying patients, Browning poignantly reminds us of our responsibility to understand our personal reservoirs of suffering. Working with a therapist and through poetry writing, he began to find meaning in his mother's death and this discovery, in turn, helped him to enter fully and faithfully into relationships with clients experiencing significant loss.

Art and healing

In his book, *The Emotional Cancer Journey*, Michele Angelo Petrone (2003) describes his harrowing experience of cancer treatment. He died in 2007, aged 43, after 13 years of struggling with Hodgkin's disease and involvement in programmes that promoted awareness of the healing power of art. As an artist in residence for a group of hospices in the south of England, he taught fellow patients and their carers about using art to promote spiritual and emotional wellbeing. He believed that the journey of illness was not only about the physical illness but also about the emotional response. It was the human face of care and not just treatment that contributed to the healing of what he described as his 'tortured soul' (Petrone 2003: 26). He also wrote about having a 'guardian angel ... a sense of faith in the invisible inner strength, perhaps a combination of everyone who has helped' (Petrone 2003: 34).

Robert Pope was a Canadian artist who died of Hodgkin's lymphoma in 1992 at the age of 36 after a 10-year battle with the illness. He also described his experience in his paintings, many of which have been used extensively in medical education since his death. In 'Sparrow' Pope painted a man lying in bed gazing through a window at a sparrow sitting on the branch of a tree:

> One haunting memory of my illness is spring. From my window all I could see were the tops of horse-chestnut trees, covered with beautiful blossoms. These blossoms seemed to say to me all I was feeling. They became for me encouragement to persevere, a symbol of recovery. This image also shows the sparrow. I have tried to contrast a number of opposites: outside and inside, the horizontal man with the vertical bird and trees, passiveness and activity, illness and health. The man and the bird share the same vulnerability and strength.
>
> (in Stewart 2005: 794)

Metaphors and symbolic language

Listening with a third ear to symbolic language is very important when working with dying and bereaved people. The capacity to tune in and to be moved by something that is profound and meaningful has been referred to in the expressive arts therapy literature as 'empathic attunement' (Kossak 2015: 3). Attunement is described as an immersion in the present moment and a sensory awareness of ourselves, others and the spaces we inhabit. Being attuned to our own 'sensory presence and internal pulse' (Kossak 2015: 105) is regarded as very important in establishing rapport and working empathically with patients in end-of-life care. Being fully present in this way requires a more imaginative and heart-felt involvement than traditional psychosocial assessment and intervention-based on the biomedical model.

It has been more as an art therapist than as a social worker that I have become aware of opportunities for this kind of empathic attunement through art making, non-verbal communication and connectedness through symbols and metaphors. The word metaphor is derived from the Greek *meta* meaning above and beyond, and *phorein*, meaning to carry from one place to another. Metaphor can be regarded as a way of knowing that engages the imagination. Art therapy and other expressive arts approaches such as poetry, movement and creative writing are not always recognised as tools for healing and spiritual development, and yet there is growing evidence of the need for a more imaginative approach to suffering, or what Levine (1997: 2) refers to as 'the healing *of* the imagination *by* the imagination'. Allen (1995: 3) goes even further when she says that our imagination is the most important faculty that we possess and that it is through our imagination that we discern possibilities and options. It represents the 'deepest voice of the soul'.

Art therapy in palliative care

The following vignettes show that art therapy can lift patients' spirits when they are very ill. An art-making opportunity with a trained therapist can provide respite from a focus on medical problems and on everything that is 'wrong'. Drawing and painting can be used for reminiscence and life review as patients recall happier times. Sometimes the colours, materials and actions that are chosen can convey strong feelings of anger, sadness and regret. The process of creating the image is seen as an end in itself and its meaning is not necessarily interpreted nor discussed.

James was an 85-year-old man with lung cancer who was very distressed about his shortness of breath. As I accompanied the doctor on her daily round, I heard James say, 'What happens now, doctor. If I can't breathe there's nowhere to go, is there?' In other words, if I can't breathe I will die. He was afraid of running out of breath. As a sensitive palliative care physician, the doctor was able to listen to James who began to weep as he spoke of his fears and sadness about leaving his wife behind. She was very frail and he had been her carer. He never expected to be the first to 'go'. Not having picked up a coloured pencil since childhood, James was not sure about doing any kind of art activity. However, when he told me that he had always been interested in black and white photography I suggested that he might try drawing with a stick of charcoal. After I showed James how to make simple squiggles to get the feel of the charcoal on paper, he spent many hours sketching the tree outside his window and various objects in his room. He said that 'it took his mind off things' and he felt more at peace. He proudly showed his sketch book to his visitors.

Audrey, a 65-year-old woman whose husband had died two years previously in the same unit confided in me: 'No one thinks I'm capable any more. I feel so useless.' Her adult children were very protective and highly anxious given that they had already lost one parent and were facing the death of another. She had been on a cruise when she became ill and the next thing she knew she was dying from ovarian cancer. When offered an opportunity to do some painting, she began to make cards for her grandchildren and chose an image for each child. A horse for one child, a boy playing cricket for another and a dancing ballerina for her granddaughter. She was able to lose herself in this activity and said, 'This is fun!' When the grandchildren came to visit her, I provided materials for them and they created cards and drawings for her in return. These were attached to the wall in front of her hospital bed to remind her of this very special family connection.

Jan, 68, used watercolour crayons to draw and paint a number of her favourite holiday places. She had become ill just before moving into a retirement village with her husband and derived great pleasure from quietly creating and reminiscing. She and her husband had planned their retirement very carefully and were both very sad that the dream would not now be realised. Watercolour crayons are particularly suitable for people who are frail as they are able to use a light touch to draw something on paper and by adding water with a brush there is a flowing movement of colour on the page. It is often experienced as a soothing and pleasurable activity and patients often take delight in seeing a crayon line drawing transform into a watercolour painting with a few brush strokes.

Paul, a 56-year-old architect, enjoyed drawing ships when he felt well enough to join other patients in the main lounge room of the palliative care unit. He was always critical of his artwork and struggled to get the sails 'right'. Despite all efforts to relieve his symptoms he was in constant pain and was often bad tempered or withdrawn with the nursing staff and with his visitors. One day he invited me to bring some art materials to his room. Choosing dark blue pastel paper and various coloured soft pastels, Paul swiftly and purposefully drew a scene that he described as 'the cosmos'. He then proudly drew a TARDIS, the time machine from the BBC *Doctor Who* television series. With tears running down his cheeks he said, 'I don't know where I'm going ... but I know that I am not staying'. Paul was able to return to his home for a short time before returning to the palliative care unit to die. The name he gave to his drawing was 'The Journey'.

Fragmentation in bereavement

The idea that grief and bereavement are fragmenting experiences is reflected in the language that is used by bereaved people after the death of someone they have loved deeply. Terms such as 'falling apart', 'broken', 'shattered' and 'in pieces' are frequently used to convey the intensity of their grief. Levine (1997: xvi) believes that it is 'essential for human being (sic) to fall apart, fragment, disintegrate, and to experience the despair that comes with lack of wholeness' and that it is by moving into the experience of the void that the possibilities for creative living arise and a new form of existence begins to emerge. One of the ways in which grieving and bereaved people can 'put themselves together again' creatively is through collage. Moon (2001a: 18) defines the creation of collage as 'a structured activity that engages a client in making choices and organising materials, and can be symbolic of creating order out of fragmented aspects of life or chaotic feelings'.

Sharon Strouse, an art therapist whose 17-year-old daughter died by 'falling' off the roof of her college dormitory, created collages for 'transformation and healing' and to 'reaffirm and construct a world of meaning that had been challenged by the loss' (Strouse 2015: 187). The name Strouse (2013) has given to this process is 'artful grief' and she has published her collages and story in a book by that name. She also conducts workshops for other bereaved people. Strouse (2015: 192) describes her creative process as 'unlocking doors to unexplored feelings' and made the discovery that she felt empowered through the act of creating. A further example of the use of collage and creativity for healing of grief and bereavement is offered as follows. It is a fine example of 'artful grief'.

Cat among the leaves

Emma was a participant in a workshop I conducted for counsellors and therapists on the theme of 'Loss, Grief and Bereavement: An Arts-Based Exploration'. In the workshop Emma had engaged in a collage activity, which she later described as 'meditative and therapeutic' although she had struggled with the set task. I had invited participants to bring a copy of a photograph of a person or place that they associated with loss and grief and had spoken about the fragmentation inherent in bereavement experience. It was an attempt to symbolically explore what was lost or broken and to try to do some repairing and healing through cutting and pasting in a photomontage or collage activity.

I did not know that Emma's mother had recently died and it was not until we corresponded after the workshop that I learned more about her experience of grief and the creative process she had engaged in. She had been very quiet and fully absorbed in her creative task on that day and had been reluctant to share thoughts with fellow participants after the art-making activity. I had been deeply moved by the image she had created of a small black cat nestling in among golden leaves that she had painstakingly cut out of some wrapping paper.

Emma's description of the process of creating the collage conveys something of the mystery and beauty that often surprises people when they allow themselves to enter into the unknown or as Allen (2005: 2) puts it, the 'place of all possibilities'. Emma's grief about her mother's death, her own vulnerability, her love of cats and their attachment to her all seemed to converge as she struggled to begin:

How could I even start to put something so big into such a small space? ... Then I saw the fabric with the little black cat prints and something clicked in. It tugged at an edge of something I was feeling, though I didn't try to make sense of it and the creative process had started. Anyway, when I saw the fabric with the little black cat I intuitively picked it up. Then I saw that golden leaf paper and I knew that the cat needed to be inside among them, it was a feeling. Cutting it all out until it fitted my felt sense of it all felt very meditative and therapeutic. Like something was settling into place. I think it was certainly a process that allowed me to symbolise my experience into something tangible. ... the grief often feels bigger than me and it has a magical, transpersonal or spiritual element to it. I don't have ideas to attach to it. I often feel deep sadness. But often I also find myself sitting with a sense of awe at the vastness and intricate nature of it all. I can't control it ... it's scary and beautiful all at once. I breathe and be and try not to get too overwhelmed. Making it turned out to be a very honest moment for me.

Emma's feeling about the spiritual element in her art making resonates with Farrelly-Hansen's (2001) suggestion that art making is inherently spiritual, and spirituality is an important ingredient in therapy or in becoming whole. It is essentially a search for meaning, new answers and fresh perspectives. Allen (2005:2) believes that art making can be a 'spiritual path' and can lead us to 'new places in ourselves, our work, our relationships and our communities'. Through art making Emma was able to develop new insights and a greater acceptance of the grief she was experiencing following her mother's death. Her love for her cat was a source of sustenance because this was the cat that had 'rescued her' when she was at her most lost and vulnerable. For some reason Emma's collage had moved me deeply and when we exchanged email messages about the process it was interesting to learn that far from being a small vulnerable figure her cat in among the leaves was in fact quite a powerful creature. It was an assumption or projection on my part and a reminder to keep one's own experience separate even when others' images trigger our own feelings and thoughts. I began to wonder about strength and vulnerability and the connection between them. Social workers who enter into the places of pain when people are dying or grieving will need to embrace this kind of ambiguity.

Arts-based research

While the interrelationships between research, theory and practice in the field of social work are now well established, there was a time when social workers found it difficult to articulate the complex nature of their interventions with vulnerable populations. Ethical issues aside it was not always possible to capture the uniqueness and efficacy of the helping encounter. Arts-based practitioner-researchers face a similar dilemma in that they struggle to define what they do and what it means. As Hartley (2008: 51) explains, 'There is about the creative process and the object that is created something of the wordless; no group of words can accurately describe what is seen or heard'.

Arts-based research practices offer qualitative researchers alternatives to traditional research methods (Leavy 2009). They draw on such things as literary writing, poetry, music, dance, visual art and collage, and these media may be used in all phases of the research endeavour, not just in its final representation. McNiff argues that art-making by the researcher should be included in an inquiry and that we need to be able to distinguish between artistic knowing and scientific understanding. He also believes that research methods and questions need to arise from the unique character of the art experience because 'art is a way of knowing, problem solving, healing and transformation that we marginalize if we do not embrace it as a vehicle for research' (McNiff 2013: xiii).

Collage, a word derived from the French, *coller*, meaning to stick, refers to a genre in which 'found' materials that are either natural or made up are cut up and pasted onto a flat surface. The use of collage as a form of visual inquiry is particularly appropriate in bereavement given the often shattering and fragmented nature of grief experience. Butler-Kisber describes three approaches for using collage. Collage can be used in a memoing/reflective process, to conceptualise or to elicit writing or discussion or perhaps all three. As she goes on to explain, 'the researcher works in an intuitive and non linear way using disparate fragments and joining them in ways that can produce associations and connections that might otherwise remain unconscious' (Butler-Kisber 2008: 270.

Collage can be used to both formulate and respond to a research question, for example by creating art cards or small-scale collages to express themes. In writing an autobiographical dissertation and narrative inquiry, one arts-based researcher made a collage before beginning a new section. Evaluation of arts-informed research using images as well as writing poses further challenges for the field including those related to copyright. It might be helpful for practitioners and researchers (Moon 2001b: 50) to keep an art journal to 'capture images of daily life' without analysing or judging them. The images can be about experiences, objects or emotions and Moon suggests working in the art journal for a short time each day.

Conclusion

As social workers in end-of-life care, we will be required to enter into the spiritual domain as we empathise, seek to understand and assist patients and their families at the most vulnerable of times. We will be called on to witness their suffering, confront our own mortality and ultimately, try to find meaning in these experiences. I believe that it is through remaining open and connected that the answers will come. I would like to urge readers to explore the potential of the expressive and creative arts to literally make sense of difficult experiences through the senses, through art making and soulful practices that nourish our own spirits as we try to nourish those of others.

References

Allen, P. (1995) *Art Is a Way of Knowing*, Boston: Shambhala Publications.

Allen, P. (2005) *Art Is a Spiritual Path*, Boston: Shambhala Publications.

Browning, D. (2004) 'Fragments of love: explorations in the ethnography of suffering and professional caregiving', in J. Berzoff and P. Silverman (eds) *Living with Dying: a handbook for end-of-life health care practitioners*, New York: Columbia University Press.

Butler-Kisber, L. (2008) 'Collage as inquiry', in J.G. Knowles and A.L. Cole (eds) *Handbook of the Arts in Qualitative Research: perspectives, methodologies, examples and issues*, Los Angeles: Sage Publications.

Clark, D. (2002) 'Between hope and acceptance: the medicalisation of dying', *British Medical Journal*, 324(7342): 905–7.

Eckersley, R.M. (2007) 'Culture, spirituality, religion and health: looking at the big picture', *Medical Journal of Australia*, 186(10): S54–6.

Farrelly-Hansen, M. (ed) (2001) *Spirituality and Art Therapy: living the connection*, London: Jessica Kingsley Publishers.

Hartley, N. (2008) 'The palliative care community: using the arts in different settings', in N. Hartley and M. Payne (eds) *The Creative Arts in Palliative Care*, London: Jessica Kingsley Publishers.

Holloway, R. (2005) *Looking into the Distance*, Edinburgh: Canongate.

Kearney, M. (1996) *Mortally Wounded: stories of soul pain, death and healing*, New York: Scribner.

Kossak, M. (2015) *Attunement in Expressive Arts Therapy: toward an understanding of embodied empathy*, Springfield, IL: Charles C. Thomas Publisher.

Kushner, H.S. (2004) *When Bad Things Happen to Good People*, New York: Anchor.

Larkin, P.J. (2016) *Compassion: the essence of palliative and end-of-life care*, Oxford: Oxford University Press.

Leavy, P. (2009) *Method Meets Art: arts-based research practice*, New York: The Guilford Press.

Levine, S.K. (1997) *Poiesis: the language of psychology and speech of the soul*, London: Jessica Kingsley Publishers.

Moon, C. (2001a) *Studio Art Therapy: cultivating the artist identity in the art therapist*, London: Jessica Kingsley Publishers.

Moon, C. (2001b) 'Prayer, sacraments, grace', in M. Farrelly-Hansen (ed) *Spirituality and Art Therapy: living the connection*, London: Jessica Kingsley Publishers.

McNiff, S. (2013) *Art as Research: opportunities and challenges*, Bristol: Intellect.

Parkes, C.M. (1972) *Bereavement: studies of grief in adult life*, Harmondsworth: Pelican.

Patchen, K. (1957) *Selected Poems*, New York: New Directions Books.

Petrone, M.A. (2003) *The Emotional Cancer Journey*, London: MAP Foundation.

Puchalski, C.M., Ferrell, B., Virani, R., Otis-Green, S., Baird, P., Bull, J., Chochinov, H., Handzo, G., Nelson-Becker, H., Prince-Paul, M., Pugliese, K. and Sulmasy, D. (2009) 'Improving the quality of spiritual care as a dimension of palliative care: the report of the Consensus Conference', *Journal of Palliative Medicine*, 12(10): 885–904.

Saunders, C. (1988) *Spiritual Pain*, London: St. Christopher's Hospice.

Stewart, M. (2005) 'Reflections on the doctor-patient relationship: from evidence and experience', *British Journal of General Practice*, 55(519): 793–801.

Strouse, S. (2013) *Artful Grief: a diary of healing*, Bloomington, IN: Balboa Press.

Strouse, S. (2015) 'Collage: integrating the torn pieces', in B.E. Thompson and R.A. Neimeyer (eds) *Grief and the Expressive Arts: practices for creating meaning*, New York: Routledge.

Tolle, E. (2003) *Stillness Speaks*, Novato, CA: New World Library.

Part VI
Social work practice

28

Religious literacy in public and professional settings

Adam Dinham

Introduction

Religious literacy is a term that has been in use for some years (Wright 2016), though it has been used relatively rarely and vaguely. More recently it has grown in use and popularity, and it has been observed that it has growing traction anywhere that people encounter increasingly plural landscapes of religion and belief (Davie 2015). This makes it an issue for everyone, regardless of personal religion or belief. After all, billions of people around the world remain religious, despite the assumptions of secularity, which had expected religion and belief to decline in social significance and eventually to disappear to a vanishing point. Indeed, sociology had predicted exactly this disappearance by the year 2000 (Berger 1967), though this statement has been challenged and revised since (Berger 1999). Eighty-four per cent of the global population reports a religious affiliation, according to the Pew Research Center (2012). Millions of these religious people are in Britain, Europe and the West. Globalisation and migration mean we encounter religion on a daily basis; however, the crisis is that, after decades in which we have barely talked about religion and belief, society has largely lost the ability to do so. In many cases, it has largely lost the understanding of why it might be legitimate and pressing to discuss religion in the first place.

Religious literacy in health and social care

It has been argued that this discussion is urgent and pressing in every public setting (Dinham and Francis 2015). This chapter explores ways in which religion might have a particular significance within health and social care. This appears to be one of the most populated front lines for religious literacy, where public professionals meet great numbers of individuals and a growing diversity of spiritual beliefs and needs: in England there are 13.9 million users of emergency rooms and 70,000 children in care each year. Furthermore, 25 per cent of English adults have a mental illness (UK Government 2014).

It is also the case that health and social care professions frequently claim to embody a systemic understanding of the person as physical, mental, social and spiritual, and in England and Wales, for example, have recently re-emphasised the importance of practitioners considering their work as care in a context of compassion (Cummings and Bennett 2012). At the same time, many health and social care providers and educators employ chaplaincies as a resource for all, and in some cases these are legally mandated (for example, in UK hospitals). Yet curricula for training and education of health and social care professionals appear largely to neglect religion and belief, and the resources (such as chaplaincies) associated with them. Curricula instead reflect a wider secularised sensibility in higher education, which over-emphasises natural scientific paradigms and epistemologies at the expense of the wisdoms of care that reside in traditions of spirituality, religion and belief (Dinham and Jones 2010a). Within this scope, health and social care education tends especially towards medical models and social scientific accounts of the person, which can obscure the spiritual (Furness and Gilligan 2014).

At the same time, because health and social care is a public issue, these settings find themselves on a front line with public policy-making too, which is itself heavily inflected with secular assumptions that militate against engagement with the issue of religiously literate practices of health and social care (Dinham and Francis 2015). Conversely, a range of policy documents, regulations, benchmarks and professional guidelines hint at a role for spirituality in health and social care, referring to 'wellbeing' and the 'holistic person'. However, these references tend to be minimal, largely undefined and non-operationalised, as, for example, the so-called 'health and wellbeing boards' established by the UK Health and Social Care Act 2012.

Thus, research on religion in nursing education is limited to a focus on encouraging spiritual sensitivity (Catanzaro and McMullen 2001). The limited research on the relationship between religion and counselling and psychotherapy education has tended to focus on attitudes and capabilities of practitioners (Carlson et al. 2002; Walker et al. 2004). While the role of religion in social work education is slightly better established, this research has tended to focus on the attitudes of staff (Sheridan et al. 1994) or students (Sheridan and Amato-von Hemert 1999) as to whether or not religion or spirituality should be involved in social work education. Where work has focused on the need for better teaching on the connections between religion and social work (Gilligan and Furness 2006; Russel 1998), there is a neglect of the diverse belief and practice contexts in which practitioners will work, and little is offered by way of exactly what kinds of knowledge are required, and for which contexts.

With researchers tending to use the term 'spirituality' as a proxy for religion and belief, a clear link has been established between spirituality and mortality, coping and recovery (Puchalski 2001; Yates et al. 1981), counselling and psychotherapy (Powell and Cook 2006) and social care needs (Gilligan and Furness 2006; Pentaris 2012). Yet the implications of this link for practitioners are extremely demanding in the context of the radically and increasingly diverse array of religious and nonreligious beliefs and practices found in the UK. It also elides the distinctions between spirituality, religion and belief, which have overlaps but are not the same things. The use of proxies may itself be indicative of the religious literacy problem, reflecting the inability to talk well about religion and belief, which is identified as a core starting point of the problem. In any case, there is no evidence of how this manifests, if at all, in lecture halls in professional training, and students' opportunities for formation in this area are largely unknown.

This adds up to a health and social care environment of intense religious diversity alongside an emphasis on the restoration of compassion and care, and little or no capacity or language for connecting or engaging them. Very little is understood about the role, legitimacy, impacts and meanings of religion and belief in public and professional life in general, and in health and social care in particular. In this context, the question of how to prepare practitioners to engage with the real religious landscape becomes fundamental to providing holistic and effective care.

The religious literacy problem

At the root of the religious literacy critique is the observation that there is a lamentable lack of conversation about religion and belief, just as we need it most (Davie 2015). There are similarities with the state of public discourse on race in the 1960s and gender in the 1970s – that is to say, with some prominent voices, and large numbers of stakeholders, but a generally unformed popular way of talking about it. In the cases of race and gender, many people thought that because people were not talking about being black or being a woman, there was not really a problem. This applied (and in many cases continues to apply) to same-sex relationships too. As Furness and Gilligan (2014) suggest, for a long time this has also been the case on religion or belief. We have tended to end up hearing about them only when things go wrong. Developing a discourse for everyone seems like a pressing task, therefore, and it needs to be both thoughtful and theorised on the one hand, and publicly accessible and practical on the other.

As I have observed elsewhere, the conversation has revolved around four key elements that make religious literacy widely relevant and pressing (Dinham 2015). First there is diversity, which is a matter of cohesion. Second is globalisation, which is a matter of the export and import of trade and culture. Third is equality, which is a matter of good employee practice and service user experience. Fourth is extremism, which is a matter of security. This is a lot for religious literacy to be handling, and part of success is knowing which you are handling, and when. It cannot all be done at once, in one place, with one purpose. It is context specific. And as the concept of religious literacy grows in usage and popularity, it is also increasingly contested.

Part of this contested nature lies in differing ideas of its purpose. Versions include better faith to faith engagement (Barnes and Smith 2015), biblical literacy in various forms, especially in the US (Prothero 2007) – about regaining a sense of a Christian West in the context of growing plurality – a strand that is committed to peace-building (Moore 2015), and versions that are interested in the relationships between religion and non-religious people (Dinham and Francis 2015). It is also important to pay attention to the interface between spaces that are religious and those that are not – and especially of workplaces and other everyday shared spaces, such as medical settings, and social, cultural and educational institutions.

Another aspect of religious literacy that is contested is who needs to be doing it – both the talking and the listening. A tempting answer for many in the West has been that it is best done in some kind of secular way, which reflects a wider idea that secularity somehow equals neutrality, and that this is an essential condition for the impartial inclusion of all. But nobody starts from nowhere and there is no such thing as neutrality. The secular is a normative notion, and is as much misunderstood as religion itself. Secular literacy is an inescapable part of religious literacy because secularity is the assumed context of religiousness. Religious literacy requires clarity about what both concepts could mean. Thus, Wilson's (1966) proposal that religion is losing its social significance is taken on by Berger's (1967) suggestion that religion will disappear to a vanishing point. Davie (1994) counters with the observation that people believe without belonging, and Hervieu-Leger (2000) inverts this to add that people are also belonging without believing. Woodhead (2013) concludes that while traditional religion may be in decline, new spiritual and informal forms are thriving. Bruce (2013) dismisses this, saying that all this religion talk is nothing but a last gasp before it finally disappears, as originally predicted.

The Religious Literacy Programme

In my conception of it, the religious literacy idea has evolved out of the Religious Literacy Leadership in Higher Education Programme [RLLPHE], established in 2009, which has since worked with more than 600 participants across 130 universities (Dinham and Jones 2010a, 2010b, 2010c). This came initially out of anxiety about extremism on university campuses. I started by challenging the focus on the issue of extremism itself. I argued that no approach to religious literacy would start well from there. It was also important to point out that extremism, on campuses and elsewhere, is not only rare but also difficult to define and judge. Universities are supposed to be places for the exploration of difficult ideas, including radical ones. Where one draws the line is an obvious and highly fraught question. I argued that it would be much more effective and realistic to set religion and belief in their proper contexts as normal, mainstream and widespread. Universities were a good place to start because, as these assumptions are produced and reproduced in university settings, they are presumed to become part of the formation of minds that underpins the public conversation in wider society.

We carried out semi-structured interviews with 21 university vice chancellors and/or their deputies and determined what sort of stances they thought their universities took in relation to religion and belief. We also asked what concerns them in relation to religion and belief.

In relation to the first question, we identified four university stances, or 'types', which appear to be translatable into a range of other sectors and settings across wider society (Dinham and Jones 2012). In the first type, the university is conceived of as a secular space where public institutions remain neutral as far as possible and education avoids mentioning religions or belief. We called this group 'soft neutral'. A similar but firmer line we identified seeks the protection of public space from religious faith, asserting a duty to preserve public bodies, such as universities, as secular. We called this group 'hard neutral'. Others saw religious faith as a source of learning and formation and a larger number of the VCs we spoke to took this view, with many stressing that their campus is friendly to religions and religious people, and comfortable with religious diversity. We called this group 'repositories and resources'. The fourth approach we identified aims to offer education 'for the whole person', incorporating religious or belief dimensions. This perspective was more common in universities that were founded as religious institutions, and we called this group 'formative-collegial'.

The second issue we asked about was what sorts of matters about religion preoccupy vice chancellors and other university leaders. Here we found that practical and policy concerns inflected the debate. Vice chancellors were concerned about issues in four key areas. First, they were focused on legal action arising out of possible discrimination on the grounds of religion and belief; second, on campus extremism and violence; third, on being able to market their universities to students of all religious and belief backgrounds and none; and fourth, especially about appealing to international students, including those from all parts of the world, and from all religious and belief traditions, identities and backgrounds. These were very concrete and practical concerns, and could be primarily characterised in terms of anxieties detectable in wider society, about being sued and being bombed. On the other hand they were interested in the potential opportunities, as well as the risks, in terms of 'widening participation' and attracting international students. This too reflects an interest in faith groups in wider society for what they can bring to the table, in welfare and in the provision of schools particularly.

We also conducted case study research in three universities to understand the narratives of religious faith as experienced by students and staff. This enabled us to dig down into the many practical ways in which faith plays out in universities much more widely (Dinham and Jones 2012). We found students who had not felt able to attend interviews, or exams Saturday lectures because of clashes with religious events. There were anxieties regarding public speakers and what to 'allow' them to say on topics such as Israel and Zionism. Timetabling staff were worried about how to handle the years after 2014 when Ramadan coincides with exam periods. Canteens and bars were taking all sorts of stands for or against halal food, alcohol-free events and single-sex socials, and there were bitter rumours in one institution that the Muslims were receiving subsidised lunches. There were sports societies whose members were ribbing a Sikh for wearing the 5 Ks (worn by orthodox Sikhs: kesh – uncut hair; kara – armband; kangha – comb; kacchera – knee length shorts; and kirpan – sword). Residences were struggling with kosher kitchens and women-only halls. Campus banks either could or could not handle the requests of Muslim students for halal borrowing for student fees, while counselling services felt they could not discuss religion with religious students.

The theoretical and empirical work would never be useful if it was not also linked to action, and the programme had an action orientation built in from the outset. The intention was to translate what we found theoretically and empirically into training, and this was developed in a wide range of areas. We devised training workshops for vice chancellors and their senior delegates, designed to draw their attention to the critique and analysis we had undertaken and to stimulate university leaderships to consider their own stances and how these affected the tone and practice of their institutions. We also delivered training workshops to upwards of 600 HE staff – academic and administrative – from more than 100 universities. These workshops explored the analyses and stances evolved from the leadership work, but also strove to induce bottom-up solutions to concrete dilemmas in student services, timetabling, accommodation, food and alcohol, dress and etiquette, and a whole range of practical issues and settings. This included our devising specialist workshops on religion and belief law and in conflict resolution, in partnership with expert bodies in these areas.

A religious literacy framework

The experience of this process of thinking, researching, training and reflecting has led to the development of a religious literacy framework that is intended as a way of thinking about religion and belief, not only in university spaces, but across wider society. It is presented as a journey in four parts: categorisation, disposition, knowledge and skills.

This begins with conceptualising religion and belief and why they matter (Dinham and Jones 2012). This stage is called 'categorisation'. It asks 'what do we mean by religion and how can we think about it?' There is limited understanding of how much religion and belief have changed over the past century. The dominance of the idea of secularity in sociology as the primary lens through which to understand religion has translated into its social dominance more broadly. So understanding the real religious landscape, and the idea of the secular that frames it, is just as important as understanding the religion and belief within it. While we know that the religious and the secular are hugely debatable categories, the trends are clear enough, pointing to how religious forms have been changing in this period, as well as the religious mix and the mix of religion and non-religion. To do religion justice, therefore, religious literacy requires a stretchy understanding of religion to include religious traditions, such as Baha'i, Buddhism, Christianity, Hinduism, Islam, Jainism, Judaism, Sikhism and Zoroastrianism; informal, non-traditional religion, to do with nature, goddesses, angels and afterlife; non-religion, including secularism, atheism and humanism; and non-religious beliefs, such as environmentalism and veganism. At the same time it demands an understanding that European societies continue to be secular but also Christian and plural, and that moreover, all of these things are happening together. Knowing which religion and beliefs we think count, what we mean by secular, and what purpose we are pursuing – security, cohesion or something else – is key.

The second phase is 'disposition'. This asks 'what emotional and atavistic assumptions are brought to the conversation and what are the affects of people's own emotional positions in relation to religion or belief?' Like politics, almost everybody feels they know something about religion and belief, and often this is experienced highly personally. This emotional dimension is important not least because religion or belief deal in things that deeply matter, such as values, life, death and sex. It is also important because there may be significant gaps between what people feel, what they think, and what they know in relation to religion and belief, and this can hinder religious literacy when ideas and emotions unintentionally conflate. Indeed, not addressing our feelings about religion or belief is likely to be part of why the conversation is often ill-informed and grumpy – obsessed with the ways in which religion and belief clash or oppress people. People feel strongly. What we tend to end up with is a muddled conversation, often mired in anxiety about violence and sex, and leading to knee-jerk reactions. Controversies abound, often about same-sex marriage and violence. Media reflects and sometimes inflates them. Such muddles demand that we get to grips with religion as it is lived in the public sphere. Moving from the sub-textual and emotional – the largely untested assumptions and emotions that underpin so much experience – to the expressly understood will be crucial if citizens and students are to engage thoughtfully with the religion and belief they encounter.

The third phase of religious literacy is rooted in 'knowledge'; but not comprehensive knowledge – that is obviously impossible. The Religious Literacy Programme talks about 'a degree of general knowledge about at least some religious traditions and beliefs' and the confidence to find out about others. The knowledge that is needed is about the shape of religion and belief you find yourself. This is referred to as 'the real religious landscape' (Dinham and Shaw 2015), and it obviously varies from place to place and time to time. An engagement with religion and belief as identity, rather than tradition, is required, which releases us from the notion that we can and ought to learn the A–Z of a tradition, as though this is always the same, everywhere, in every person. Rather, it is about recognising that the same religions and beliefs are different and differently lived by different people in different places. Sometimes they differ within the same person, from one day to the next.

This leads directly to the fourth and final aspect of religious literacy, which is 'skills'. This is where clarity about religion and belief as a category, along with an open disposition, and *some* knowledge of *some* religious practices and beliefs, translates into what to *do* in practice, especially in public and work places. The Religious Literacy Programme usually does this in two stages: first, by auditing the challenges and needs, sometimes through a highly formal research process; at others through a lighter touch, depending on the time and resources available to the setting. Second, those findings are translated into training that fits, often through facilitated co-production with people in those settings. This recognises that religions and beliefs cannot be understood as monolithic blocks of unchanging tradition, the same for everyone, but are lived, contingent and fluid. Responses must fit needs and opportunities where they are made.

Conclusion

This approach makes religious literacy a framework, not a recipe. You cannot say 'do this' and religious literacy will result. It has different purposes, contents and outcomes in different settings. In relation to training for the public professions, students have come to almost entirely lack a framework for thinking or engaging well with religion and belief, yet globalisation, migration, equality and human rights discourses put them in daily contact with the greatest religious and belief diversity in history. Challenging the post-religious and secular assumptions that characterise universities in general, and health and social care training in particular, will be key to unlocking the conversation. Discovering the challenges, needs and opportunities is a pressing task for research. Responding in ways that do not collapse into more comfortable proxies, like spirituality, is crucial if we are to socialise professionals and citizens in the distinctions as well as the overlaps between religious and other aspects of identity.

References

Barnes, M. and Smith, J. (2015) 'Religious Literacy as Lokahi: social harmony through diversity', in A. Dinham and M. Francis (eds) *Religious Literacy in Policy and Practice*, Bristol: Policy Press.

Berger, P. (1967) *The Sacred Canopy: elements of a sociological theory of religion*, New York: Doubleday.

Berger, P. (1999) 'The desecularization of the world: a global overview', in P. Berger (ed) *The Desecularization of the World: resurgent religion and world politics*, Michigan: William B. Eerdmans.

Bruce, S. (2013) *Secularisation: in defence of an unfashionable theory*, Oxford: Oxford University Press.

Carlson, T.D., Kirkpatrick, D., Hecker, L. and Killmer, M. (2002) 'Religion, spirituality, and marriage and family therapy: a study of family therapists' beliefs about the appropriateness of addressing religious and spiritual issues in therapy', *The American Journal of Family Therapy*, 30(2): 157–71.

Catanzaro, A.M. and McMullen, K.A. (2001) 'Increasing nursing students' spiritual sensitivity', *Nurse Educator* 26(5): 221–6.

Cummings, J. and Bennett, V. (2012) *Compassion in Practice: nursing, midwifery and care staff – our vision and strategy*. Online. Available HTTP: www.england.nhs.uk/wp-content/uploads/2012/12/compassion-in-practice.pdf (accessed 9 August 2016).

Davie, G. (1994) *Religion in Britain since 1945: believing without belonging*, Oxford: Blackwell Publishing.

Davie, G. (2015) 'Foreword', in A. Dinham and M. Francis (eds) *Religious Literacy in Policy and Practice*, Bristol: Policy Press.

Dinham, A. (2015) *What Is the Future for Religion in Britain?* Online. Available HTTP: www.theosthinktank.co.uk/comment/2015/02/04/what-is-the-future-for-religion-in-britain-1 (accessed 9 August 2016).

Dinham, A. and Francis, M. (2015) (eds) *Religious Literacy in Policy and Practice*, Bristol: Policy Press.

Dinham, A. and Jones, S.H. (2010a) *Religious Literacy Leadership in Higher Education: an analysis of challenges of religious faith, and resources for meeting them, for university leaders*. Online. Available HTTP: https://research.gold.ac.uk/3916/1/RLLP_Analysis_AW_email.pdf (accessed 3 September 2016).

Dinham, A. and Jones, S.H. (2010b) *Religious Literacy Leadership in Higher Education: leadership challenges – case studies*. Online. Available HTTP: http://religiousliteracyhe.org/wp-content/uploads/2010/11/RLLP-Case-Studies.pdf (accessed 3 September 2016).

Dinham, A. and Jones, S.H. (2010c) *Religious Literacy Leadership in Higher Education: programme evaluation. Phase 1: September 2010–February 2011*. Online. Available HTTP: http://religiousliteracyhe.org/wp-content/uploads/2010/11/RLLP%20Evaluative%20Summary%20(final).pdf (accessed 3 September 2016).

Dinham, A. and Jones, S.H. (2012) 'Religion, public policy, and the academy: brokering public faith in a context of ambivalence?', *Journal of Contemporary Religion*, 27(2): 185–201.

Dinham, A. and Shaw, M. (2015) *REforREal: the future of teaching and learning about religion and belief*, London: Goldsmiths University of London. Online. Available HTTP: www.gold.ac.uk/media/goldsmiths/169-images/departments/research-units/faiths-unit/REforREal-web-b.pdf (accessed 9 August 2016).

Furness, S. and Gilligan, P. (2014) '"It never came up": encouragements and discouragements to addressing religion and belief in professional practice. What do social work students have to say?', *The British Journal of Social Work*, 44(3): 763–81.

Gilligan, P. and Furness, S. (2006) 'The role of religion and spirituality in social work practice: views and experiences of social workers and students', *The British Journal of Social Work*, 36(4): 617–37.

Hervieu-Leger, D. (2000) *Religion as a Chain of Memory*, New Brunswick: Rutgers University Press.

Moore, D.L. (2015) 'Diminishing religious literacy: methodological assumptions and analytical frameworks for promoting the public understanding of religion', in A. Dinham and M. Francis (eds) *Religious Literacy in Policy and Practice*, Bristol: Policy Press.

Pentaris, P. (2012) 'Religious competence in social work practice: the UK picture', *Social Work and Society*, 10(2). Online. Available HTTP: www.socwork.net/sws/article/view/344/681 (accessed 3 September 2016).

Pew Research Center (2012) *The Global Religious Landscape: a report on the size and distribution of the world's major religious groups as of 2010*, Washington DC: Pew Research Center. Online. Available HTTP: www.pewforum.org/files/2014/01/global-religion-full.pdf (accessed 18 April 2016).

Powell, A. and Cook, C. (2006) Spirituality and Psychiatry Special Interest Group of the Royal College of Psychiatrists ID – 1855.

Prothero, S. (2007) *Religious Literacy: what every American needs to know – and doesn't*, Boston: Barnes and Noble.

Puchalski, C. (2001) 'The role of spirituality in healthcare', *Baylor University Medical Center Proceedings*, 14(4): 352–7.

Russel, R. (1998) 'Spirituality and religion in graduate social work education', *Social Thought*, 18(2): 15–29.

Sheridan, M.J. and Amato-von Hemert, K. (1999) 'The role of religion and spirituality in social work education and practice: a survey of student views and experiences', *Journal of Social Work Education*, 35(1): 125–41.

Sheridan, M.J., Wilmer, C.M. and Atcheson, L. (1994) 'Inclusion of content on religion and spirituality in the social work curriculum: a study of faculty views', *Journal of Social Work Education*, 30(3): 363–76.

UK Government (2014) Statistics. Online. Available HTTP: www.statistics.gov.uk/hub/index.html (accessed April 2014).

Walker, D.F., Gorsuch, R.L. and Tan, S-Y. (2004) 'Therapists' integration of religion and spirituality in counseling: a meta-analysis', *Counseling and Values*, 49(1): 69–80.

Wilson, B.R. (1966) *Religion in Secular Society*, Oxford: Oxford University Press.

Woodhead, L. (2013) *Religion in Britain has Changed, Our Categories Haven't*. Online. Available HTTP: http://faithdebates.org.uk/wp-content/uploads/2013/09/1335118113_Woodhead-FINAL-copy.pdf (accessed 3 September 2013).

Wright, A. (2016) *Religious Education and Critical Realism: knowledge, reality and religious literacy*, London: Routledge.

Yates, J.W., Chalmer B.J., St James, P., Follansbee, M. and McKegney, F.P. (1981) 'Religion in patients with advanced cancer', *Medical and Pediatric Oncology*, 9(2): 121–8.

29

Spirituality and sexuality

Exploring tensions in everyday relationship-based practice

Janet Melville-Wiseman

Introduction

Contemporary social work practice in the United Kingdom is characterised by inherent tensions, whether at the heart of decisions about removing children from abusive situations, or depriving people with mental health needs of their liberty if they pose an unacceptable risk to themselves or others. Perhaps less obvious tensions exist for social workers at the intersection of religion or spirituality and sexuality.

It would be strange if such tensions did not exist in social work given that they exist and present apparently insurmountable problems in wider society. For example, the largely unresolved schism in the Anglican Communion about same-gender marriage or lesbian or gay clergy has taxed some of the most eminent theologians and thinkers including the current Archbishop of Canterbury Justin Welby, and his predecessor Dr Rowan Williams. However, faith leaders have a specific duty to lead their congregations and to discern the meaning of religious texts, whether popular or not. On the other hand, social work, as a profession, has greater freedom to position itself wherever it thinks fit in these debates, with certain limitations.

In reality social workers in the UK are trained to follow the law and to practice within the professional values of inclusion and anti-oppressive practice. But that means towards all people at all times including towards people who may be homophobic; people of a similar or opposing faith to individual practitioners; and people who may have perpetrated gender- or child-based violence that disturbs and upsets us. In essence social workers work equally with people who may hold a range of diverse views and values that the profession itself may not share. In that sense there are permanent tensions and challenges for social workers in their relationships with people who need services. However, tensions at the interface between religion and sexuality have not been well explored.

There have been advances in our understanding of the interface between religion and sexuality through studies that examine what it is like to be Christian and gay (Subhi and Geelan 2012), critiques of therapy designed to change people from gay to straight (Sacks 2011) and the distinctions between different religions and their attitudes to sexuality (Moon 2014). However, to date there has been very little specific insight or guidance for social workers on how to resolve such tensions in their everyday practice or how to train them in order to address such tensions

(Melville-Wiseman 2013). One reason for lack of recognition of the need for expertise in this area may be the increased secularisation of the profession (Furman *et al.* 2005). In this study the authors looked at differences in views between members of the British Association of Social Workers in the UK and the National Association of Social Workers in the US in terms of the role of religion and spirituality in practice and education. The majority in each group indicated a lack of inclusion of spirituality and religion in their education and training. However, social work as a profession has a long and distinguished history underpinned by religious or faith-based values.

The move to secularisation in social work

Early founders of social work in the UK often brought their religious-based values to their ideas and work. For example, Elizabeth Fry, who reformed the prison service, was a Quaker; Octavia Hill, who transformed social housing, was inspired by her Anglicanism; and Eileen Younghusband, who developed social work education, was influenced by her membership of the congregation of St Martins-in-the-Fields in London at a time when social reform was an intrinsic part of the preaching there (Jones 1984). Boyd (1982) emphasises these intrinsic links in her biography of Octavia Hill:

> The spirituality which directed this life of great activity and its almost incredible record of accomplishments was deep and, though free from inner conflicts, highly complex. Octavia Hill was a born pantheist. In the beauty of the countryside at Finchley, she saw the spirit of God: flowers, trees, and other objects of the created world she perceived as tokens of a transcendent reality. At the same time her affections taught her that spiritual reality is conveyed as authentically through human relationships as in the mystic's vision. When she and her family moved to London and undertook the responsibility of working with and for the poor, she found in the Anglicanism of E.D. Maurice a theology that gave concrete form to her strongly felt but dimly articulated views on the value of community and service.
>
> (Boyd 1982: 121)

However, in contemporary social work practice and social work education there is little evidence that religion or spirituality and their consequential values are influential drivers. Instead, the profession is dominated by its professionalisation, the search for empirical evidence and the management of care (Furman *et al.* 2005). One perhaps inadvertent consequence of this shift is that social workers do not develop their skills and knowledge base to address everyday spiritual tensions in practice or in their relationships with people who need services (Melville-Wiseman 2013).

Relational work

Our personal sexual and spiritual identity can shape and influence the way we understand the sexual and spiritual identity and needs of others. In social work this can happen at many levels including at an interpersonal level with individual service users; how services are planned, shaped and delivered; and our choices of research areas and knowledge development for the profession. However, at an interpersonal level, social workers are more often driven by imperatives to address physical risk and potential harm than by concerns about relational risk or need (Melville-Wiseman 2012).

Relationship-based social work is increasingly recognised as a discrete area of study, knowledge and skills but it is often based on a psychodynamic theoretical perspective (Ruch *et al.* 2010). This can be useful in terms of understanding some aspects of relational work but it can also lead to a negative or pathologising view of conflicts or tensions such as those in relation to sexuality and spirituality. If opposing views are in conflict then that equates to a problem in or for one side that has to be solved. An alternative perspective is given that we are a diverse group, diversity and the ensuing conflict and tensions could in fact be relationship enhancing (Spano and Koenig 2007).

Recourse to legal intercession

The *UK Equality Act* came into force in 2010. The aim of the legislation was to bring together and enhance all previous laws relating to discrimination in an attempt to protect individuals from unfair treatment, harassment and victimisation (Equality Act 2010). The provisions of the act cover nine protected characteristics: age; disability; gender reassignment; marriage and civil partnership; pregnancy and maternity; race; religion or belief; sex; and sexual orientation (usually listed alphabetically). Within the *Equality Act*, religion and belief (including no religion or belief) and sexual orientation (including heterosexuality) are equally protected by the law. However, more than any other combination of characteristics, these two have come into direct conflict with each other where a particular religion or belief teaches that homosexuality is wrong.

As a consequence there has been a steady stream of UK case law to determine whose rights take precedence. In general terms rulings have supported the position that the right to hold a religion or faith-based view that homosexuality is wrong does not extend to the translation of that view into a refusal to provide equal goods and services. For example, an owner of a hotel was deemed to have discriminated against a gay couple by not permitting them to share a double bed. The owners argued that, based on their religious views that the only acceptable sexual relationships are within heterosexual marriage, they would not have permitted a non-married heterosexual couple to share a double bed either. However, they still lost the case.

Within social work practice the law may help to determine some solutions but it does not necessarily help practitioners to resolve the real world tensions in such situations or to use them transformationally to enhance their practice. The following real life case vignette provides an opportunity to explore an alternative approach.

Case example

A recent much-publicised case in the UK involved Eunice and Owen Johns, who wished to return to foster caring for Derby City Council. To summarise, the couple were applying to become short-term respite foster carers. Eunice Johns was a retired nurse and the couple, who had brought up four children of their own, had previously fostered 15 children. They had applied to return to fostering but when the assessing social worker identified that they were Evangelical Christians, and that they had indicated that they believed homosexuality was wrong, their application was not taken forward. The couple then sought judicial review in the High Court of this decision and the approach of the council towards their religion. Their application was refused and the judges in the case stated:

> While as between the protected rights concerning religion and sexual orientation there is no hierarchy of rights, there may, as this case shows, be a tension between equality

provisions concerning religious discrimination and those concerning sexual orientation. Where this is so, Standard 7 of the National Minimum Standards for Fostering and the Statutory Guidance indicate that it must be taken into account and in this limited sense the equality provisions concerning sexual orientation should take precedence.

(Johns & Anor, R (on the application of) v Derby City Council & Anor [2011] EWHC 375: para. 93)

The couple had been interviewed several times by the assessing social worker and had indicated that, should it arise, they would be compelled by their religious belief to tell a child, should they ask, that homosexuality was wrong. This was therefore adjudged to indicate that the couple would not be able to meet the local authority's requirements to safeguard and promote the welfare of the child.

The case raises several questions in terms of how social workers can practice at the interface and tensions between religion or spirituality and sexuality. For example, it is not unlawful in the UK to belong to a religion or faith that simply preaches that homosexuality is wrong or to raise children in that faith. However, once a child comes into the care of a local authority, different standards for their protection and welfare apply. This is to ensure that any previous harm to a child, which has led to the local authority becoming the parent, is neither replicated nor increased by their new care setting.

In theory, if all foster carers can meet the standards, any child could be placed with any foster carer. In practice this does not happen, and is not expected to happen. Significant resources are usually invested in the often lengthy processes of 'matching' children with specific foster carers. The criteria for matching has traditionally been based on finding carers who are similar to the child in terms of background, culture or ethnicity. The ideal of matching children with alternative carers of similar identities, or the idealism that underpins this approach, has to be weighed against the need to place a child with someone who is available and approved, sometimes at short notice. Inevitably decisions are often made on the basis of the best available person or family to care for the child.

The outcome of the previous legal determination is important for the couple involved and the social work team who were involved in the assessment of the couple. However, there are many problems involved in relying on such a legal judgement to guide practice. Instead, a broader approach may support a more comprehensive exploration of the risks and possible benefits of taking one approach or another. Risk in this context refers to aspects of relational care that are not simply based on narrowly defined assumptions about what good enough care looks like. Instead it describes the limitations that we create when we do not look and look again for better solutions beyond what or who is right or wrong. In addition there may have been many potential benefits in the Johns' case that were never fully explored as the case faltered on the single dimension of the tension between spirituality and sexuality.

The anti-discriminatory imperative is well established in social work practice. However, it has been argued previously that a claim to have achieved that in full can only ever be partial (Melville-Wiseman 2012). The reasons are that we have yet to know all there is to know about discrimination and how it affects individuals, groups and yet to emerge marginalised groups. One of those yet to be fully understood groups may be children who are struggling to understand their religion or how to give meaning or a spiritual dimension to their lives alongside fearing that they may be homosexual or even homophobic. It is highly likely that all those involved in the case described here, including the social workers, the couple and the judges, had some aspects of their attitudes that were, albeit unconsciously, discriminatory.

The context of social work practice, and the provision of alternative care for children, is ever changing as society develops new approaches to such personal and crucial aspects of our identities. Until as late as 2003, local authorities in the UK (who provided foster care) were prohibited from promoting homosexuality by Section 28 of the Local Government Act 1988, which stated:

> A local authority shall not—
> (a) intentionally promote homosexuality or publish material with the intention of promoting homosexuality;
> (b) promote the teaching in any maintained school of the acceptability of homosexuality as a pretended family relationship.
>
> (Office of Public Service Information 1988: c.9 Section 28 1a & b)

During this time many children and young people struggling with their sexuality were left with no support from their teachers, social workers or foster carers for fear that their employment could be terminated by the local authority under this section. Foster carers who were approved before 2003 have had to make a seismic shift in their care of foster children to ensure that they were compliant with the law and are now compliant with the law that states the opposite.

Risk and benefit assessment framework

Using the Johns' case as an example, and thinking about it in relational terms, it is possible to look at a number of possible risks and benefits.

Recruitment of carers

First, by denying the application the council risked losing potential foster carers from the Christian faith. This was at a time when there was a shortage of foster carers and when they could not predict whether any children requiring care would be from the same faith or benefit from care grounded in that faith. In the legal hearing, Derby Council argued that Mr and Mrs Johns were applying to be respite carers and they did not currently have a shortage of such carers so did not need to take a more inclusive approach. However, it was inevitable that such a case would attract much publicity and possibly deter other Christians, or people from other faiths or no faith, from coming forward to provide other types of foster care. We know that Mr and Mrs Johns were unambiguously honest about their views and their values, and the surrounding negative publicity and refusal of their application may encourage other applicants to be far less candid. This carries risks in terms of those carrying out assessments not truly knowing applicants but also diminishes the possibility of difference, and conflict within difference, being seen and modelled in a positive way.

The role of personal and professional identity

The decision also calls into question how much those who work directly with children should be expected to disclose of their own personal information and for what purpose. For example, it is not a requirement for applicants for places on social work training courses to disclose either their sexuality, their religion or faith, or their attitude to people of the same or different sexuality or faith. The profession prides itself on inclusivity and is predicated on an assumption that a diverse workforce can best meet the needs of diverse service users. Social workers work directly and indirectly with children and may have many conversations with them about their concerns relating to either sexuality or spirituality. It is assumed that training will ensure that individual social workers will know how to practice in an anti-oppressive and anti-discriminatory way. However, it is still not a requirement for social workers to abandon their faith or religion in order to practice effectively. The need for effective training and more robust selection may be even more significant for foster carers who provide 24 hour care as opposed to social workers who may only occasionally meet with children; but are such dual standards reasonable or necessary?

The importance of religion, spirituality and sexuality

Next, this decision could be viewed as giving primacy to the struggles looked-after children may have with their sexuality over concerns about their religion or their spiritual lives. Social workers and other statutory bodies may need to intervene where children may be harmed in the context of a religion such as sexual abuse by clergy or lay leaders in the church or where children may be encouraged to mistreat others as a result of their faith. However, understanding the emerging or already formed spiritual needs of children is equally important.

In a study to measure the correlation between spirituality and happiness, Holder *et al.* (2010) found that, as with adults, spirituality enhanced the happiness of children especially in the areas of individual and personal meaning and meaningful relationships with others. This suggests that foster carers need to be skilled at supporting spiritual growth and experience for children especially where they may have been through experiences that make them doubt their personal worth or meaning. In a recent report on the 'matching' process for permanent alternative care for children, the Children's Rights Commissioner for England consulted several young people who had experienced the matching process. They were asked their views on the following:

> When looking for a placement, how important is it to match young people and carers on the basis of religion, race and culture etc?
>
> (Office of the Children's Rights Director 2013: 12)

The group were asked to vote on this issue and unanimously agreed that those factors were not as important as feeling cared about by the foster carers or adopters; however, it should not be assumed that they are completely unimportant (Office of the Children's Rights Director 2013).

Faith-based views about sexuality

The decision by the court was based primarily on the imperative of foster carers to promote diversity as enshrined in the national minimum standards for foster care (Department for Education 2011). However, it was accepted by the court and Derby Council that foster carers of a particular religious faith, working for a private agency, could positively discriminate and agree to only foster children of the same faith. The reason for this is that the Equality Act 2010 placed an overarching equality duty on the provision of goods and services by local authorities. However, a distinction was also drawn between whether the decision to not allow Mr and Mrs Johns' application was based on their objection to homosexuality or their religious views. Either way it appears that they were subject to high levels of scrutiny once their religious views were known. The court maintained though that the local authority was entitled to probe the couple once their views about sexuality were known and would in fact be negligent if it had not done so. In return the couple argued that they should not have been so highly scrutinised and judged other than in relation to a specific child and a specific potential placement with them. This was also rejected by the court. However, this approach and the judgement carries additional risks, specifically for a potential foster child who may also believe that homosexuality is wrong, and that view may be based on their own religious views. How could that child receive the right level of support that they need if placed with foster carers who may have been approved specifically because they believe that homosexuality is not wrong?

The assessment of the suitability of foster carers

Another risk from the judgement is that local authorities appear to not be able to accommodate a pluralistic approach to either spirituality or sexuality. The judgement has indicated that foster carers cannot hold views that homosexuality is wrong however careful or sensitive they may be about how or where that view is expressed. The couple were subjected to intensive scrutiny, including being asked to comment on different possible scenarios. The assessing social worker informed the court:

> Mrs Johns stated, "I will not lie and tell you I will say it is ok to be a homosexual. I will love and respect, no matter what sexuality. I cannot lie and I cannot hate, but I cannot tell a child that it is ok to be homosexual. Then you will not be able to trust me. There has got to be different ways of going through this without having to compromise my faith."
> (Johns & Anor, R (on the application of) v Derby City Council & Anor [2011] EWHC 375: para. 11)

An alternative option could have been for the council to focus additional support or training on the couple to give them tools they needed to provide the right care without compromising their beliefs. For example, telling a child that homosexuality is wrong is quite different to telling a child that people have many different views about homosexuality and it happens to be the case that their faith teaches them that it is wrong – but that is just one view and they are happy to support them to speak with people who believe it is right. It appears that Mr and Mrs Johns were looking for a solution to the conflict but that the social workers were not able to go beyond the legal interpretation of the policy and guidance.

The Anglican Church has recently published guidance for Church schools on how to tackle homophobic bullying (Church of England Archbishops' Council Education Division 2014) and this could have helped in this case. This advisory policy recognises the need for an inclusive approach, i.e. that faith-based views about sexuality have to accommodate alternative views if homophobic bullying is to be eradicated in schools. This guidance may have provided a useful tool for both the council and the couple.

Conclusions

The fundamental challenge for social work practitioners remains one of understanding how far it is a social work task to discern seriously-held religious belief or whether we should instead be skilled at discernment of the complex tensions when working at the interface between religion, spirituality, heteronormativity and sexuality equality.

The case example given in this chapter provides an opportunity to explore alternative ways of resolving sexuality and spirituality tensions in everyday practice. Key points include the following.

- Such conflicts and tensions could provide unique opportunities for transformation of individuals and services.

- However, this means looking for alternative solutions that are not just driven by interpretations of policy and law.
- Children are diverse and of changing identities and characteristics. As such they need adults, including social workers and foster carers, to model diversity, to be comfortable with diversity and to have the temerity to work with tensions and conflicts that may arise between people and in relationships until they can alight on common ground.

Finally, there are decisions to be made by the social work profession including those charged with judging the suitability of others to work in the field in terms of the sexuality and spirituality tensions described here. If we require openness and transparency by foster carers in terms of their faith-based views on sexuality then perhaps those assessing them should also be encouraged to be completely open. The reasons to do this would not be to subject them to the type of legal scrutiny that befell Mr and Mrs Johns, but instead to support the possibility of transformation of their practice and, ultimately, services. This is best achieved not by getting rid of tensions and conflicts inherent in difference, but by embracing them to deepen our understanding of individual experience.

The societies in which we live change, and sometimes they change rapidly. In the UK, during the eight years between the repeal of Section 28 of the Local Government Act 1988 and the Johns case in 2011, social workers have had to transform their practice from not being permitted to promote homosexuality to pro-actively ensuring that the needs of lesbian and gay people of any age are fully supported. It is inevitable that some people will adjust more quickly than others. However, it would be a shame if we did not pause to ensure we take all those interested in the care of vulnerable people with us through supportive training and a relational focus rather than harsh and excluding processes or proceedings. In that way we may also reclaim some of the authentic spiritual reality of Octavia Hills's vision of human relationships.

References

Boyd, N. (1982) *Josephine Butler, Octavia Hill, Florence Nightingale: three Victorian women who changed their world*, London: Macmillan.

Church of England Archbishops' Council Education Division (2014) *Valuing All God's Children: guidance for Church of England schools on challenging homophobic bullying*. Online. Available HTTP: www.churchofengland.org/media/1988293/valuing%20all%20god's%20children%20web%20final.pdf (accessed 8 January 2016).

Department for Education (2011) *Fostering Services: national minimum standards*. Online. Available HTTP: www.fosteringsupport.co.uk/documents/National%20minimum%20standards.pdf (accessed 8 January 2016).

Equality Act (2010) London: HMSO. Online. Available HTTP: www.legislation.gov.uk/ukpga/2010/15/contents (accessed 8 January 2016).

Furman, L.D., Benson, P.W., Canda, E.R. and Grimwood, C. (2005). 'A comparative international analysis of religion and spirituality in social work: a survey of UK and US social workers', *Social Work Education*, 24(8): 813–39.

Holder, M.D., Coleman, B. and Wallace, J.M. (2010) 'Spirituality, religiousness, and happiness in children aged 8–12 years', *Journal of Happiness Studies*, 11(2): 131–50.

Johns & Anor, R (on the application of) v Derby City Council & Anor [2011] EWHC 375 (Admin). Online. Available HTTP: www.bailii.org/ew/cases/EWHC/Admin/2011/375.html (accessed 8 January 2016).

Jones, K. (1984) *Eileen Younghusband: a biography*, London: Bedford Square Press.

Melville-Wiseman, J. (2012) 'Taking relationships into account in mental health services', in G. Koubel and Bungay, H. (eds) *Rights, Risks and Responsibilities: interprofessional perspectives*, Basingstoke: Palgrave.

Melville-Wiseman, J. (2013) 'Teaching through the tension: resolving religious and sexuality based schism in social work education', *International Social Work*, 56(3): 290–309.

Moon, D. (2014) 'Beyond the dichotomy: six religious views of homosexuality', *Journal of Homosexuality*, 61(9): 1215–41.

Office of the Children's Rights Director (2013) *Improving Adoption and Permanent Placements: children's views to the Select Committee on Adoption Legislation*. Online. Available HTTP: www.parliament.uk/documents/lords-committees/adoption-legislation/Report%20of%20Children's%20Groups.pdf (accessed 8 January 2016).

Office of Public Service Information (1988) *Local Government Act 1988 c.9*. Online. Available HTTP: www.legislation.gov.uk/ukpga/1988/9 (accessed 8 January 2016).

Ruch, G., Turney, D. and Ward, A. (2010) *Relationship-Based Social Work: getting to the heart of practice*, London: Jessica Kingsley Publishers.

Sacks, J. (2011) '"Pray away the gay?" An analysis of the legality of conversion therapy by homophobic religious organizations', *Rutgers Journal of Law and Religion*, 13(1): 67–86.

Spano, R. and Koenig, T. (2007) 'What is sacred when personal and professional values collide?', *Journal of Social Work Values and Ethics*, 4(3): 91–104.

Subhi, N. and Geelan, D. (2012) 'When Christianity and homosexuality collide: understanding the potential intrapersonal conflict', *Journal of Homosexuality*, 59(10): 1382–402.

30

Mindfulness for professional resilience

James Lucas

Introduction

Professional resilience is essential for social workers and other health professionals who, on an almost daily basis, expose themselves to their clients' and colleagues' life stresses while also managing their own. The development of professional resilience starts with cultivating a mindfulness of the state energy and information flow within and between one's mind, body and relationships (Baldini *et al.* 2014; McGarrigle and Walsh 2011; Shier and Graham 2010). Mindfulness sheds light on areas of this mind–body–relationship triangle of wellbeing (Siegel 2010) that requires healing through targeted self-care strategies. Without mindfulness social workers leave themselves vulnerable to the negative effects of stress and trauma, potentially, transferring those effects onto their clients and colleagues (Epstein and Krasner 2013; Pidgeon *et al.* 2014; Thomas and Otis 2010). The aim in this chapter is to discuss the role and benefit of mindfulness in the development and maintenance of professional resilience with a particular focus on the links between the mind, body and relationships.

Mind, body and relationships: energy and information flow

In his Interpersonal Neurobiological (IPNB) framework, Siegel (2015) argued that the mind, brain/body and relationships are part of one system of energy and information flow within and between people. Energy is the capacity to do something, while information is the symbolic representation of something other than itself. Siegel (2015: 160) defined the mind as 'an emergent, self-organising, embodied and relational process that regulates the flow of energy and information'. The mind is an emergent and embodied process as it is distributed throughout the brain and broader nervous system (the body) within which energy and information flows, but cannot itself be found within that body, the energy, or the information. The body is the primary, physical mechanism through which the mind's energy and information is embodied and flows. Relationships are the basis for the sharing of energy and information in the form of behaviour, and verbal and non-verbal communication. From these IPNB-based definitions, it becomes apparent how a person's mind and body are inextricably linked and this has an impact on the mind and body of others through their relationships.

These three elements, (1) mind, (2) body and (3) relationships, represent the three aspects of what Siegel (2010, 2012, 2015) termed the 'triangle of wellbeing'. The state of energy and information flow between each of these three aspects is indicative of a person's resilience and wellbeing and can be viewed like the flow of a river. Under certain conditions, such as in rocky terrain, a river can flow chaotically in the form of white-water rapids; while under other conditions, such as during a Siberian winter, the flow of the river is rigid or completely frozen. When chaotic, the river flow is uncontrollable, disorganised and potentially dangerous. When rigid, the river flow is slow, sluggish and inflexible.

In the case of energy and information flow within and between the mind, body and relationships, a person's wellbeing is the attainment of balance between chaos and rigidity where the three aspects of the triangle of wellbeing are integrated and the flow of energy and information is Flexible, Adaptive, Coherent, Energised and Stable. Siegel (2010) utilised the acronym 'FACES' to remember these five characteristics of an integrated flow distinctive of a positive state of wellbeing.

In order to attain such a state of integration or wellbeing, Siegel (2015) argued that the mind uses its ability to see itself, or mindsight, to consciously monitor and regulate the flow of energy and information accordingly. Mindsight, according to Siegel, involves a presence that is grounded in the present moment, which discerns or senses the state of one's mind, body and relationships. This presence necessarily involves a mental defusion between the person as the observer and their mind, body and relationships as the observed. Without this defusion and subsequent present-moment presence, a person's sense of self or 'I' remains fused with the content of that self (i.e. the mind, body and relationships) and as a consequence they are unable to exert a great deal of control or regulation over habitual ways of thinking, feeling and acting. In Buddhist spiritual traditions, such as Zen, Mahayana and Mahamudra traditions, this inability to exert control over the mind due to a lack of defusion and presence is not dissimilar to being swept through life by the force of one's Karma, that is the effects of one's actions, due to a lack of mindfulness (Flanagan 2011).

Mindfulness, discussed later in this chapter, is an aspect of mind, that functions to hold a person's mindsight on a particular object, for example their state of mind, body and relationships, in their awareness (Black 2011; Siegel 2009). It is important to note here that mindfulness is not mindsight. It is only when people's mindsight is held focused on an object in awareness by their mindfulness that they can effectively monitor and regulate the flow of energy and information within and between people.

Siegel (2012) highlighted the link between mindfulness and mindsight in terms of a camera set upon a tripod. A person's mindsight can be viewed as a camera, the lens of which can be stabilised and focused when set upon a tripod, the three legs corresponding to three outcomes of effective mindfulness: (1) openness to experiences as they are, as opposed to the way they should be; (2) observation of the self as the experiencer; and (3) objectivity from the content of experiences of which are inherently transient. In the same way that a person can take a photo with a camera without the use of a tripod, so too can they use their mindsight to monitor and regulate energy and information flow without the effective use of mindfulness. Their mindsight, however, might not be very stable, leading to photos being taken (i.e. snapshots of their experiences of energy and information flow) that are out of focus thus creating a distorted or irrational image of reality. The effective application of mindfulness would foster the person's openness, observation and objectivity (the tripod) to create a stable and more focused picture of reality.

The use of mindfulness appears to have an important role in stabilising the mind and allowing people to focus their mindsight on the flow of energy and information within their mind, body and relationships. This stabilisation and focus would then allow people to have increased awareness and control over their thinking, feelings and actions and more space to choose courses of action that are aligned with their life values (Baldini *et al.* 2014; Purser and Milillo 2015; Siegel *et al.* 2011; Thompson *et al.* 2011). Mindfulness, however, is not a product of Western psychology, but has its origins in Buddhist spiritual traditions where it is utilised primarily for the attainment of Enlightenment or Buddhahood (Flanagan 2011).

Mindfulness

The word, mindfulness, is an English translation of the Pali[1] word 'sati'. References to sati can be found in some of the early Buddhist scriptural texts, such as the Abhidhamma and the Vishuddimagga, which originated some 2,600 years ago from the senior disciples of the Buddha, Gautama Siddhartha, in ancient India. The meaning of sati connotes an interrelation between remembering, attention and awareness and can be defined as remembering to pay attention to something in one's awareness (Chiesa and Malinowski 2011; Dreyfus 2011; Siegel *et al.* 2011). Grossman and van Dam (2011), however, have argued that sati/mindfulness is better considered in terms of its adjectival form, (being) mindful, to highlight the state-like or fluctuating nature of mindfulness.

In an everyday illustration of this definition of mindfulness, or being mindful, imagine your work supervisor advising you to be mindful of how you speak to clients in the workplace. You would then continue with your work, but now you find you are remembering to pay attention to, or being mindful of, the way you speak to each client you interact with for the rest of the day. In this way, your mindfulness is functioning to keep your attention on the object or thought – 'how am I am speaking with my clients?' – like a type of mental glue. The utilisation of mindfulness in this way maintains your awareness focused on what you are experiencing in the present moment and choosing a course of action, for example how you interact with clients, that is in accordance with the values of your workplace or profession.

The role of mindfulness in Buddhism, like in the previous workplace example, is essentially to remember to pay attention to the Dharma (Buddha's teachings) so they become integrated into your everyday actions and life generally (Tenzin 2014). The main difference lies in what the person is being mindful of: (a) how they are speaking to their clients at work or (b) the Dharma. Therefore, Buddhists and non-Buddhists alike can utilise techniques to strengthen and consequently benefit from mindfulness. The primary method in Buddhism that people utilise to exercise and strengthen their mindfulness is meditation (Kornfield 2008).

Buddhist meditation practices generally fall into two types: (1) Shamatha and (2) Vipassana (Tenzin 2014). The role of Shamatha meditation is for people to practice regulating their attention so that they are able to concentrate or pay attention single-pointedly on an object such as their breath, body, feelings or thoughts. This concentration or attention training requires people to exercise their mindfulness so as to anchor their attention on a chosen object continually without distraction. The second type of meditation, Vipassana, involves people applying their mindfulness and single-pointed concentrative abilities developed in Shamatha meditation to gain insight into the true nature of reality (the mind, body and all other phenomena), which is interdependent and insubstantial.

The ultimate goal of gaining such insight through Vipassana mediation, which is dependent on applying the techniques of Shamatha mediation, is to attain a permanent state of Enlightenment or Buddhahood. Tenzin (2014) argued, however, that without training their mindfulness people will be unable to attain Buddhahood as their mind will continue to be attached to objects it considers attractive, avoidant of those it considers aversive, and indifferent to everything else. In other words, a person's state of mind remains dependent on external conditions. It is through meditation that people train their minds to find happiness and peace internally.

We can see from the discussion that a person's mindfulness is essential in keeping their mind stabilised and focused on a chosen object that, when directly realised, will eventually lead them to a permanently peaceful and happy state of Enlightenment. Faith in a spiritual or religious tradition such as Buddhism, however, is not a requirement for people to possess, develop and benefit from mindfulness. The largely positive outcomes that have resulted from the integration of mindfulness into Cognitive-Behavioural Therapies (CBT), such as Hayes' (2004) Acceptance and Commitment Therapy (ACT) and Linehan's (1987) Dialectical Behaviour Therapy (DBT), is an example of where the development of mindfulness can be of benefit to people who might hold a more secular worldview.

In traditional CBTs, for example in Beck's (1976) Cognitive Therapy (CT) and Ellis' (1962, 1970, 1993) Rational-Emotive Behaviour Therapy (REBT), the mental suffering people experience is due to their thoughts and thinking processes, their cognitions, becoming distorted and rigid. Some of the common cognitive distortions Beck and Weishaar (1989) identified include: (a) all-or-nothing/black and white thinking, (b) maximisation/minimisation of importance, (c) personalisation and (d) tunnel vision. Rigidity in such cognitive distortions becomes evident when the words 'I should' or 'I must' are involved as they create a blanket or generalised nature to cognitions in the form of, what Ellis (1962, 1970, 1993) termed, core beliefs. Core beliefs are arranged with all other experiential information in mental structures that Piaget (1950, 1963, 1970) termed schemas.

Piaget argued that, as new experiential information is perceived, people try initially to assimilate new information into their established schemas as assimilation is often found to require less effort and involves less internal conflict or stress. If the new information cannot be assimilated, then a process of accommodation is undertaken to change established schemas. When the new information is either assimilated or accommodated then the person, according to Piaget, is said to have attained a higher level of cognitive development. These processes, however, can become inhibited if the cognitions that make up the structure of people's schemas become distorted and rigid. The goal of traditional CBT, therefore, is to help people in challenging, changing and replacing these distorted or rigid cognitions with those that are more realistic and flexible.

The concepts of cognitive distortions and rigidity are not unlike Siegel's (2010, 2012) IPNB-based river of integration, where either chaotic or rigid energy and information flow throughout a person's mind, body and relationships has a negative impact on their overall wellbeing. The central difference between IPNB and traditional CBT, however, is in the former's positive focus on developing mindfulness and integration instead of the deficit focus in traditional CBT on distortions and rigidity. For example, the emphasis of Hayes and colleagues (2006) is that ACT is for people to develop their psychological flexibility through the application of mindfulness directed towards reducing experiential avoidance and increasing their commitment to courses of action that are in-line with their life values.

Harris (2008: 41) defined psychological flexibility as 'the ability to adapt to a situation with awareness, openness, and focus and to take effective action, guided by your values'. Harris' reference to awareness, openness and focus is parallel to the core outcomes of effective mindfulness discussed earlier. Through the application of mindfulness, people are encouraged to accept all experiences that arise in the form of thoughts (including mental images and sounds), feelings and bodily sensations and become fully present in the 'Now'. Once fully present, the person is better able to reduce any mindless reacting to external situations, reconnect with their life values, what is important to them, and commit to actions in-line with those life values.

Empirical research on outcomes associated with ACT has been largely positive. For example, in a review comparing the effects of ACT with traditional CBT, Ruiz (2012) found that people who received ACT reported a greater reduction in the severity of their depression and a greater increase in their quality of life compared with those who received traditional CBT. In a similar review, Sharp (2012) found that people who received ACT reported significant reductions in the severity of their anxiety. Additionally, in a sample of people with chronic pain, Lee *et al.* (2015) found participation in ACT reduced the intensity of their pain. Furthermore, Yadavaia *et al.* (2014) found significantly greater reductions in reported stress, anxiety and depression in a sample of adults who participated in an ACT-based workshop compared to a control group that did not participate in the workshop. The ACT group also had significantly greater increases in reported self-compassion than the control group. As the cultivation of mindfulness is a central aspect of ACT, these empirical results provide some support for the positive effect of increasing mindfulness on alleviating distress and increasing wellbeing. Social workers and other health professionals might also benefit from applying mindfulness in the context of maintaining their resilience in the face of continual stress, trauma and conflict.

Mindfulness for professional resilience

Epstein and Krasner (2013: 301) defined resilience as 'the ability of an individual to respond to stress in a healthy, adaptive way such that personal goals are achieved at minimal psychological and physical cost' and that resilient people 'not only "bounce back" rapidly after challenges but also grow stronger in the process'. Given the inherent stress involved in social work, how might social workers utilise mindfulness to foster their resilience against the negative effects of vicarious trauma and burnout?

First, social workers could benefit by putting aside regular time in the day or night for formal meditation practice. This meditation practice need not be long, in the beginning; a social worker might put aside 10 minutes each day to sit down and train their mindfulness accordingly. The duration of this formal mediation can be increased incrementally much like increasing the size of the weights lifted or the speed of the treadmill at the gym. This type of practice is similar to initial Shamatha meditation emphasised in Buddhism, whereby the practitioner starts to develop their concentrative abilities through continual exercising of their mindfulness.

As mindfulness requires an object of which to be mindful of, meditation practice necessarily involves a meditation object. One example of a meditation object is the breath. In their meditation practice, the social worker would try to remember (be mindful of) focusing on their breath as it enters and leaves their nostrils, or the rise and fall of their abdomen as they inhale and exhale. It is natural for the mind to wander from the meditation object, the breath in this instance, to other objects such as the events of the day or plans for tomorrow, but by being alert the meditator calls their mind back to the meditation object and applies their mindfulness to hold their attention on that object for as long as possible. With regular practice, like the regular exercise of the body, the ability of the person's mindfulness to hold their attention on the meditation object will gradually increase until their mind remains firmly stabilised without distraction. Social workers could expand their mindfulness practice to include additional meditation objects such as the five senses of the body, affect or emotions, thoughts and mental images, and relational phenomena such as equanimity and compassion. These objects are commonly utilised in Buddhist meditation practices (Kornfield 2008) and reflect the three aspects of Siegel's (2012, 2015) IPNB-based triangle of wellbeing discussed earlier.

Daily meditation practice with a focus on being mindful of the energy and information flow within and between the mind, body and relationships that make up the triangle of wellbeing could just as effectively be applied during professional practice. For example, the social worker could practice being mindful of any bodily sensations of fear they might be experiencing prior to walking into an Intensive Care Unit to see a distressed family in order to ground themselves and present. The social worker could also practice being mindful of their thoughts and emotions arising when consulting with a colleague to foster more assertive, instead of aggressive, communication. Social workers could also be mindful of the way they are communicating or relating with their clients to ensure they create a safe and compassionate counselling space. In each example the mindfulness developed during formal meditation practice can be integrated into everyday professional situations, where it could be said that the real practice begins, resulting in a greater resilience to life stressors and trauma (Flanagan 2011; Harris 2009; Kabat-Zinn 2005).

Furthermore, the daily exercising of mindfulness creates the possibility for social workers to have greater control over regulating the energy and information flow within and between their body, mind and relationships towards a state of health that fosters their resilience (Baldini et al. 2014; Thompson et al. 2011). Siegel (2009, 2012, 2015) stated that a mindful regulation of energy and information flow leads to enhanced bodily regulation, attuned communication, emotional balance, response flexibility, fear modulation, empathy, insight, moral awareness and intuition. These health functions are not dissimilar to what social workers might try to foster in their clients, but are not necessarily the best at fostering in themselves (Baldini et al. 2014; Dombo and Gray 2013). In order to thrive in the stressful environment inherent to social work practice, it is crucial that social workers commit themselves to cultivating these health functions in themselves, through their use of mindfulness, and therefore maintain an effective and ethical practice.

Conclusion

Professional resilience is invaluable to social workers and other health professionals who work closely with people often facing extreme life stressors and trauma. In order to avoid vicarious traumatisation and burnout, social workers could benefit from a continual mindfulness of the flow of energy and information within and between their mind, body and relationships. Mindfulness originates from Buddhist traditions and is like a mental glue that stabilises the mind and keeps the person's mindsight on the flow of energy and information so as to then regulate that flow in a healthy way characterised by enhanced bodily regulation, attuned communication, emotional balance, response flexibility, fear modulation, empathy, insight, moral awareness and intuition. The ability to be mindful is, like exercise, dependent on practice and with the primary practice method in Buddhist traditions being meditation. The integration of formal, daily meditation practice into everyday professional practice would allow social workers to strengthen their professional resilience and maintain an effective and ethical practice.

Note

1 Pali is the language in which the teachings of the Buddha were originally written.

References

Baldini, L.L., Parker, S.C., Nelson, B.W. and Siegel, D.J. (2014) 'The clinician as neuroarchitect: the importance of mindfulness and presence in clinical practice', *Clinical Social Work Journal*, 42(3): 218–27.

Beck, A.T. (1976) *Cognitive Therapy and the Emotional Disorders*, London: Penguin Books.

Beck, A.T. and Weishaar, M. (1989) 'Cognitive therapy', in A. Freeman, K. M. Simon, L. E. Beutler and H. Arkowitz (eds) *Comprehensive Handbook of Cognitive Therapy*, New York: Plenum.

Black, D.S. (2011) 'A brief definition of mindfulness', *Mindfulness Research Guide*. Online. Available HTTP: http://citeseerx.ist.psu.edu/viewdoc/download?doi=10.1.1.362.6829&rep=rep1&type=pdf (accessed 2 December 2015).

Chiesa, A. and Malinowski, P. (2011) 'Mindfulness-based approaches: are they all the same?', *Journal of Clinical Psychology*, 67(4): 404–24.

Dombo, E.A. and Gray, C. (2013) 'Engaging spirituality in addressing vicarious trauma in clinical social workers: a self-care model', *Social Work and Christianity*, 40(1): 89–104.

Dreyfus, G. (2011) 'Is mindfulness present-centred and non-judgmental? A discussion of the cognitive dimensions of mindfulness', *Contemporary Buddhism*, 12(1): 41–54.

Ellis, A. (1962) *Reason and Emotion in Psychotherapy*, New York: Lyle Stuart.

Ellis, A. (1970) *The Essence of Rational Psychotherapy: a comprehensive approach in treatment*, New York: Institute for Rational Living.

Ellis, A. (1994) 'Changing rational-emotive therapy (RET) to rational emotive behaviour therapy (REBT)', *The Behaviour Therapist*, 16(10): 1–2.

Epstein, R.M. and Krasner, M.S. (2013) 'Physician resilience: what it means, why it matters, and how to promote it', *Academic Medicine*, 88(3): 301–3.

Flanagan, O. (2011) *The Bodhisattva's Brain: Buddhism naturalized*, London: The MIT Press.

Grossman, P. and van Dam, N.T. (2011) 'Mindfulness, by any other name…: trials and tribulations of *sati* in western psychology and science', *Contemporary Buddhism*, 12(1): 219–39.

Harris, R. (2008) *The Happiness Trap*, London: Robinson.

Harris, R. (2009) 'Mindfulness without meditation', *Healthcare Counselling and Psychotherapy Journal*, 9(4): 21–4.

Hayes, S.C. (2004) 'Acceptance and commitment therapy, relational frame theory, and the third wave of behavioural and cognitive therapies', *Behavior Therapy*, 35(4): 639–65.

Hayes, S.C., Luoma, J.B., Bond, F.W., Mauda, A. and Lillis, J. (2006) 'Acceptance and commitment therapy: model, processes and outcomes', *Behaviour Research and Therapy*, 44(1): 1–25.

Kabat-Zinn, J. (2005) *Wherever You Go, There You Are: mindfulness meditation in everyday life*, New York: Hyperion.

Kornfield, J. (2008) *The Wise Heart: Buddhist psychology for the West*, London: Rider Books.

Lee, E.B., An, W., Levin, M.E. and Twohig, M. P. (2015) 'An initial meta-analysis of acceptance and commitment therapy for treating substance use disorders', *Drug and Alcohol Dependence*, 155: 1–7.

Linehan, M.M. (1987) 'Dialectical behaviour therapy: a cognitive-behavioural approach to parasuicide', *Journal of Personality Disorders*, 1(4): 328–33.

McGarrigle, T. and Walsh, C.A. (2011) 'Mindfulness, self-care, and wellness in social work: effects of contemplative training', *Journal of Religion and Spirituality in Social Work*, 30(3): 212–33.

Piaget, J. (1950) *The Psychology of Intelligence*, London: Routledge & Keagan Paul.

Piaget, J. (1963) *The Origins of Intelligence in Children*, New York: Norton.

Piaget, J. (1970) 'Piaget's theory', in P.H. Mussen (ed) *Carmichael's Manual of Child Psychology*, 3rd edn, New York: Wiley.

Pidgeon, A.M., O'Brien, B., Hanna, A. and Klaasen, F. (2014) 'Cultivating a resilient response to stress through mindfulness and cognitive re-appraisal: a pilot randomised control trial', *Global Science and Technology Forum Journal of Psychology*, 1(2): 8–13.

Purser, R. E. and Milillo, J. (2015) 'Mindfulness revisited: a Buddhist-based conceptualization', *Journal of Management Inquiry*, 24(1): 3–24.

Ruiz, F.J. (2012) 'Acceptance and commitment therapy versus traditional cognitive behavioural therapy: a systematic review and meta-analysis of current empirical evidence', *International Journal of Psychology and Psychological Therapy*, 12(2): 333–57.

Sharp, K. (2012) 'A review of acceptance and commitment therapy with anxiety disorders', *International Journal of Psychology and Psychological Therapy*, 12(3): 359–72.

Shier, M.L. and Graham, J.R. (2010) 'Mindfulness, subjective wellbeing, and social work: insight into their interconnection from social work practitioners', *Social Work Education*, 30(1): 29–44.

Siegel, D.J. (2009) 'Mindful awareness, mindsight, and neural integration', *The Humanistic Psychologist*, 37(2): 137–58.

Siegel, D.J. (2010) *The Mindful Therapist: a clinician's guide to mindsight and neural integration*, New York: Norton & Company.

Siegel, D.J. (2012) *The Developing Mind: how relationships and the brain interact to shape who we are*, New York: Guilford.

Siegel, D.J. (2015) 'Interpersonal neurobiology as a lens into the development of wellbeing and resilience', *Children Australia*, 40(2): 160–4.

Siegel, R.D., Germer, C.K. and Olendzki, A. (2011) 'Mindfulness: What is it? Where did it come from?', in F. Didonna (ed) *Clinical Handbook of Mindfulness*, New York: Springer.

Tenzin, N.K. (2014) *The Royal Seal of Mahamudra, vol. 1: a guidebook for the realization of coemergence*, London: Snow Lion.

Thomas, J.T. and Otis, M.D. (2010) 'Intrapsychic correlates of professional quality of life: mindfulness, empathy, and emotional separation', *Journal of the Society for Social Work and Research*, 1(2): 83–98.

Thompson, R.W., Arnkoff, D.B. and Glass, C.R. (2011) 'Conceptualising mindfulness and acceptance as components of psychological resilience to trauma', *Trauma, Violence, and Abuse*, 12(4): 220–35.

Yadavaia, J.E., Hayes, S.C. and Vilardaga, R. (2014) 'Using acceptance and commitment therapy to increase self-compassion: a randomised controlled trial', *Journal of Contextual Behavioral Science*, 3(4): 248–57.

31

Spiritual competence

The key to effective practice with people from diverse religious backgrounds

David R. Hodge

Introduction

It is increasingly recognised that spirituality is an important dimension of human existence that frequently intersects service provision (Hodge 2015a). For example, a substantial and growing body of research indicates that spirituality tends to facilitate health and wellness (Koenig *et al.* 2012; Koenig and Shohaib 2014). As a result, social work practitioners frequently seek to identify and operationalise clients' spiritual assets to help them cope with, and overcome, the challenges they face.

In the process of addressing client spirituality, social workers often encounter people from diverse religious backgrounds. Such differences can represent an obstacle to effective service provision (Sue and Sue 2013). Clients' spirituality typically informs a diverse array of beliefs and values that intersect service provision, from communication styles to gender and marital interactions to medical care (Richards and Bergin 2014). Dissimilarity in beliefs and values can negatively impact service provision. Indeed, such differences – if not addressed appropriately – can even accentuate clients' problems.

To provide effective services with such clients, sufficient levels of spiritual competence are necessary (Hodge 2015a). Spiritual competence is the vehicle that allows practitioners to overcome the obstacles presented by dissimilar value systems. Although working across different value systems is typically a complex endeavour, developing one's level of spiritual competence can position practitioners to successfully navigate this potentially challenging task.

What is spiritual competence? Spiritual competence can be understood as a form of cultural competence that deals with spirituality and religion, specifically clients' individually constructed spiritual worldviews (Hodge and Bushfield 2006). In a manner analogous to cultural competence, spiritual competence is characterised by three, interrelated dimensions: 1) an awareness of one's own value-informed worldview along with its associated assumptions, limitations and biases; 2) an empathic, strengths-based understanding of the client's spiritual worldview; and 3) the ability to design and implement interventions that resonate with the client's spiritual worldview.

Spiritual competence is not a fixed entity. Rather, it is an ability that can be developed over time (Furness and Gilligan 2010). More specifically, spiritual competence is a dynamic set of attitudes, knowledge and skills that practitioners can acquire regarding different religious groups or traditions (Sue and Sue 2013).

To help practitioners understand and implement spiritual competence in their work with clients, each dimension of spiritual competence is discussed. Before beginning with the first dimension, however, the concepts of spirituality, religion and culture are defined. Sketching out some general definitions for these terms may help readers understand the subsequent content.

Spirituality, religion and culture

It is important to note that clients define spirituality and religion – and the relationship between these two constructs – in a variety of ways (Hodge 2015b). Some view spirituality as the broader construct, while others view religion as the more encompassing construct (Crisp 2010). Still others use the terms interchangeably (Ammerman 2013; Gallup and Jones 2000). This diversity of views should be kept in mind in work with clients. Practitioners should seek to avoid imposing their own definitional constructs on client narratives and attempt to work within the parameters of clients' definitional understandings.

For the purposes of this paper, however, the concepts of spirituality and religion are defined as distinct but overlapping constructs. Spirituality is conceptualised as an individual's subjective connection or relationship with the sacred or transcendent (Hodge 2013), often manifested in the form of a relationship with God (Wuthnow 2007). Religion is defined as a culturally-shared set of beliefs, values and practices that have been developed over time by those who share similar experiences of transcendent reality (Praglin 2004). Thus, religion is one manifestation of culture, which can be defined as a value system or worldview shared by a relatively large group of people (Scollon *et al.* 2012). Put differently, religion is a spiritually animated culture, or a culture that is characterised by certain ideals, principles and practices that have a spiritual purpose.

Understood in this manner, spirituality is an individually-constructed entity while religion is a communally-constructed entity (Derezotes 2006). People develop their own spiritual value system that tends to be informed by their participation in religion. Put differently, religion tends to mediate spirituality. In many cases, full mediation occurs. In other words, individuals' spirituality is essentially completely shaped by their religion. In addition to religious participation, other factors inform individuals' relationship with the sacred, such as race or ethnicity. These thumbnail definitions provide a foundation for understanding the three dimensions of spiritual competence, the first of which pertains to one's personal worldview or value system.

Awareness of one's own value-informed worldview and biases

The first dimension of spiritual competence is developing an understanding of one's own value-informed worldview, in tandem with its assumptions, limitations and biases. Everyone views reality through the prism of an individually-distinct worldview. These worldviews serve important functions, such as helping adherents understand and interpret life experiences (Soenke *et al.* 2013).

Although personal worldviews play an essential role in making sense of life experiences, they also function to refract reality. Every worldview rests upon certain assumptions, which, in turn, serve to highlight particular information while simultaneously obscuring other data (Kuhn 1970). People tend to be unaware of this process. It is a dynamic that largely occurs at an unconscious level (Scollon *et al.* 2012). Consequently, it is important to engage in self-examination to develop awareness of the limitations of one's worldview and its potential biases.

Perhaps the most prevalent worldview in Western nations is secularism (Hodge 2002). As the

Table 31.1 Values commonly affirmed in Western secular culture and Islamic culture

Western secular culture	Islamic culture
Material/naturalistic orientation	Spiritual/eternal orientation
Individualism	Community
Separateness	Connectedness
Self-determination	Consensus
Independence	Interdependence
Self-actualisation	Community actualisation
Personal achievement and success	Group achievement and success
Self-reliance	Community reliance
Respect for individual rights	Respect for community rights
Self-expression	Self-control
Clothing used to accentuate individual beauty and sexuality	Clothing used to operationalise modesty and spirituality
Sensitivity to individual oppression	Sensitivity to group oppression
Identity rooted in sexuality and work	Identity rooted in culture and God
Egalitarian gender roles	Complementary gender roles
Pro-choice	Pro-life
Sexuality expressed based on individual choice	Sexuality expressed in marriage
Explicit communication that clearly expresses individual opinion	Implicit communication that safeguards others' opinions
Spirituality and morality individually constructed	Spirituality and morality derived from the *shari'a*
Food consumed in accordance with individual tastes and preferences	Food consumed in accordance with Islamic values to honour God and community

Adapted from Hodge (2005)

dominant worldview in Western societies, it serves as the cultural default (Smith 2003). Other worldviews are implicitly judged in terms of how they compare to secularism.

To be clear, many other worldviews exist in addition to secularism. Religions can also serve as worldviews for devout adherents (Pargament 2013). Common examples in Western nations include charismatic or pentecostal Protestantism, traditional or orthodox Roman Catholicism, Islam, Hinduism and, in certain manifestations, the New Age or syncretistic spirituality movement. These cultural belief systems often provide adherents with a unique value system that serves to guide and shape adherents' personal beliefs and practices. Nevertheless, these value systems tend to function as subordinate worldviews in Western nations where secularism dominates discourse (Smith 2003).

Due to secularism's status as the cultural default, it can be difficult to comprehend its influence. Because secularism permeates contemporary Western discourse, its values are implicitly assumed to be normative (Sue and Sue 2013). Table 31.1 depicts values that are commonly affirmed in Western secular culture. The origins of this culture can be traced to the Enlightenment, an eighteenth-century movement that originated in Western Europe. Enlightenment thinkers explicitly rejected transcendent worldviews. In their place, they affirmed worldviews characterised by materialistic value systems that privileged the notion of the autonomous, secular individual (Gellner 1992).

The values delineated in the first column of Table 31.1 are likely familiar to most readers. To be clear, this is not to say that readers will necessarily personally affirm all the values listed. Rather, the point is that social workers will likely have some degree of familiarity with the listed values. In addition to being widely disseminated in popular culture, they animate educational programmes throughout the helping professions. In such forums, they are also implicitly associated with healthy functioning (Jafari 1993). As noted previously, however, no worldview is neutral. Every worldview has an associated set of limitations (Lyotard 1979/1984).

Take, for instance, the value of explicit communication that is commonly operationalised in the form of 'I statements'. Social workers are frequently taught to accept the assumption that explicit communication that clearly expresses individual opinion engenders salutary functioning. While this may be true among many secular adults in Western societies, it is not a universally affirmed value in all cultural contexts (Yarhouse and Johnson 2013). In some cultural value systems, explicit forms of communication are viewed unfavourably. For instance, some Hindus may prefer more indirect communication styles that safeguard others' feelings (Hodge 2004). Direct communication may be perceived as self-centred and lacking in respect for others.

In addition to helping address more overt value conflicts, developing an awareness of one's personal beliefs and biases assists practitioners deal with potential conflicts that are of a more covert nature. Take, for instance, the issue of spiritual countertransference (Vogel *et al.* 2013). Countertransference biases can damage therapeutic relationships by distorting perceptions, creating blind spots and engendering detrimental emotional responses (Hepworth *et al.* 2013). To cite a common example, marriage and family practitioners from divorced families may attempt to work through any unaddressed negative experiences in their work with conflicted couples.

In a similar manner, negative feelings about past spiritual events can result in spiritual countertransference (Vogel *et al.* 2013). Practitioners may attempt to resolve deleterious spiritual experiences with their clients. Attempts may be made unconsciously, or even consciously, to use therapeutic relationships to address unresolved spiritual needs to the detriment of clients.

Working with clients from traditions practitioners have personally rejected may trigger spiritual countertransference biases. Although people leave the religious traditions of their family of origin for a variety of reasons, some leave due to what are perceived to be negative experiences (Chaves 2011). For instance, some data suggests a significant percentage of therapists reject the theistic beliefs of their family of origin and report negative sentiments regarding their childhood religious experiences (Hodge 2003; Shafranske and Cummings 2013).

In much the same way that practitioners from a divorced family may experience countertransference biases when working with couples considering a divorce, the unresolved sentiments associated with negative childhood experiences can elicit spiritual countertransference biases. Animosities rooted in childhood experiences may be projected onto clients, resulting in increased negative appraisals and a less empathic posture. Practitioners may attempt to pathologise clients' values, implicitly frame them as unhelpful or attempt to convert them to the values affirmed by the dominant culture. In some cases, these biases may be projected upon all clients who affirm values that differ from those affirmed in the dominant secular culture (Yancey 2014; Yancey and Williamson 2012).

To help mitigate such biases, self-examination is necessary. It provides a vehicle to identify the ways in which one's values may impact the therapeutic conversation. Identification is the first step in the process of ensuring that one does not impose one's values in detrimental ways. Developing awareness of one's beliefs and values is the first step in developing spiritual competence. It also aids in the process of developing the second dimension of spiritual competence.

An empathic understanding of the client's spiritual worldview

The second dimension of spiritual competence is to develop an empathic, strengths-based understanding of the client's spiritual worldview. To be clear, this understanding goes beyond mere knowledge of clients' beliefs and values. Rather, the goal is to develop some degree of psychological appreciation for, and identification with, the client's value system.

Clients' spiritual worldviews can affect a host of areas that intersect with service provision (Richards and Bergin 2014). These areas include beliefs and practices that stretch from birth to death, including child birth and care, schooling, gender interactions, diet, clothing, communication styles, marital relations, emotional expressiveness, celebrations, finances, recreation, coping practices, health, healing, wellness, medical care, burial practices and grieving. As this list implies, spirituality can inform virtually every facet of existence across the lifespan.

Given that values permeate social work practice, it is to be expected that differences in values will emerge between practitioners and clients. Indeed, such value conflicts can be expected to occur with some frequency when working with clients from different religious backgrounds. In some cases, practitioners may strongly disagree with clients' spiritual values.

It is important to note that agreement with clients' values is not a prerequisite for effective service provision. For instance, the American-based National Association of Social Workers' [NASW] (2001) *Standards for Cultural Competence in Social Work Practice* state that it is not necessary to personally concur with the values of clients who affirm culturally different worldviews. It is, however, essential that practitioners appreciate clients' worldviews as legitimate understandings of reality. The goal is not agreement, but to understand the worldview's internal logic and why adherents find the value system so compelling, at both a rational and affective level.

Developing this type of emphatic resonance can be particularly challenging when clients' spiritual values differ from those affirmed in the broader secular culture (Snyder *et al.* 2008). As the dominant cultural worldview, secularism is understood to represent the natural state of affairs. It is often implicitly assumed that all reasonable, intelligent people share the values depicted in the first column of Table 31.1. Western secularism is assumed to represent the cultural centre. As a result, its values are typically viewed as normal, legitimate and health-promoting.

To the extent that other cultural value systems deviate from the cultural centre, they tend to be viewed as abnormal, illegitimate and even detrimental to clients' welfare. Since practitioners have typically been socialised to see Western secular values as normative, it is often difficult to see the strengths of other worldviews (Smith 2014). Indeed, the more religious cultures depart from the conventions of Western secularism, the greater the difficulty practitioners can have in developing an empathetic understanding of culturally different worldviews.

The potential difference in values between the dominant and alternative cultures is illustrated by comparing the first and second columns in Table 31.1. In addition to depicting Western secular values, the table features common Islamic values. As can be seen, Muslims often affirm values that differ substantially from those affirmed in the dominant secular culture (Husain and Ross-Sheriff 2011). For instance, Islam places a relatively greater stress upon values such as community, complementary gender roles and modesty.

Given this difference in value systems, what might an emphatic understanding look like in practice? The value of modesty may serve as a helpful case example. Modesty is operationalised by many Muslim females through the practice of veiling or hijab (Sloan 2011). From within the worldview of Western secularism, it can appear that this value is oppressive to women by, for example, restricting their ability to express themselves. Indeed, veiling is often understood to symbolise the oppression that women are assumed to experience within Islam.

From within the vantage point of an Islamic worldview, however, things can look radically different (Graham *et al.* 2010). From the perspective of many Muslim women, it is not Islamic values, but Western secular values that lead to the oppression of women. In support of this position, these Muslims highlight how women are treated in secular Western societies. To cite some examples, they might point to the commodification of women as sexual objects in

Western discourse, elevated levels of eating disorders among females, popular music that extols the humiliation of women and high rates of physical and sexual violence targeting women on universities and other secular settings (Hodge 2005).

Muslim women argue that such oppression is comparatively rare in Islamic societies where women, they contend, are treated with respect and dignity. In Qatar, for example, humiliating sexualised depictions of women are virtually non-existent, as are instances of rape (Sloan 2011). Moreover, hijab can also have a protective effect in Western societies. In Britain, research suggests Muslims who wear the hijab have more positive body images, place less importance upon appearance and are less reliant on Western media messages regarding beauty ideals (Swami *et al.* 2014). Even in the ideological surround of oppressive Western secularism, Islam is emancipatory for women.

Recognition of the limitations of one's worldview helps in the process of developing an emphatic understanding of culturally different worldviews. To follow up on the previous example, recognising how the secular culture can oppress women tends to free up cognitive space to acknowledge, and then appreciate, that Islam can have a liberating effect upon women. It is at this point – when one develops an emphatic understanding of the client's construction of reality – that one is equipped to operationalise the third dimension of spiritual competence.

The ability to design interventions that resonate with clients' spiritual worldview

The third dimension of spiritual competence is the ability to design and implement interventions that resonate with clients' spiritual worldview. This dimension is intertwined with the other two dimensions. For instance, the creation of therapeutic strategies that resonate with clients' values is typically contingent upon developing an empathic understanding of the internal logic of clients' value system.

It may be helpful at this junction to reiterate that, for the purposes of this chapter, spirituality is an individually constructed entity while religion is a communally constructed entity. Accordingly, formalised religious value systems are rarely adopted without some qualification. In other words, individuals rarely incorporate every facet of their religion's teachings into their personal spiritual worldview. Rather, their worldviews are typically individualised to some extent. An individual's unique impulse to connect with the sacred or transcendent shapes the specific religious values that are incorporated into their personal spiritual value system. Other factors that shape the construction of clients' personal spiritual worldview include ethnicity, nation of origin and perhaps most importantly, the degree of assimilation to the dominant secular culture (Loewenthal 2013). These factors, in tandem with clients' religion, all serve to shape and influence the parameters of clients' unique spiritual value system.

Accordingly, when considering interventions it is important to focus on clients' individualised spiritual worldview as opposed to their reported religious affiliation. Therapeutic strategies should make sense within the matrix of clients' personal belief system. Such interventions are associated with a number of potential benefits (Hepworth *et al.* 2013). Included among these are the protection of client autonomy, enhanced therapeutic rapport, increased likelihood of intervention adoption and implementation, and reduced likelihood of perpetrating harm.

What does an intervention that resonates with clients' spirituality look like? To some extent the answer to this question will depend upon the specific therapeutic context. A variety of factors influence the selection and construction of interventions, including the nature of the presenting problem, practitioners' theoretical orientation, and of course, clients' spiritual values.

Bearing these qualifications in mind, Table 31.2 provides a couple of examples that might

Table 31.2 Islamically-modified CBT protocols

Therapeutic concept	Secular self-statements	Islamically-modified statements
Self-acceptance	If I fail at school, work or some other setting, it is not a reflection on my whole being. (My whole being includes how I am as a friend, daughter, etc. as well as qualities of helpfulness, kindness, etc.) Further, failure is not a permanent condition	Allah knows us better than we know ourselves. Allah knows our weakness. Allah knows we make mistakes. Consequently, we can take comfort in Allah's mercy and accept ourselves with our strengths and weaknesses
Self-worth	I am a worthwhile person with positive and negative traits	We have worth because we are created by Allah. We are created with strengths and weaknesses

Adapted from Hodge and Nadir (2008)

be used with a Muslim client dealing with issues related to self-worth and self-acceptance. The examples are based upon a cognitive behavioural theoretical (CBT) framework, one of the most widely used evidence-based modalities (Hepworth *et al.* 2013). The table features three key components: 1) secular self-statements drawn from the work of Ellis (2000), a prominent founder of CBT in Western discourse; 2) the therapeutic issue the self-statement is designed to address; and 3) statements that have been modified to incorporate Islamic values.

As can be seen in Table 31.2, the underlying therapeutic concept reflected in the secular self-statements has been 'repackaged' in terminology drawn from an Islamic worldview. Practitioners work with clients to express a salutary therapeutic concept in language that makes sense within the context of their Islamic value system. The end result is the creation of an intervention that resonates with the beliefs and values of the Muslim client. Additional information on spiritually modified CBT is available from a number of sources (Hodge 2008; Hodge and Nadir 2008; Nielsen 2004).

Conclusion

As noted previously, spiritual competence is not a fixed entity, but a dynamic set of attitudes, knowledge and skills regarding different religious worldviews that can be developed over time. Toward that end, practitioners might consider obtaining some of the various texts developed to assist practitioners in understanding the internal logic of various religious cultures (Koenig 1998; Koenig 2013; Pargament 2013; Richards and Bergin 2014; Van Hook *et al.* 2001). Similarly, self-assessment can be facilitated through introspection and consultation with spiritually competent supervisors (Furness and Gilligan 2010). This process can be facilitated through the administration of self-assessments using various diagrammatic assessment tools, such as spiritual lifemaps, genograms, eco-maps and ecograms (Hodge 2015a).

Like other important practice attributes, it takes time and effort to develop spiritual competence with the various groups practitioners regularly encounter in their work. This expenditure is well worth it, however, as it lays the foundation for ethical and effective practice with religiously different clients. Spirituality is often a touchy subject and even the most well-intentioned social workers can inadvertently offend clients. Spiritual competence assists practitioners in circumventing these potential minefields, establishing therapeutic rapport, and developing effective interventions that are more likely to be implemented. Indeed, it is the key to effective practice with clients from different religious backgrounds.

References

Ammerman, N.T. (2013) 'Spiritual but not religious? Beyond binary choices in the study of religion', *Journal for the Scientific Study of Religion*, 52(2): 258–78.

Chaves, M. (2011) *American Religion: contemporary trends*, Princeton, NJ: Princeton University Press.

Crisp, B.R. (2010) *Spirituality and Social Work*, Farnham: Ashgate.

Derezotes, D.S. (2006) *Spiritually Oriented Social Work Practice*, Boston: Pearson Education.

Ellis, A. (2000) 'Can rational emotive behavior therapy be effectively used with people who have devout beliefs in God and religion?', *Professional Psychology: Research and Practice*, 31(1): 29–33.

Furness, S. and Gilligan, P. (2010) *Religion, Belief and Social Work: making a difference*, Bristol: Policy Press.

Gallup, G.J. and Jones, T. (2000) *The Next American Spirituality: finding God in the twenty-first century*, Colorado Springs, CO: Victor.

Gellner, E. (1992) *Postmodernism, Reason and Religion*, New York: Routledge.

Graham, J.R., Bradshaw, C. and Trew, J.L. (2010) 'Cultural considerations for social service agencies working with Muslim clients', *Social Work*, 55(4): 337–46.

Hepworth, D.H., Rooney, R.H., Rooney, G.D. and Strom-Gottfried, K. (2013) *Direct Social Work Practice: theory and skills*, 9th edn, Belmont, CA: Brooks/Cole.

Hodge, D.R. (2002) 'Equally devout, but do they speak the same language? Comparing the religious beliefs and practices of social workers and the general public', *Families in Society*, 83(5-6): 573–84.

Hodge, D.R. (2003) 'The challenge of spiritual diversity: can social work facilitate an inclusive environment?', *Families in Society*, 84(3): 348–58.

Hodge, D.R. (2004) 'Working with Hindu clients in a spiritually sensitive manner', *Social Work*, 49(1), 27–38.

Hodge, D.R. (2005) 'Social work and the house of Islam: orienting practitioners to the beliefs and values of Muslims in the United States', *Social Work*, 50(2): 162–73.

Hodge, D.R. (2008) 'Constructing spiritually modified interventions: cognitive therapy with diverse populations', *International Social Work*, 51(2): 178–92.

Hodge, D.R. (2013) 'Implicit spiritual assessment: an alternative approach for assessing client spirituality', *Social Work*, 58(3): 223–30.

Hodge, D.R. (2015a) *Spiritual Assessment in Social Work and Mental Health Practice*, New York: Columbia University Press.

Hodge, D.R. (2015b) 'Spirituality and religion among the general public: Implications for social work discourse', *Social Work*, 60(3): 219–27.

Hodge, D.R. and Bushfield, S. (2006) 'Developing spiritual competence in practice', *Journal of Ethnic and Cultural Diversity in Social Work*, 15(3–4): 101–27.

Hodge, D.R. and Nadir, A. (2008) 'Moving toward culturally competent practice with Muslims: modifying cognitive therapy with Islamic tenets', *Social Work*, 53(1): 31–41.

Husain, A. and Ross-Sheriff, F. (2011) 'Cultural competence with Muslim Americans', in D. Lum (ed) *Culturally Competent Practice: a framework for understanding diverse groups and justice issues*, 4th edn, Belmont, CA: Brooks/Cole.

Jafari, M.F. (1993) 'Counseling values and objectives: a comparison of western and Islamic perspectives', *The American Journal of Islamic Social Sciences*, 10(3): 326–39.

Koenig, H.G. (ed) (1998) *Handbook of Religion and Mental Health*, San Diego, CA: Academic Press.

Koenig, H.G. (2013) *Spirituality in Patient Care: why, how, when, and what*, 3rd edn, West Conshohocken, PA: Templeton Press.

Koenig, H.G. and Shohaib, S.A. (2014) *Health and Wellbeing in Islamic Societies: background, research, and applications*, New York: Springer.

Koenig, H.G., King, D. and Carson, V.B. (2012) *Handbook of Religion and Health*, 2nd edn, New York: Oxford University Press.

Kuhn, T.S. (1970) *The Structure of Scientific Revolutions*, 2nd edn, Chicago: University of Chicago Press.

Loewenthal, K.M. (2013) 'Religion, spirituality, and culture: clarifying the direction and effects', in K.I. Pargament (ed) *APA Handbook of Psychology, Religion, and Spirituality: vol. 1. context, theory, and research*, Washington, DC: American Psychological Association.

Lyotard, J-F. (1979/1984) *The Postmodern Condition: a report on knowledge* (G. Bennington and B. Massumi, Trans), Minneapolis, MA: University of Minnesota Press.

National Association of Social Workers [NASW] (2001). *Standards for Cultural Competence in Social Work*

Practice, Washington, DC: NASW. Online. Available HTTP: www.socialworkers.org/practice/standards/NASWCulturalStandards.pdf (accessed 14 December 2014).

Nielsen, S.L. (2004) 'A Mormon rational emotive behavior therapist attempts Qur'anic rational emotive behavior therapy', in P.S. Richards and A.E. Bergin (eds) *Casebook for a Spiritual Strategy in Counseling and Psychotherapy*, Washington, DC: American Psychological Association.

Pargament, K.I. (ed) (2013) *APA Handbook of Psychology, Religion, and Spirituality: vol. 1. context, theory, and research*, Washington, DC: American Psychological Association.

Praglin, L.J. (2004) 'Spirituality, religion, and social work: an effort towards interdisciplinary conversation', *Journal for Religion and Spirituality in Social Work*, 23(4): 67–84.

Richards, P.S. and Bergin, A.E. (eds) (2014) *Handbook of Psychotherapy and Religious Diversity*, 2nd edn, Washington, DC: American Psychological Association.

Scollon, R., Schollon, S.W. and Jones, R.H. (2012) *Intercultural Communication: a discourse approach*, 3rd edn, Malden, MA: John Wiley & Sons.

Shafranske, E.P. and Cummings, J.P. (2013) 'Religious and spiritual beliefs, affiliations, and practices of psychologists', in K.I. Pargament (ed) *APA Handbook of Psychology, Religion, and Spirituality: vol. 2. an applied psychology of religion and spirituality*, Washington, DC: American Psychological Association.

Sloan, L. (2011) 'Women's oppression or choice? One American's view on wearing the hijab', *Affilia*, 26(2): 218–21.

Smith, C. (2003) *The Secular Revolution*, Berkeley, CA: University of California Press.

Smith, C. (2014) *The Sacred Project of American Sociology*, New York: Oxford University Press.

Snyder, C., May, J.D. and Peeler, J. (2008) 'Combining human diversity and social justice education: a conceptual framework', *Journal of Social Work Education*, 44(1): 145–61.

Soenke, M., Landau, M.J. and Greenberg, J. (2013) 'Sacred armor: religion's role as a buffer against the anxieties of life and the fear of death', in K.I. Pargament (ed) *APA Handbook of Psychology, Religion, and Spirituality: vol. 1. context, theory, and research*, Washington, DC: American Psychological Association.

Sue, D. and Sue, D. (2013) *Counseling the Culturally Diverse: theory and practice*, 6th edn, Hoboken, NJ: John Wiley & Sons.

Swami, V., Miah, J., Noorani, N. and Taylor, D. (2014) 'Is the hijab protective? An investigation of the body image and related constructs among British Muslim women', *British Journal of Psychology*, 105(3): 352–63.

Van Hook, M., Hugen, B. and Aguilar, M.A. (eds) (2001) *Spirituality within Religious Traditions in Social Work Practice*, Pacific Grove, CA: Brooks/Cole.

Vogel, M.J., McMinn, M.R., Peterson, M.A. and Gatherecoal, K.A. (2013) 'Examining religion and spirituality as diversity training: a multidimensional look at training in the American Psychological Association', *Professional Psychology: Research and Practice*, 44(3): 158–67.

Wuthnow, R. (2007) *After the Baby Boomers: how twenty- and thirty-somethings are shaping the future of American religion*, Princeton, NJ: Princeton University Press.

Yancey, G.A. (2014) *Dehumanizing Christians: cultural competition in a multicultural world*, New Brunswick, NJ: Transaction Publishers.

Yancey, G.A. and Williamson, D.A. (2012) *What Motivates Cultural Progressives? Understanding opposition to the political and Christian right*, Waco, TX: Baylor University Press.

Yarhouse, M.A. and Johnson, V. (2013) 'Values and ethical issues: the interface between psychology and religion', in K.I. Pargament (ed) *APA Handbook of Psychology, Religion, and Spirituality: vol. 2. an applied psychology of religion and spirituality*, Washington, DC: American Psychological Association.

32

A spiritual approach to social work practice

Ann M. Carrington

Introduction

There has been much debate regarding spirituality's role in social work over the past three decades. The dust has settled and there appears to be a general acceptance now that not only can there be a role for spirituality in social work, but that it is an important inclusion in order to work with the whole person. However, when it comes to guides to, or consensus on, how one should practice when integrating spirituality, gaps remain. In order to contribute to the discipline's attempts to address such gaps, a research journey was embarked upon. The research explored different spiritual paradigms, theories and practices with a view to establishing the contribution these may provide in the process of, not only including spirituality in social work practice, but doing so from an authentic spiritual perspective (see publications from this research program: Carrington 2010a, 2010b, 2013, 2014).

This chapter suggests a spiritual approach to social work practice reflective of one of the key overarching findings of this research programme – the importance of linking paradigmatic positioning with practice (Carrington 2010b). Before we explore the approach, it is important to examine the current context of spirituality in social work and some of the relevant discussions unfolding in this arena.

Spirituality and social work

Although social work has its historical roots firmly planted in religion, specifically Judo–Christian (Lynn and Mensinga 2015; Senreich 2013), social work successfully engaged in a process of marginalising and excluding religion and spirituality in response to the scientific modernist agenda (Lynn and Mensinga 2015; Martinez-Brawley and Zorita 2007; Rice and McAuliffe 2009). In an attempt to be recognised as a professional discipline, it opted to conform with the scientific push that began with the Enlightenment and became focused on empirical, evidenced-based practice, informed by a positivist secular and modernist paradigm (Martinez-Brawley and Zorita 2007; Rice 2002), excluding other ways of knowing and doing in the process (Barker and Floersch 2010; Hodge 2009). We now see a resurgence of interest in the religious and spiritual dimensions within social work (Crisp 2008), but there are many tensions (Edwards 2002; Gilham

2012; Rice 2002) in attempting to bring a dimension of spirituality and other ways of knowing back within the fold of social work.

This shift again to embrace religious or spiritual dimensions has tended to be assisted by a focus more on spirituality than on religion (Barker and Floersch 2010; Senreich 2013; Wong and Vinsky 2009). Given the historical context, and the links between religion and colonisation processes across the world, spirituality, it seems, is more palatable to the new modernist and secular social work (Lindsay 2002; Wong and Vinsky 2009). To this end, as social work looks to re-embrace a spiritual dimension, there has been a distinction made between religion and spirituality (Barker and Floersch 2010), although Wong and Vinsky (2009) suggest that this distinction may well reproduce colonial othering and marginalisation. While many (Holloway and Moss 2010; Lindsay 2002; Senreich 2013; Tacey 2000) have engaged in the debate and process of defining both religion and spirituality, the definitions provided by Canda and Furman (2010) tend to be those that have become the cornerstone of this discussion. The key distinction is that religion is a pattern of beliefs or rules shared by communities or groups that are transmitted or reinforced over time, while spirituality is experienced at a more individual level in relation to the creation of meaning and purpose. Further, there is recognition that there is, or can be, a level of overlap between religion and spirituality as some may house their spiritual experience within the construct of an organised religion (Barker and Floersch 2010; Hodge 2015).

In an effort to further remove itself from past mistakes, social work seems to be focusing on the argument that spirituality should be included because it is important to some clients and meets clients' needs with little consideration being given to the practitioner's position or needs (Buckey 2012; Crisp 2008; Gilham 2012; Hodge 2015; Senreich 2013). This was often argued as a form of anti-oppressive practice (Gilham 2012; Lynn *et al.* 2015; Wong and Vinsky 2009) and has been found in the past predominantly within the area of culturally appropriate practice (Hodge 2015; Rice 2002; Rice and McAuliffe 2009). Although it now seems to be expanding to a more general or broader position, spirituality still seems to be associated mostly in working with 'others' (Rice and McAuliffe 2009; Senreich 2013).

Despite some authors mentioning the importance of including spirituality in acknowledgement of the practitioner's spiritual dimension, this has not been a central focus of the argument (Gilham 2012; Rice and McAuliffe 2009). In fact, this seems to be one of the key ethical concerns for many as there is a fear that practitioners will use their position as a social worker to indoctrinate, impose upon or convert vulnerable clients to their specific religious ideology, directly contravening client self-determination (Gilham 2012; Rice 2002; Sheridan 2009). It is interesting, however, to recognise that within such arguments there is little acknowledgement that such a process is already occurring in regard to imposing secular ideologies and beliefs upon practitioners, clients and the discipline. This, for the most part, continues to go on unquestioned and is illustrative of the secular's position as the dominant and unchallenged norm (Hodge 2009). This chapter begins to challenge this position by putting forth an approach to practice that focuses on the practitioner's spiritual paradigmatic positioning as the foundation of a spiritual approach to social work practice.

A paradigmatic chasm

The pressure to conform to the dominant discourse is not specific to social work and has occurred across the board; as Wilber (2006) argues, the spiritual perspectives have been the largest casualty of this process, as the spiritual perspectives were in direct opposition to that of the secular. As the secular humanist perspective's view of reality and what can be known is limited only to that which exists within the temporal and tangible physical world, all ontological, epistemological and methodological methods, measures and practices that fell outside of this were delegitimised (Hodge 2009). With the scientific secular discourse positioning itself as the valid authority and 'owners' of the 'truth' (Hodge 2009), social work fell in line with its demands and made every attempt to satisfy requirements with a keen focus on evidence-based practice (Rice 2002; Rice and McAuliffe 2009). This process not only rejected spirituality but largely discarded 'the art' of social work in the form of tacit knowledge and practice wisdom (Martinez-Brawley and Zorita 2007; Osmond 2006).

It is perhaps this pressure to align with the dominant discourse that has created the chasm between spiritual paradigm and spiritual practice. As social work has endeavoured to include spirituality, many practitioners and scholars have done so with a focus on practice, with little consideration of the paradigmatic foundations that inform these practices. Further, in attempts to make such techniques palatable and valid within the current context of the secular, scientific discourse, there has been, I would suggest, a conscious tendency to strip away the underlying spiritual beliefs and theories. As Lynn *et al.* (2015) highlight, this has led to a process of secularisation of spiritual practices such as 'mindfulness'. This process of secularisation extends to the process of evidencing the effects of such practices by applying secular scientific methods and measures within research, in order to establish it as a viable practice, again further distancing it from its origins within the Buddhist tradition. Although research shows that this process has positive effects (Birnbaum and Birnbaum 2008; Holzel *et al.* 2011), the rationale regarding such outcomes are now couched in psychological neurological terms rather than understood and experienced in spiritual terms.

A spiritual approach to practice is paradigmatic

The spiritual approach to practice put forth in this chapter is not a complicated model or framework but rather a call for that which already guides practice to be acknowledged – one's individual paradigmatic position! All practice is guided by the individual social worker's paradigmatic positioning. It is these paradigmatic values, beliefs and worldview that inform an individual's overall practice, how they engage with clients and from which theory and practice models they draw. This is not only inescapable but something that, as educators, we strive to foster in students before they enter practice. Assisting students and new practitioners to identify, articulate and implement their individual professional practice framework is a core component of social work education. Therefore, in order to achieve this, students and new practitioners are encouraged to identify their paradigmatic position or worldview and to recognise how this links with theory and practice models from which they draw – exploring not just the alignment between their paradigmatic position and theory and practice, but also in understanding any tensions and how their paradigmatic position aids in negotiating such tensions.

Critical reflection (Fook 2012; Gardner 2011) is a core component of this process and an essential skill in social work practice, as supported by the research of Barker and Floersch (2010). Perhaps the key difference here, as illustrated in a further example that will follow, is that, within the secular scientific environment of academia, there is an assumption students will articulate their practice frameworks drawing from secular paradigms, ideologies, theories and practices. This practice is not only acceptable, but core to basic practice, with ethical concerns only arising if alternative paradigms and ways of knowing and doing, such as the spiritual, are included.

A truly spiritual approach, therefore, is paradigmatic – resolutely positioned within and informed by a spiritual perspective. It is not spiritual practice techniques that have been secularised and made palatable to the secular, such as 'mindfulness' (Lynn *et al.* 2015; Lynn and

Mensigna 2015), or secular practices labelled as 'spiritual' under the guise of culturally appropriate practice. A truly authentic spiritual approach to practice is just that: practice informed by a spiritual perspective, steadfastly and foundationally, not something that can be picked up or left out, depending on the client or the circumstances. A spiritual approach is unapologetically guided by the ontological, epistemological and methodological understandings of the spiritual paradigm and recognises its value and validity irrespective of the dominant discourse's attempts to undermine, exclude and marginalise.

The foundations of any spiritual practice or spiritual approach to social work is one's paradigmatic positioning. Conversely, this argument would suggest that if one is practicing from a spiritually paradigmatic position, then secular practice methods could be drawn upon and executed from a spiritual perspective. Although some might argue that one cannot draw practice from that which are ideologically or paradigmatically opposed, others would hold to the above argument, suggesting that the paradigmatic perspective influences how one executes the practice. For the purposes of this chapter, it does not matter upon which side of the argument one may fall. What is essential is the recognition that paradigmatic positioning directly impacts and influences practice, whether this be via electing only to work from theory and practice models aligned with one's paradigmatic position, or by applying theory or practice models through the lens of one's paradigmatic positioning. This affirms that any form of spiritual practice starts with paradigmatic positioning, whether utilising secular theory and practice, and spiritualising it through the paradigmatic lens, or whether utilising spiritual practices in their authentic form.

A paradigmatic approach in practice

To illustrate the importance of paradigm to practice, I will demonstrate how the Integrated Spiritual Paradigm (Carrington 2010a, 2010b) that is the foundation of my professional practice framework has influenced my practice as a social worker. It is hoped that drawing on my experiences in practice may help others, who may be grappling with tensions, to help guide a practice approach that has a level of authentic spirituality within it and to allow them to practice authentically.

Before exploring the experiences from practice, it is important to outline the basic paradigmatic assumptions of the Integrated Spiritual Paradigm. The Integrated Spiritual Paradigm holds the ontological position that there are multiple physical and spiritual realities of which the ultimate reality is the sum. Physical reality is a reflection of the spiritual. Epistemologically, it holds that knowledge is understood via the varying existing perspectives. They all exist at once and each reflects aspects of the 'Ultimate Truth'. Methodologically, the Integrated Spiritual Paradigm aims to discover, remember or unite with God or the absolute truth through the acknowledgement, exploration and integration of all aspects of reality, both physical and spiritual (Carrington 2010b). As supported by these foundational beliefs, the Integrated Spiritual draws from methods of knowing both physical and spiritual; however, it values the spiritual over the physical. It is, therefore, important to mention the spiritual methods that are seen as valid from this perspective. They include: pure rationale, knowing and intuition guided by pure consciousness, drawn from spiritual positivism; sensing, feeling and intuiting, from spiritual constructivism; and being, contemplation and experience, drawn from the conscious spiritual (Carrington 2014).

To begin the illustration of how the Integrated Spiritual Paradigm informs a spiritual approach within my practice, I will first articulate my professional practice framework, absent of the spiritual component. My professional practice framework consists of feminist, critical and postmodern ideologies, theories and practices. These are the foundation that informs other theories and practices from which I draw and how I implement them. Others from which I draw include cognitive and behavioural theories and psychodynamic theories. Additional specific practice models I utilise include expressive therapies, narrative and strengths. This framework is entirely secular and I would suggest could be implemented without question within most mainstream organisations. Looking at this framework, it is fairly easy to see connections between most of these components and to appreciate that, although some level of tension exists between different aspects, overall there is a level of internal consistency present. The assumption here, also, is that each of the components of this framework are secular and hold to secular principles as highlighted earlier when discussing the development of students' practice frameworks. There is an absence of the spiritual dimension – perhaps with the exception of the expressive therapies, which allude to such a dimension.

When the Integrated Spiritual Paradigm is introduced as the foundation, it changes the lens through which each of these components is interpreted and therefore applied. For example, gender analysis is a key component of feminist theory (Dominelli 2002; Payne 2014) and practice and, although I utilise a gendered analysis in my work, the Integrated Spiritual Paradigm reminds me that ultimately there is no distinction between genders, that we are all one and that we each hold both masculine and feminine qualities. This has helped me to respond to gender issues present within social and political structures and in the lived experience of individual clients in a form aligned with critical and feminist theory, yet which has encouraged me to recognise a bigger picture beyond gender and this moment in time. This has helped me not to fall into the trap of polarising the genders, although at times, when immersed in the theory and sector, this has been somewhat difficult to maintain.

Critical and feminist principles have also influenced my spiritual practice by encouraging me, not only to work with people to raise consciousness (Dominelli 2002; Payne 2014) in regard to gender or structural issues, but also to work with people to raise consciousness about that which is not physical. For example, with women who have experienced sexual assault or domestic violence, in addition to raising consciousness regarding gender and structural issues, I have encouraged them to find something higher than themselves to support them through the trauma and ongoing associated difficulties, e.g. dealing with police, court system, etc. I do not impose a view of what this might be but I encourage them to identify what it is for them. Those who do not have specific religious or spiritual beliefs, or who may identify as atheists, I invite to explore where or what makes them feel safe, strong and nurtured. I have often found that when encouraged to explore this, many of those who do not identify as having religious or spiritual beliefs will identify nature as a place in which they feel the presence of something bigger, higher or other than themselves. With others, I have encouraged them to find that part within that is wise and untouchable, that is a well of peace and strength.

My foundational paradigmatic positioning has also influenced the types of practice approaches and models I use. I draw from the expressive therapies (Pearson 2004; Pearson and Nolan 2004), as they work with that which is beyond the mind; in my view, the spiritual. They allow space for the person to connect with inner or spiritual parts of themselves and yet do not require them consciously to engage in this process, while still reaping the rewards of such practices. This approach allows me to bring in the spiritual component within practice more authentically, supported by an approach that has a level of mainstream acceptance.

Yet even cognitive and behavioural therapy, which is strongly situated within the secular scientific or positivist paradigm (Payne 2014), aligns with aspects of the spiritual foundations of my professional practice framework. In the most basic sense, it aligns with the Integrated Spiritual Paradigm because the paradigm itself recognises all that exists and that different people at different times will require different approaches. In addition, it aligns because the spiritual paradigm recognises that it is the mind which causes disconnection from the Divine or 'Ultimate Truth' and that, if the mind is controlled or managed, the 'Ultimate Truth', God or whatever the label may be, can be found. Therefore, by learning to control the mind, even if using psychology methods as opposed to spiritual techniques, still allows the person the opportunity, should they choose to, to engage at a spiritual level.

This is somewhat in contradiction to arguments I have previously made, where I have said paradigm is important because meditation, taken out of the spiritual context, will not reap the spiritual results intended, which, overall, I still believe to be true, as often meditation within the secular is actually visualisation and relaxation rather than an attempt to commune with God. My argument here is that the spiritual that has been secularised and enacted from a physical or secular perspective has limitations pertaining to meeting spiritual goals. However, the same is not true in reverse. If the secular is practiced from the spiritual perspective, the methods can yield the physical result but also allow an opening for further spiritual movement because they are enacted from a spiritual perspective.

Further to this, the methods through which such practices are engaged are also guided by the spiritual paradigm. In the case of the Integrated Spiritual Paradigm, all those methods mentioned (Carrington 2014) previously are at the disposal of the practitioner. For me, my practice was strongly guided by intuition in every moment. I would rarely have a plan in advance for a client session as I would respond to the person in the moment, as guided by my intuition. What was discussed, and different practice exercises, were allowed to develop within each individual session rather than having a pre-established session plan. This approach required me to trust in the knowledge and skills I had and to allow them to be drawn upon as needed in the moment, rather than through some false intellectual process or timeline outlined in a text book. Sometimes this meant saying something that made no sense to me but that not only resonated with the person, but was integral to their journey. This could be linked to tacit knowledge or practice wisdom, something that has a long and valuable history within social work (Martinez-Brawley and Zorita 2007; Zeira and Rosen 2000). If so, perhaps spiritual practice is really not as far from social work's grasp as some would believe.

This predominantly is the spiritual approach I have taken in practice and am suggesting here that if practice is informed by a spiritual foundation then everything about one's practice becomes spiritual. Although this is not explicitly so now, one day, when the space is created, this too may change. This spiritual approach is not explicitly about meeting client needs, or being culturally appropriate; it is about practicing authentically by not only integrating my foundational spiritual paradigm, but by allowing it to guide my understanding and application of other ideological and theoretical understandings attained through social work education. As with the use of intuition, this overall approach may not be as foreign to social work as one might expect. It strongly aligns with a Rogerian client-centred approach that recognises the relationship between worker and client directly impacts outcomes and that dissonance, disingenuousness or internal conflict within the worker may negatively impact this relationship (Payne 2014).

Having said that, perhaps some of the limitations and restrictions present are required in order not only to maintain ethical social work practice, but also to ensure clear roles are maintained. As social workers, we can draw from spiritual theories to inform our practice with clients to aid in the therapeutic process, but is there not a line that, once crossed, means you are no longer acting in the role of a social worker? Perhaps for those wishing to cross this line, there is another calling to which they need to respond, one that takes them on a journey towards becoming a spiritual or religious practitioner and not a social worker? Although as a social worker my practice may be guided by a spiritual paradigm, and I may utilise spiritual theories and practices, or even discuss spiritual or religious concepts with people, it is not within my role to give spiritual instruction. For that I would suggest there is a need for appropriate referral to a suitable spiritual practitioner.

Reflecting further, I see that much of this approach relies on spiritualising the secular due to the current scientific secular context in which we practice. However, there were some spiritual practices I was able to include and remained authentically spiritual because the foundational paradigm guiding the practice was spiritual, rather than the secularised version often seen in practice today under the guise of culturally appropriate practice. These included the use of spiritual visualisation, energy work, working with the breath and the present moment, cleansing processes, prayer and calling in or upon the Divine. Although these practices remained spiritual, they did not impose a spiritual or religious ideology onto clients. For example, the spiritual visualisations worked either with the spiritual symbology clients had already identified, or encouraged them to connect with their 'inner selves', however that presented for them. In terms of cleansing processes, prayer and calling in the Divine, this was my practice for me, done before and after seeing each client, where I asked for the presence of God to guide my practice, or I used incense, oils or other methods to cleanse the room.

I would suggest that conscious (Carrington 2010a) or critically reflective practice (Gardner 2011) is of paramount importance in applying this spiritual approach to practice as it allows for the exploration and management of tensions or ethical issues. In fact, conscious reflection is a core component of my spiritual practice that goes beyond critical reflection and encourages me to be ever present in practice and in life and to maintain a constant reflective or 'mindful' stance. The following questions are put forward as an aid in the process of adopting such a spiritual approach to social work practice, ethically and consciously.

1   What is your spiritual paradigm and what are the values, beliefs and assumptions it holds?
2   Is your spiritual paradigm foundational to your professional practice framework or simply a component of it?
3   How does your spiritual paradigm inform other paradigms, ideologies, theories and practice approaches within your framework?
4   What tensions are present and how do you deal with these?
5   How does your paradigm inform how you are with people interpersonally?
6   Do the values and beliefs of your spiritual paradigm conflict or cause tensions with social work values, ethics and standards?

Conclusion

We do not explicitly practice secularly, or try to coerce, recruit or indoctrinate clients into believing or following our secular paradigms and ideologies that guide our individual practice; why, then, would we do so with spiritual paradigms? Some would argue that we do, in fact, do this and that, because the secular is the dominant discourse, this goes unchallenged as the norm. If this is so, then should not the spiritual be allowed the same freedom? Or further still, should individuals be allowed to have self-determination or free will, as ascribed to by social work values, and select workers based on being informed explicitly of the worker's practice framework? Is it not more dangerous to have workers implicitly or unconsciously allowing their spiritual or religious beliefs to inform their practice?

If spirituality is included as a valid component of one's practice framework within the discipline, individual practitioners will be able to engage in conscious or critical reflection in regard to their spiritual paradigm and their practice, assisting in ensuring ethical best practice. I would suggest that introducing such a reflective process in the classroom (Barker and Floersch 2010;

Buckey 2012; Senreich 2013) and then continuing it in practice through professional supervision (Gilham 2012) would aid greatly in addressing the valid ethical concerns that have been raised within social work. One's personal paradigms, values and beliefs inform practice, whether we like it or not. By bringing this aspect out of the shadow, we can not only start to 'manage' it ethically, but we can begin to learn and develop new practices from this 'silenced knowledge' (Osmond 2006).

References

Barker, S. L. and Floersch, J. (2010) 'Practitioners' understandings of spirituality: implications for social work education', *Journal of Social Work Education*, 46(3): 357–70.

Birnbaum, L. and Birnbaum, A. (2008) 'Mindful social work: from theory to practice', *Journal of Religion and Spirituality in Social Work*, 27(1–2): 87–104.

Buckey, J.W. (2012) 'Empirically based spirituality education: implications for social work research and practice', *Journal of Social Service Research*, 38(2): 260–71.

Canda, E.R., and Furman, L.D. (2010) *Spiritual Diversity in Social Work Practice: the heart of helping*, 2nd edn, New York: Oxford University Press.

Carrington, A.M. (2010a) 'Spiritual paradigms: a response to concerns within social work in relation to the inclusion of spirituality', *Journal of Religion and Spirituality in Social Work*, 29(4): 300–20.

Carrington, A.M. (2010b) 'A researcher in wonderland: a spiritual approach from paradigm to practice', unpublished doctorate thesis, James Cook University.

Carrington, A.M. (2013) 'An integrated spiritual practice framework for use within social work', *Journal of Religion & Spirituality in Social Work*, 32(4): 287–312.

Carrington, A.M. (2014) 'Expanding the debate', *Qualitative Research Journal*, 14(2): 179–96.

Crisp, B.R. (2008) 'Social work and spirituality in a secular society', *Journal of Social Work*, 8(4): 363–75.

Dominelli, L. (2002) *Feminist Social Work Theory and Practice*, Basingstoke: Palgrave.

Edwards, P.B. (2002) 'Spiritual themes in social work counselling: facilitating the search for meaning', *Australian Social Work*, 55(1): 78–87.

Fook, J. (2012) *Social Work: a critical approach to practice*, 2nd edn, London: Sage.

Gardner, F. (2011) *Critical Spirituality: a holistic approach to contemporary practice*, Farnham: Ashgate.

Gilham, J.M. (2012) 'The ethical use of supervision to facilitate the integration of spirituality in social work practice, *Social Work and Christianity*, 39(3): 255–72.

Hodge, D.R. (2009) 'Secular privilege: deconstructing the invisible rose-tinted sunglasses', *Journal of Religion and Spirituality in Social Work*, 28(1–2): 8–34.

Hodge, D.R. (2015) 'Administering a two-stage spiritual assessment in healthcare settings: a necessary component of ethical and effective care', *Journal of Nursing Management*, 23(1): 27–38.

Holloway, M. and Moss, B. (2010) *Spirituality and Social Work*, London: Palgrave MacMillan.

Holzel, B.K., Carmody, J., Vangel, M., Congleton, C., Yerramsetti, S.M., Gard, T. and Lazar, S.W. (2011) 'Mindfulness practice leads to increases in regional brain gray matter density', *Psychiatry Research: Neuroimaging*, 191(1): 36–43.

Lindsay, R. (2002) *Recognizing Spirituality: the interface between faith and social work*, Crawley: University of Western Australia Press.

Lynn, R. and Mensinga, J. (2015) 'Social workers' narratives of integrating mindfulness into practice', *Journal of Social Work Practice*, 29(3): 255–70.

Lynn, R., Mensinga, J., Tinning, B. and Lundman, K. (2015) 'Is mindfulness value free? Tip toeing through the mindfield of mindfulness', in L. Pyles and G. Adam (eds) *Holistic Social Work Education in the 21st Century*, New York: Oxford University Press.

Martinez-Brawley, E.E. and Zorita, P. (2007) 'Tacit and codified knowledge in social work: a critique of standardization in education and practice', *Families in Society*, 88(4): 534–42.

Osmond, J. (2006) 'A quest for form: the tacit dimension of social work practice', *European Journal of Social Work*, 9(2): 159–81.

Payne, M. (2014) *Modern Social Work Theory*, 4th edn, Basingstoke: Palgrave MacMillan.

Pearson, M. (2004) *Emotional Healing and Self-Esteem: inner-life skills of relaxation, visualisation and meditation for children and adolescents*, London: Jessica Kingsley Publishers.

Pearson, M. and Nolan, P. (2004) *Emotional Release for Children: repairing the past, preparing the future*, London: Jessica Kingsley Publishers.

Rice, S. (2002) 'Magic happens: revisiting the spirituality and social work debate', *Australian Social Work*, 55(4): 303–12.

Rice, S. and McAuliffe, D. (2009) 'Ethics of the spirit: comparing ethical views and usages of spiritually influenced interventions', *Australian Social Work*, 62(3): 403–20.

Senreich, E. (2013) 'An inclusive definition of spirituality for social work education and practice', *Journal of Social Work Education*, 49(4): 548–63.

Sheridan, M.J. (2009) 'Ethical issues in the use of spiritually based interventions in social work practice: what are we doing and why?', *Journal of Religion and Spirituality in Social Work*, 28(1–2): 99–126.

Tacey, D. (2000) *Reenchantment: the new Australian spirituality*, Sydney: HarperCollins.

Wilber, K. (2006) *Integral Spirituality: a startling new role for religion in the modern and postmodern world*, Boston: Integral Books.

Wong, Y.L.R. and Vinsky, J. (2009) 'Speaking from the margins: a critical reflection on the "spiritual-but-not-religious" discourse in social work', *The British Journal of Social Work*, 39(7): 1343–59.

Zeira, A. and Rosen, A. (2000) 'Unraveling "Tacit Knowledge": what social workers do and why they do it', *Social Service Review*, 74(1): 103–23.

33

Critical spirituality and social work practice

Fiona Gardner

Introduction

This chapter begins by exploring the impetus for developing a framework for including spirituality in practice, called 'Critical Spirituality'. The framework was influenced by my experiences as a practitioner, social work educator and trainer, and from research with health and social care professionals who wanted to actively include the 'spiritual' in their professional practice. The process of articulating underlying theory and values from practice contributed to the formation of principles for practice outlined here. The chapter finishes by giving examples to ground understanding of how these principles might influence practice.

My interest in this was triggered by several experiences as a beginning social work academic. One of the students, who I will call Sarah, expressed her frustration in a seminar group with the attitude of her 'fundamentalist Christian church' (her words) to her sexuality. She wanted to remain part of this church community, which in other ways had supported her and her family through many crises, but felt undermined and despairing about their attitude to her as a lesbian. What Sarah (and I) found challenging was the attitude of several members of her seminar group; they simply could not understand where she was coming from. Instead they saw the answer as simply to remove herself from the church: they asked with genuine concern and incredulity, 'why would you want to stay somewhere that made you feel like that?' This effectively silenced Sarah, who felt her desire to explore the complexities of her situation were simply not being heard.

When I pointed out to the class that they might be working with someone in the same situation as Sarah who wanted them to understand what this meant for her, the class members had quite different reactions. Some felt a client's religious background was irrelevant, connected to their private life, not relevant to practice. Others expressed confusion about how they could understand religion when it wasn't part of their experience. Somehow it was possible to stand in the shoes of another person, or at least attempt to, with other life experiences, but not when it came to religion. Some students reacted from the pain of their own church experience, which meant they had also rejected religion. Conversely, some of the students who could understand about the desire for religious connection were also members of religious traditions negative about homosexuality and struggled to accept Sarah being same-sex attracted. Two said that they thought someone's religion was an important part of who they were even though they saw themselves as spiritual rather than religious.

So how to make sense of this experience in training social work students for professional practice? It seemed there were some key themes:

- the value of a broad and inclusive definition of spirituality that people with such different views could connect with
- the subjectivity of the spiritual experience and the challenge of generating mutual understanding
- the strength of people's different views and emotions related to spirituality
- the value of understanding how your own and the broader social context and history influenced views about spirituality
- being able to actively reflect critically on these
- the importance of the spiritual community.

I began to explore this more in other classes but also in practice, related research and workshops with practitioners. For part of this time, I worked half a day a week at a faith-based agency as a social worker in relationship counselling. Two research projects were particularly relevant: the first (the Pastoral Care Networks Project) involved developing training for those working and volunteering in palliative care to foster inclusion of spirituality in practice. Another (Health Promoting Palliative Care) encouraged communities to increase their comfort in supporting those who were dying and their families, which often related to understanding what was meaningful in people's lives. Similarly, in workshops called Spirituality and Work, it became clear that there was a need to make more explicit some ideas about working with spirituality. In critical reflection workshops, professionals affirmed the importance of unearthing what really mattered to them related to underlying values. The themes elicited from my teaching example were reinforced by these later experiences. Practitioners, as well as students, were struggling with what it meant to include the spiritual in practice. While many affirmed the value of this in principle, in practice, they agreed it was challenging and potentially divisive.

Development of a framework

The difficulties expressed by students and practitioners in including the spiritual in practice led to the development of a framework 'Critical Spirituality', which can be used to argue for the integration of the critical, the reflective and the spiritual into a coherent approach to practice that is holistic, inclusive and addresses issues of social justice. More specifically, 'Critical Spirituality' means seeing people and communities holistically, seeking to understand where they are coming from and what matters to them at a fundamental level; the level that is part of the everyday but also transcends it. The expectation is to combine postmodern valuing of the diversity of individual and/or community spiritual experience with a critical perspective that asserts the importance of living harmoniously and respectfully at an individual, family and community level (Gardner 2011).

In beginning to develop the framework, the first issue to be addressed was how spirituality was to be defined. It was clear that there were many definitions in the literature and little agreement (Swinton 2012). This has a positive aspect; Cobb *et al.* (2012: 487) say spirituality 'rejoices in ambiguity and by avoiding simple resolutions maintain the elusive qualities of the human condition'. Similarly, practitioners varied in their reactions to language and definition; some responded negatively to the word spiritual or wellbeing, seeing these as too vague, but equally, others reacted against pastoral care or religion, saying these evoked narrow and unhelpful ways of being that only suited some of their clients. What seemed to be important in reaching agreement was to talk through what was meant and to have a broad and inclusive definition that could encapsulate all of these possible meanings. What I decided to use is spirituality defined as 'that which gives life meaning that includes a sense of something beyond or greater than the self' (Gardner 2011: 24), a definition that can clearly include religious traditions. The critical aspect of critical spirituality makes it explicit that this sense of meaning is understood to be influenced by the broader social context. As Kamitsuka (2007: 22) says, 'spirituality can (not) be abstracted from embodied and cultural experience', while Sorajjakool *et al.* (2010: 170) suggest religion and culture 'constantly modify each other'.

Second, in the process of developing the framework, it was helpful to articulate the many theoretical perspectives that underpinned the workshops, training and research. What I found was that there were two overlapping sets of theories: those that related specifically to spirituality and religion and those that underpinned the critical reflection approach I had used in all of the areas of practice and research. Critical reflection is both a theory and process that fosters deeper understanding of the links between:

- a specific experience
- the emotions, thoughts and actions related to that experience
- the meaning of that experience, including underlying assumptions and values
- the influence of social context and history both individually and collectively with an expectation that this will lead to socially just change.

(Gardner 2014: 24)

In the first stage of critical reflection, the person whose experience it is might explore such questions as: how did I react and why? What underlying values, beliefs, assumptions were there for me? What sense of meaning is there? How does this connect to my family history and social context and to the society in which I live? Similarly, these questions might be explored (in theory) from the perspective of others involved. In the second stage, they would ask, given my new understanding of this experience and why it matters, how would I react differently now; what would I change or do differently?

Theories

The four theories combined in critical reflection are outlined as follows, combined with their connection to spiritual and religious thinking. Making these links explicit reinforced their connections to practice and the value of including the spiritual in practice, for practitioners as well as their clients. As one practitioner said, 'I can use critical reflection to be aware of my own deeper meaning and spirit, so that my spirit feeds my practice'.

Critical social theory and liberation theology

The critical in critical spirituality relates to critical social theory, which links liberation theology and critical social work practice. Critical social theory makes explicit how individuals and communities are influenced by their social, economic, historical and political context both individually through internalising social expectations and structurally in institutional arrangements. Both of these theories analyse the world in terms of power and oppression, critiquing the structures that embed social, political, economic and more latterly, environmental injustice and seeking a more socially just, accepting and inclusive world. This is not to suggest that there is agreement about how to do this, but more that it is important to do it (Brookfield 2005). Both see the combining of individual experience and political understanding as central whatever the starting point is – being of different religious background, class, sexuality or gender or a combination of these.

Critical social theory is particularly helpful in identifying how what we take for granted as important is internalised, i.e. unconsciously influenced by the prevailing ways of thinking in our society. This might include such assumptions as everyone should conform to prevailing secular norms or that certain religions are accepted but not others. Brookfield (2011: 6) points out that these kinds of assumptions are 'particularly hard to uncover, precisely because these ideologies are everywhere, so common as to be thought blindingly obvious and therefore not worthy of sustained questioning'. Therefore, he suggests 'part of critical thinking is making sure that the actions that flow from our assumptions are justifiable according to some notion of goodness or desirability', including the spiritual. The challenge then in professional practice is to be aware of the dominating ideologies and how we and those we work with are unconsciously influenced by these, make them conscious and to actively choose the values we want to operate from that reinforce a 'good' and socially just approach.

Postmodern understandings of spirituality and practice

The development of postmodernism as a reaction to modernism has influenced Western culture significantly and, in turn, both spiritual expression and professional practice. Modernist expectations still also permeate the culture: valuing of scientifically determined objectivity, the belief there is one right solution to every issue and the prevalence of dichotomous thinking, so that ideas, people, values are perceived in polar opposites – spiritual or not, religious or not. In a more traditional or even a more modernist perspective, communities would have been more likely to share the same religious convictions, but now each community is likely to have a variety of beliefs from atheist to religious and those who are religious might range across a continuum from fundamentalist to mystical. This reflects a more postmodern way of thinking about the spiritual, what Heelas and Woodhead (2005) describe as a move for many people from the religious institution providing an external form of authority to valuing of subjective experience, with the inner authority of the self. This, they suggest, might be expressed through religion but equally through holistic healing or practices such as yoga.

However, I also want to explicitly avoid here the modernist trap of polarised thinking such as spirituality versus religion. It is important to recognise that much religious writing is about being spiritual and affirms there are many paths. This might be in what are often called stages of faith or religious development (Wilber 1996), which can be connected to development of professional practice (Trelfa 2005), such as the movement from a more literal and concrete perspective to a more reflexive and inclusive understanding of self and others. Fox (1991: 18) identifies four spiritual paths, which again can relate to professional practice, from the via positiva, the seeing of God in everyday life to the via transformativa: 'in the combating of injustice ... and in the celebration that happens when persons struggling for justice and trying to live in mutuality come together to praise and give thanks.'

In professional practice, postmodern thinking reinforces that there are many ways of seeing things, many ways of being rather than the 'one way' of modernist thinking. This can feel both inspiring and challenging to professionals expected to move from a sense of finding the 'right' path to the lack of clarity of many paths. As Lartey (2003: 39) says, 'the postmodern condition into which we have been ushered is characterized on the one hand by ephemerality and uncertainty – a situation that has been criticized by many – and on the other hand by endless possibilities for new ways of being'. He suggests valuing both what is common in our experience of the spiritual and what is different, which fits with the postmodern valuing of diversity.

Reflexivity

Reflexivity reinforces the importance of understanding the individual's subjective sense of how to express their spirituality, encouraging us to 'identify and challenge our own underlying assumptions with the theoretical, cultural and psychological positions of others in mind' (Bager-Charleson (2010: 2). Critical reflexivity then means questioning the connections to our own social context and history, understanding the links between the two: how does our own individual and family history interact with the broader social context to influence our reactions to spirituality? This suggests the centrality of reflexivity in articulating where you are coming from, but then standing back from it so that this is not assumed to be the same for others. Sneed (2010: 179) points out that as a gay, black Christian, what is most challenging in the church community for him is being gay; that is where he feels least accepted, but the church sees being black as the central issue. He questions liberation theology's assumption of oppressor and oppressed, suggesting this is an unhelpful binary and what is more helpful is advocating an 'ethic of openness' or 'human flourishing'.

Reflection or reflective practice and experiencing the spiritual

Finally, reflective practice makes explicit the value of building knowledge from experience. This reinforces both the professional wisdom aspect of professional practice, and also the learning that comes from the experiential nature of spirituality. This theory encourages articulating underlying assumptions that influence practice and the importance of ensuring that what we espouse as our values is what we are actually using in practice. Reflective practice validates intuitive and creative responses to the person, working in ways that value their uniqueness.

Combined, these theories encourage spiritually sensitive practice that 'respects the diverse religious and nonreligious forms of spirituality by working within the clients' systems of meaning and support and helping them to achieve their highest potential for development' (Robbins 2005: 387). Moving beyond the either/or of religion and spirituality means that people are redefining what the spiritual means for themselves in a more subjective, but also more complex way that can combine the two:

> Many contemporary spiritualties, even alternative ones, draw on certain traditional religious elements or historical precedents mixed with new secular and global concerns, such as the pressing environmental and ethical issues affecting the whole planet; other forms of spirituality are primarily geared to the discovery of the personal self.
>
> (King 2008: 119)

What this means for professionals, then, is the need to understand the complexity of each person's sense of meaning, which may or may not include the religious. This is challenging in practice: it means developing the capacity to engage across a wide spectrum of beliefs, preferences and understandings from the more traditional religious observance across religious traditions to those whose sense of what matters means respecting their values about relationships, activities, connections with nature. What emerged to provide a framework was the development of key aspects of critical spirituality and principles for practice. Given what students and practitioners have expressed about engaging with spirituality, I have combined each principle with an example based on my experience to make explicit what they might mean in practice. Note that details have been changed to ensure anonymity.

First, the key aspects critical spirituality were identified as:

*   recognising the influence of context, particularly history and culture on spiritual and religious experience for individuals and communities
*   actively celebrates diversity of spiritual expression with the exception of any form of violence to individuals or communities
*   requires a critically reflective attitude, the capacity to explore personal experience and reactions and the implications for practice
*   means working holistically: seeing and appreciating the person as a whole, including their spirituality.

Principles for practice

Spirituality is part of each person's experience and therefore needs to be seen as an integral part of practice

For Pat, who described herself as a sceptical atheist and worked in mental health, this was challenging. What helped was seeing spirituality and particularly religion as similar to cultural difference. Given that she had no trouble being interested and constructively curious about the influence of culture on a client's life, she could see that she could approach spirituality in the same way. She recognised that some of the general questions she asked such as 'what helped you get through other times like this?' sometimes evoked answers that reflected the person's spirituality. Previously she had ignored these; now she felt she would follow them up and ask the person to say more.

The influence of context needs to be recognised for individuals, families and communities in exploring spirituality

Ray and Daphne, both from Catholic backgrounds, came for relationship counselling. After six months, it became clear that Ray's struggles with alcohol use were significantly undermining their relationship, their financial position and their care for their children and that he wasn't ready to change. Daphne then wrestled for several months with whether to separate from Ray to provide more stability for their children. She felt this was abandoning her commitment to marriage for life and so betraying her faith, which sustained her.

When we explored these conflicting feelings, I used some critically reflective questions to explore with Daphne her family context and history and that of the community she belonged to, including what, if anything, had changed over time. She acknowledged that in her family of origin, there had been a very strong assumption that marriage must be for life, no matter how bad the experience. As she talked about one of her aunts whose husband had been consistently violent, she said how much better things were now, that in the community generally as well as in the church, it was more often made explicit that family violence was not acceptable. I asked her when she thought about her aunt's situation now, how would she want things to be for her? She responded that she would want her aunt to be able to leave if her husband couldn't or wouldn't change: 'there's a limit to what people should have to put up with' and 'I don't believe that God would want her to stay there.' That made it easy to ask, using her language: 'so what's the limit for you? Where would God be for you?' When she reflected more on this, she made explicit for herself the need to separate the church from her faith and experience of God. Her perception of God was of a loving God who would not expect her to continue in what felt like an abusive and undermining relationship and would particularly not want that for her children. She remembered too hearing from a friend that in some ways the church, although still upholding the assumption of marriage as for life, was changing in its attitude to those who were separating; things were no longer quite so clear cut. She decided to go and see her priest and explore this with him and eventually was supported in her decision to separate.

Each person is unique and their experience of their spirituality is their own

A young couple, David and Maree, came to see me as a social work relationships counsellor struggling with conflict about life priorities, money and values in caring for their children. They had come to a Catholic agency because they felt their spiritual selves were important; neither had belonged to a religious tradition, but they saw their use of colours, crystals and tarot cards as expression of their spiritual practice. Although they had mentioned these several times in the first session, I was conscious afterwards that I hadn't paid any attention, because, I realised, I felt I knew so little about the expressions of spirituality. As part of the next session, I asked them about what really mattered to them, what they saw as their most fundamental values and how this connected to their spiritual practices. What emerged was a complex and comprehensive mix of ways of trying to articulate core values and to live them out. For Maree, using colours was a way of paying attention to her state of mind and to be emotionally and spiritually present to her children and to David. For David, using the tarot cards encouraged him to constantly ask, what am I doing and why? How does this fit with what really matters? Once I understood this, we could work together much more effectively, including exploring how to have their individual practices work together to strengthen their relationship.

Practitioners need to constantly maintain consciousness of awareness

Mark is a practising Buddhist and he sees his faith is a significant and sustaining influence in his working life. As a family law court mediator he works hard at hearing all points of view, encouraging people to reach agreements and trying to be fair in recommendations to the family law court. As part of ensuring he is aware of his own reactions and how his assumptions might influence him, he participates in a monthly critical reflection group in his agency. The agency sees this as part of fostering a culture of being critically reflective: having an attitude to all of their work that embraces the expectation of reflexive and reflective awareness (Gardner 2014).

Each month, practitioners take it in turns to bring an experience and the aim is for the group to enable them to understand more deeply what this experience means for them. Mark brought a particular experience to critically reflective supervision where he felt torn between the opposing preferences of family members. As he explored this further, he identified part of the tension came from his assumption that he should be able to find solutions that pleased everyone. Underpinning this was his belief that as a Buddhist he should be loving to everyone. When asked if loving the person means you can't disagree with their preference, he could see that he needed to modify his assumption to 'I want to be loving to everyone but also combine love with truth when needed'. From this assumption, it was easier to see how to make the recommendation to the court: the fairest answer was clear, but would not make everyone equally happy. He could also acknowledge that this assumption wasn't helpful either and reminded himself to apply an existing assumption: spiritual life is about growth and can be painful.

Explicitly valuing difference as well as what is common in expression of spirituality

Hazel, a hospital social worker in a rural community, was shocked to realise she had made assumptions about how religious traditions responded to death and dying. She came from an Protestant Irish background and was used to families being able to sit with the body of a family member after death for sometimes several days, with the funeral being up to a week after death. When the Jewish mother of a client named Julia died, Hazel assumed proceedings would be the same. When Julia instead explained the need for the ceremony to be within 24 hours, Hazel realised how slow systems were to respond and was concerned about the distress this caused the family. She decided to document the death traditions of all the religious and cultural backgrounds in the rural community and to negotiate with hospital management processes and policies that would mean other people would have a better experience that validated their religious and cultural experience.

Accepting not knowing and uncertainty

Pam, who worked in palliative care, was conscious that she often avoided conversations with clients about dying because she found it so hard to live with uncertainty herself. She assumed that anyone who was dying would also find this difficult and would want definite answers from her that she would be unable to give. One day one of her clients told her that one of the joys for her of not knowing was that it encouraged her to live in the moment. She saw this as a spiritual practice she had always struggled with but was now coming to value. Another, Joan, who had been a nurse, felt that her specialist was avoiding her because he thought she wanted definite answers. Instead she wanted to know what was known and what was unknown. She also wanted to be able to express how she felt without necessarily expecting answers, just good empathic listening. These two responses changed Pam's assumptions for clients and challenged her to think about her own need for certainty given that she knew at least intellectually that certainty was simply often not possible. This connected for Pam to valuing being as important as doing.

Valuing being with as important as doing

Pam was aware another assumption was that the most important aspect of her work was to get things organised for clients, meaning coordinating service providers to minimise disruption, ensuring family were kept informed, etc. Joan also challenged this assumption, saying to her one day: 'you know if you ever had time to sit and let me talk, just be with me, that would be more use for me than all those other arrangements. They'll happen if they need to.' When Pam did sit and listen, she realised that many of the arrangements she thought were important really didn't matter to Joan; what she wanted was deeper connection about her thoughts, fears, experiences and hopes.

Recognise your limitations

Greg, a social worker in a health care facility for older people, expressed himself as spiritual but not religious. When one of his clients asked him about his beliefs about the resurrection, and the implications for life after death, he realised he was out of his depth. He admitted to the client his lack of knowledge and suggested that he contact the pastoral care worker and introduce her. The patient was pleased to have the connection made and continued to work with both practitioners on different aspects of his life.

Conclusion

This chapter has explored a framework for critical spirituality developed from the interactions of theory related to spirituality and religion as well as that underpinning critical reflection. The framework has also been influenced by students, practitioners and research participants seeking to include the spiritual in their practice. Implicit in many of the examples is how the principles of this framework might influence practice and the processes that can sustain approaching practice in this way. Partly, this means each practitioner being aware of their own spirituality and how this might influence them. However, given that our assumptions and values about the spiritual are often deeply embedded and challenging to make conscious, it can also help to use critically reflective processes to articulate them. Depending on what is possible in a given organisational and social context, this might be through individual reflection, journaling or in individual, mutually supportive pairs or group supervision. The hope is that the framework will foster practice that is spiritually inclusive and socially just as well as more deeply restoring and meaningful for both clients and workers.

References

Bager-Charleson, S. (2010) *Reflective Practice in Counselling and Psychotherapy*, Exeter: Learning Matters.

Brookfield, S.D. (2005) *The Power of Critical Theory Liberating Adult Teaching and Learning*, San Francisco: Jossey-Bass.

Brookfield, S. (2011) *Teaching for Critical Thinking Tools and Techniques to Help Students Question Their Assumptions*, San Francisco: Jossey Bass.

Cobb, M. Rumbold, C. and Pucahlski, C.M. (2012) 'The future of spirituality and healthcare', in M. Cobb, C.M. Puchalski and B. Rumbold (eds) *Spirituality in Healthcare*, Oxford: Oxford University Press.

Fox, M. (1991) *Creation Spirituality Liberating Gifts for the Peoples of the Earth*, San Francisco: Harper.

Gardner, F. (2011) *Critical Spirituality: a holistic approach to contemporary practice*, Farnham: Ashgate.

Gardner, F. (2014) *Being Critically Reflective*, Basingstoke: Palgrave Macmillan.

Heelas, P. and Woodhead, L. (2005) *The Spiritual Revolution: why religion is giving way to spirituality*, Oxford: Blackwell Publishing.

Kamitsuka, M. D. (2007) *Feminist Theology and the Challenge of Difference*, Oxford: Oxford University Press.

King, U. (2008) 'Spirituality and gender viewed through a global lens', in B. Spalek and A. Imtoual (eds) *Religion, Spirituality and the Social Sciences; challenging marginalization*, Bristol: University of Bristol.

Lartey, E.Y. (2003) *In Living Color: an intercultural approach to pastoral care and counseling*, Philadelphia: Jessica Kingsley Publishers.

Robbins, S.P. (2005) 'Transpersonal theory', in S.P. Robbins, P. Chatterjee and E.R. Canda (eds) *Contemporary Human Behavior Theory: a critical perspective for social work*, 2nd edn, Boston: Pearson.

Sneed, R.A. (2010) *Representations of Homosexuality: black liberation theology and cultural criticism*, New York: Palgrave Macmillan.

Sorajjakool, S., Carr, M.F. and Nam, J.J. (2010) *World Religions for Healthcare Professionals*, New York and London: Routledge.

Swinton, J. (2012) 'Healthcare Spirituality: a question of knowledge', in M. Cobb, C.M. Puchalski and B. Rumbold (eds) *Spirituality in Healthcare*, Oxford: Oxford University Press.

Trelfa, J. (2005) 'Faith in reflective practice', *Reflective Practice*, 6(2): 205–12.

Wilber, K. (1996) *The Atman Project: a transpersonal view of human development*, 2nd edn, Wheaton: Quest Books.

34

Spiritually informed social work within conflict-induced displacement

Malabika Das

Introduction

Globally, more than 60 million people have been forcibly displaced by conflict from places such as Syria, Afghanistan, Myanmar (Burma), Iraq, Sudan, Somalia, Eritrea and many others (UNHCR 2015). *Conflict-induced displacement* is a type of forced migration where people flee their homes from armed conflict, civil war, generalised violence or persecution on the grounds of nationality, race, religion, political opinion or social group, and where the state authorities are unable or unwilling to protect them (FMO 2012). Within these cruel, human-made disasters, displaced persons (hereafter, survivors) must leave everything they know for safety. Survivors are at risk of high degrees of traumatisation from often harrowing conditions encountered during displacement, including torture.

Spirituality and religion are frequently accessed for relief when normality becomes devastated (Worland and Vaddhanaphuti 2013). As one faith-based service provider from my research in Hong Kong has commented:

> The spiritual aspect is crucial because if you take away that you've got little hope. The hope factor is reinforced with faith. Faith, hope and trust, they are the key areas, but love is crucial to the whole of that.

This chapter emphasises *spirituality* and its expansive dimensions inclusive of faith and religion. It seeks to highlight the intersection of spirituality within conflict-induced displacement and how social workers can play a more *spiritually informed* role in the healing journey of survivors. Here, *spirituality* is conceptualised as a core human aspect, broadly encompassing meaning, purpose, wellbeing and morality in relations with self, other beings, the universe and engagement with sacred or transpersonal transcendence (Canda and Furman 2010). *Religion* refers to an organised set of beliefs and practices, and *faith* refers to the transcendent and interpretive elements of religious experience (Tuskan 2009); both embody spiritual dimensions.

Trauma and displacement

Survivors face a myriad of traumatising factors during the displacement journey. An event becomes *traumatic* when coping skills and normal stress reactions are overwhelmed and where physiological and mental functioning cannot normalise afterwards (Murakami 2015). Trauma can result from single, continuous or accrued events in life (Clervil *et al.* 2013). The stages of migration and commonly identified features generally include: Pre Flight (violence and persecution), Flight (loss of loved ones, trafficking and smuggling risks), Displacement (tents, urban areas or within country borders) and Resettlement (third country or voluntary repatriation) (Farmer 2015).

Trauma and holistic health impact

Trauma impacts psychological, physical, behavioural, social, emotional and spiritual health domains. Torture, for instance, produces physical pain, social degradation, humiliation and spiritual distress (Tuskan 2009). Fortunately, many people will recover from trauma; some, however, experience severe and devastating health and mental health consequences (Clervil *et al.* 2013). They are often not equipped to deal with the emergence of overwhelming emotions and can be consumed by negative feelings (Mollica 2006).

Post-traumatic stress, somatisation, substance misuse, headaches and chronic pain are just a few common issues. Untreated mental health problems can advance into physical health issues such as diabetes, cardiovascular disease, hypertension and cancer (Jeon *et al.* 2001). The accumulation of interacting mental, physical and behavioural health conditions can rapidly increase overall disability. The range of bio-psychosocial-spiritual health sequelae can vary; however, common features include:

1   Bio: body, head and joint pains, infectious disease, torture and violence injuries
2   Psychosocial: loss, grief, sadness, betrayal, hopelessness, weakness, anger, shame, guilt, humiliation, economic insecurity and loss of livelihood
3   Spiritual: doubting faith, questioning divine and life

Health and wellbeing research

Research and practice confirms how health deterioration associated with negative life experiences can be mediated by spiritual practices (Mollica 2006). While religious and spiritual beliefs are recognised strengths during adversity, they are under-investigated (Ai *et al.* 2003; Gozdziak 2002). Historically, the *trauma model*, focusing on pathology, dominated refugee research. It was valuable in creating reliable trauma outcome measures and documenting human rights abuses (Jeon *et al.* 2001). Later, displacement stressors, such as unemployment and family separation, also revealed mental health deterioration (Schweitzer *et al.* 2006).

Research eventually turned towards psychosocial growth (De Haene *et al.* 2010), offering a balanced understanding of trauma and positive aspects of human experience (Park and Ai 2006). Nevertheless, individual and collective psychological resources and coping strategies are often missed and underutilised by researchers, practitioners and policymakers (Puvimanasinghe *et al.* 2014). However, excitingly, the limited but emerging evidence largely supports spirituality's important role in survivors' wellbeing, including the intersection of worldviews and health, the concept of health as holistic and examples of spirituality dimensions from my research.

Convergence of cultural and spiritual worldviews for coping, health and wellbeing

Survivors exemplify diverse worldviews comprised of cultural factors, belief systems, healing traditions and help seeking behaviours and norms. This abundant diversity informs understanding of spirituality, coping, resilience, health and wellbeing (Canda and Furman 2010). Several studies illustrate these aspects. In Australia, Sudanese refugees' belief in God enabled emotional support, control and life meaning and prayer offered solace for sadness and loneliness (Schweitzer *et al.* 2007). In the US, Liberian refugee women's gratitude aided the appreciation of helpful people and new things, supported positivity and generated goodwill towards new friends (Clarke and Borders 2014). Similarly, Burundian and Sierra Leonean refugees in Australia expressed how being helped and helping others assisted in surviving displacement, adapting to Australia, helping others back home and religious-inclined meaning making (Puvimanasinghe *et al.* 2014). These facets of *altruism* related to their empathy and gratitude. For some Sierra Leoneans, beliefs of destiny and God's will supported meaning making from suffering and coping with distress.

Some Bosnian refugee women in the US viewed religion as an organised institution and spirituality as a belief in higher power (Sossou *et al.* 2008). A study of cognitive and spiritual resources for Bosnian and Kosovo refugees in the US revealed how *optimism* associated with positive religious coping and higher education and *hope* associated with education but negatively associated with negative religious coping (Ai *et al.* 2003).

In the UK, Somali refugee women accessed spiritual and religious support largely through familial and personal resources (Whittaker *et al.* 2005). Somali and Islamic beliefs informed spirit possession views. Zar possession was punishment for lacking religion, but prayer and Qur'an reading/narration offered spirit protection. In the US, Somali refugees' religious beliefs impacted health behaviours; the Qur'an was accessed prior to formal medical care and illness and wellbeing were determined by God's will (Clarkson-Freeman *et al.* 2013).

Spiritual coping factors for Tibetan refugees in India involved strong faith for protective spiritual leaders, including the belief that His Holiness Dalai Lama was the manifestation of the Bodhisattva (enlightened being) of Compassion, reborn to serve humanity (Hussain and Bhushan 2011). Faith in karma and reincarnation enabled acceptance of suffering and building of resilience. Interestingly, the Dalai Lama himself fled to India from Tibet after China annexed Tibet in 1959; afterwards, thousands of refugees followed.

Interconnection of health domains

Survivors' worldviews often embrace a holistic health perspective where health domains interconnect within the whole person. Karen refugees in the US identified health as not merely the absence of disease, but a balance between spiritual, physical and mental health, impacted by lifestyle, food and environment (Oleson *et al.* 2012). Similarly, participants of testimonial and spiritual healing ceremonies in India, Sri Lanka, Cambodia and Philippines regarded body and mind as one; conceptualised as 'embodied spirituality' (Agger *et al.* 2012: 571). This included elements of prayers, rituals, dances and symbolic pilgrimages.

Within healthcare, the interconnection of spirituality facets is emerging. Reiki, combined in a multi-disciplinary approach, accelerated torture rehabilitation (Vargas *et al.* 2004). Qigong and Tai Chi with refugees decreased psychosomatic complaints, increased body attunement, psychotherapy introspection and overall holistic wellbeing (Grodin *et al.* 2008).

Whole traditional medical systems, such as Traditional Chinese Medicine (TCM), dominated a systematic review of complementary and alternative modalities (CAM) with refugees

(MacDuff *et al.* 2011). TCM views the body, mind and spirit as a connective and interactive system (Leung *et al.* 2009). Vital energy (qi) flows freely when health is balanced but can be blocked due to physical, emotional and/or spiritual distress.

Hong Kong case illustration

Spirituality dimensions were integral for coping and wellbeing in my research regarding ecological forces impacting mental health and psychosocial wellbeing of survivors in Hong Kong (Das 2015). Research participants noted a variety of pre-flight trauma: cruel and inhuman treatment, persecution, kidnapping, violent death of loved ones and massacres. One faith-based provider shared:

> There are people who suffered significant traumas; some who have been tortured and threatened with death; some experiencing periods of imprisonment by secret police. The trauma is almost indescribable over time. How they survived and remained reasonably intact is a miracle in itself.

Case study participants experienced a cycle of holistic health deterioration linked to systemic empathic failure of humanitarian, livelihood, protection and healthcare services. Fears of refoulement (forcible return to a country where they may be subjected to persecution and violence) and living in *traumatic uncertainty* (uncertain lengthy protection processing time without livelihood options) increased health deterioration. Unaddressed mental health issues worsened. Eventually, physical and behavioural health issues also manifested, including hypertension, diabetes, chronic body pain, family violence and substance dependency.

Coping strategies revealed how participants accessed a variety of spirituality dimensions. For instance, *altruism*, helping others without expectations, was integral to a participant's wellbeing when he helped at an organisation; he shared: 'When I am helping, I am too much happy.' Also, *gratitude* emerged as a healing catalyst and daily coping strategy for another participant living in limbo for more than 11 years. His gratitude attitude comprised both spiritual and cognitive aspects; he shared:

> In life is to be grateful everyday. So at Chungking Mansion for example, I see people sleeping on the stairs or old ladies pushing the trollies just to get one or two dollars. I say "God, thank you for everything". I feel like my situation is not the worst, I am so thankful.

Features of strong *faith* and having a belief system was helpful for one participant's inner strength and daily stressors:

> My faith really helped me a lot. What I decided is God has a plan for me, no matter what. Because if you have two sides of your expectations, that's not really faith. You suffer because God is planning something better for you. That means, he's teaching you, bringing you to get that wisdom, which will lead you in a better and joyful situation.

Bio-psychosocial-spiritual approach

Research and practice has demonstrated spirituality's integral role in wellbeing. 'When the traumatized inner self is thrown into chaos by violence, spirituality can prevent a total disintegration of the person' (Mollica 2006: 176). When violence occurs, the bio-psychosocial-spiritual self-healing force is activated (Mollica 2013). However, if not appropriately supported, trauma reactions can cause holistic health deterioration.

For multi-dimensional issues such as conflict-induced displacement, integrative assessment and treatment approaches incorporating physical, cognitive, emotional, social and spiritual experiences are needed (Leung *et al.* 2009). A bio-psychosocial-spiritual approach should be used for traumatised refugees (Mollica 2008). It can aid holistic exploration inclusive of torture, stress, isolation, losses and social support (Das and Chan 2013).

Social work has long encompassed the *strengths* perspective as a fundamental pillar; this emphasises people's inherent healing and resilience capacities, as opposed to reductionism (Canda and Furman 2010). Drawing from this ideal, the bio-psychosocial-spiritual approach represents interconnected health aspects of the whole person that should be accounted for: bio (physical), psycho (mental/emotional/psychological), social (cultural/political/economic) and spiritual (life meaning) (NASW 2005). This view resonates with social work's person in environment commitment (Canda and Furman 2010).

However, professionals have not been prepared to work with cultural aspects of mental health, such as spirit possession beliefs (Whittaker *et al.* 2005). Spirituality issues have often been passed to spiritual providers (Piwowarczyk 2005). While no professional consensus around spiritual practice exists (Crisp 2010), practitioners can become more attentive to *spiritually informed* features, which can aid strengths, healing and transformation support for survivors. Table 34.1 summarises three primary features and corresponding components, each of which will be discussed in turn.

Table 34.1 Spiritually informed features

Practitioner attributes	Bio-psychosocial-spiritual assessment	Healing and transformation support
Spiritual self-awareness	Ecological system	Advocacy
Trauma informed	Holistic trauma and health impact	Strengths-based therapeutic approaches
Empathic learner	Worldviews and belief systems	Multi-disciplinary holistic healthcare support
Self-care	Spiritual protective and risk factors	Spiritual and faith-based resources

Practitioner attributes

Practitioners can build and strengthen certain attributes to heighten their awareness of spiritual matters. These include ensuring their own spiritual awareness, using a trauma informed practice approach, being an empathic learner and engaging in self-care strategies.

Spiritual self-awareness

Social workers should explore their own spirituality to effectively help in the spiritual and religious matters of others (Crisp 2010). Self-evaluating faith and belief systems, transpersonal connections, and life meaning and purpose can enhance broad self-awareness and understanding of personal and professional boundaries and limiting judgments. Bias may impede clients' posttraumatic growth potential (Piwowarczyk 2005); hence, accepting others is reliant on self-acceptance (George and Ellison 2015). Spiritual self-awareness serves as a strong foundation during trauma work enhancing grounding, meaning making and self-care.

Trauma informed

Trauma's impact can be lost amid the variety of multi-dimensional issues faced by survivors throughout displacement. Incorporating a trauma informed practice approach is recommended particularly because it emphasises safety and the intersection of culture and trauma. A trauma informed approach recognises trauma's broad impact and considers cultural factors, sharing power, supporting control and autonomy, and preventing retraumatisation (Clervil *et al.* 2013). It entails awareness of a survivor's resilience and the need for empowerment and safety (Murakami 2015).

Empathic learner

Empathy broadly entails understanding others' perspectives that can guide our own action. Empathy is both active and passive, entailing affective response (feeling and mirroring), cognitive processing (self-awareness and perspective taking) and conscious decision-making (empathic action and altruism) (Gerdes and Segal 2009). Spiritual practices, supervision and therapy can help build empathy (George and Ellison 2015).

Being an empathic learner or listener can help restore control and agency, which is often stripped away during displacement. It can allow spiritually important information for healing and treatment (McKinney 2011). The empathic learner may view mental images of trauma story as art, which enables a detached but 'deeper, more meaningful understanding of the survivor's world' (Mollica 2006: 116). Healing and survival can be learned from the trauma story (Mollica 2008).

Self-care

Often, practitioners may not be emotionally or therapeutically prepared for the high levels of distressing trauma stories heard (Farmer 2015). Experiencing overt or subtle vicarious or secondary trauma is not uncommon in trauma work. Supervision, peer groups, counselling and relevant stress reduction practices can increase strengths and decrease isolation, burden and burn out. Spiritual practices can assist when experiencing upsetting feelings and thoughts (Agger *et al.* 2012). Self-reflection and awareness of extreme human capability can increase ability to be an empathic vessel for the survivor (Piwowarczyk 2005).

Bio-psychosocial-spiritual assessment

A bio-psychosocial-spiritual assessment involves a holistic exploration of people in their environments. This includes accounting for ecological factors, trauma's holistic health impact and diverse worldviews and belief systems.

Ecological system

Ecological displacement stressors can cause immediate distress and compound prior traumatisation, which intensifies health disability (Das 2015). Starting by addressing basic needs such as food and shelter can help to build a level of trust (Piwowarczyk 2005). Then, identifying employment, livelihood, acculturation and basic social welfare needs is valuable to ongoing support needs. It is also critical to consider how systems (micro to macro) impact health empowerment or deterioration. The acronym HEALTH: Healing partnerships, Empathy, Advocacy, Livelihood, Trauma-informed care and Human rights may be helpful in remembering the various ecological components that can positively impact body–mind–spirit wellbeing and inform the bio-psychosocial-spiritual assessment (Das in press).

Holistic trauma and health impact

The holistic health impact of violence, torture and cruel treatment is vast, hence, identifying health needs is crucial to overall wellbeing. Conducting or facilitating referrals for forensic, medical and psychological evaluations and trauma assessments is usually necessary. The *Istanbul Protocol* is an internationally recognised holistic torture assessment tool (PHR 1999) and can assist in protection cases and care continuum.

Trauma-informed toolkits and holistic guidelines can help providers with assessment (Mollica 2008). The Harvard Trauma Questionnaire (HPRT 2011) is the most well-known comprehensive trauma assessment, traditionally used in refugee research and is valuable for identifying mental health disorders. Short non-diagnostic tools such as the *Refugee Health Screener 15* can quickly identify distress for further care and referral (Hollifield *et al.* 2013).

Worldviews and belief systems

Every survivor embodies unique life experiences and worldviews that inform strengths, spirituality dimensions and health aspects. 'Proper understanding of traumatic experiences and its outcomes requires knowledge of the cultural factors that affects one's worldview' (Hussain and Bhushan 2011: 575). Knowledge of cultural, indigenous and traditional healing practices and societal norms can inform human development, trauma manifestation, help-seeking behaviour and barriers and appropriate referrals. A belief system (faith, political, or otherwise) can serve as a coping mechanism and can be a clinically relevant tool (Brunea *et al.* 2002).

Spiritual protective and risk factors

Once a trusting healing partnership is established, it is necessary to explore all protective and risk factors with survivors, especially those having spiritual features. For many survivors, faith has sustained them through challenges and is critical in recovery (Farmer 2015). Previous and current spirituality and other coping facets accessed can enhance awareness of strengths. It reminds survivors of their inherent strengths and capacities through past life challenges (Lee *et al.* 2009). Questions that could be asked include: 'What thoughts, rituals or mantras were used in the past or currently during stressful times?' 'Who do they rely on for strength?' 'What gives them hope?'

While understanding how spiritual dimensions supported them in the past, practitioners can sensitively assess whether these dimensions were connected to their persecution, violence and/or torture. Traumatic events such as torture can lead to a loss of faith or changes in belief systems (Piwowarczyk 2005). Therefore assessing faith belief changes is necessary (Brunea *et al.* 2002), including the previous and current meanings for them. There are also specific spirituality assessments addressing torture and trauma available, which offer guidance and further resources (GCJFCS 2012; Piwowarczyk 2005; Tuskan 2009).

Healing and transformation support

Practitioners can promote healing and transformation from victim to survivor. Some overarching components of this feature include offering advocacy, strengths-based therapeutic approaches and access to multi-disciplinary holistic healthcare support and spiritual resources.

Advocacy

Survivors are often immersed within complex ecological contexts. Adopting an advocacy perspective can aid holistic and comprehensive support, since advocacy can bridge micro and macro practice (Das *et al.* 2013). Advocacy for this community can be broad reaching and individually tailored. Practitioners can become educated about their setting's policy and legal infrastructure as well as historical events and public sentiment around conflict-induced displacement. This can elucidate a broader and more comprehensive lens about the situational context including how resources and services are impacted. Also, understanding the survivor's protection status and legal case needs can reveal areas where practitioners can provide or refer for psychosocial support.

Survivors often face discrimination or oppression in their displacement setting. Practitioners can become advocates for change, dignity and human rights since focusing on displacement stressors may be a greater priority to the survivor than trauma from conflict or persecution. This may include advocating for dignified basic services, the right to legal employment, or a fair and just legal and protection process. Additionally, seeking mental health help can be a foreign or stigmatised concept for many since traditional counselling practice is not normative in many cultures. Therefore, becoming survivors' advocate can build trust and a bridge towards further healing and transformation support.

Strengths-based therapeutic approaches

Approaching therapeutic work from a strengths-based perspective is critical in healing and transformation. For instance, providing psychoeducation around the holistic impact of trauma and bio-psychosocial-spiritual health interconnections can heighten empowerment and awareness of health status and trauma reactions. Holistic stress reduction tools such as diaphragm breathing, body scanning and mindfulness techniques can increase relaxation and mental and physical awareness of pain and stress and decrease rumination (Agger *et al.* 2012: 572. Stress reduction techniques can be introduced early on to prevent retraumatisation and enhance wellbeing, since survivors often face a myriad of stressors. More about these techniques can be found in Chapters 10, 11, 25 and 30.

Narrative therapeutic approaches can elucidate lived experience. Through a trusting healing partnership, a survivor may share their life history and past traumatic life events. 'Facilitating the entry of the full trauma story, one of the most exciting dimensions of self-healing, into the social dialogue, is another essential goal of recovery' (Mollica 2006: 237). The survivor can share at their own pace to prevent retraumatisation. The empathic learner can emotionally support and validate the survivor's experience to combat shame and isolation (Mollica 2006).

Moreover, practitioners can help to reframe perceived deficits into a strengths outlook, validating resilience and facilitating empowerment and cognitive changes. Crisis and loss can create life imbalance but also present opportunities to discover new strengths (Leung *et al.* 2009). Meaning making can help to restore life meaning after trauma (Park and Ai 2006). This can generate new ideas for hope and resilience. The trauma story can become one of survival and strength.

Providing opportunities for altruism can be an extremely healing component. Altruism can facilitate coping while also strengthening communities and networks (Puvimanasinghe *et al.* 2014). Atruism can help restore purpose and meaning for many survivors who may be unable to legally work, or wait in traumatic uncertainty while their case is processed.

Multi-disciplinary holistic healthcare support

Survivors often have commonality within forced displacement experiences. However, trauma and healing are individualised occurrences and most people require varying levels of assistance. Practitioners can facilitate access to targeted multi-disciplinary holistic healthcare support. This can be valuable for conducting health and mental health assessments and providing specialised care for trauma and torture. Integrative services inclusive of health, mental health, bodywork, mind–body practitioners and spiritual providers can be effective to address complex healthcare needs. For some, traditional healing practices are beneficial; therefore, seeking appropriate and available indigenous healers may be necessary.

Spiritual and faith-based resources

Connecting service users to spiritual resources enhances a diverse collective care network. Appropriate assessment and consent can enable referral to a 'spiritually-relevant resource that expands the fabric of care for the person' (McKinney 2011: 65). Faith-based resources have traditionally supported survivors' psychosocial–spiritual services, and while many provide genuine support, it needs to be recognised that some religious institutions hold beliefs towards women, shame and sexual abuse that may be harmful to some survivors (Mollica 2006). Further information about faith-based care and good practices with survivors include information from UNHCR (2014) and Vine (2014).

Conclusion

As conflict-induced displacement continues to accelerate globally, millions of people affected by this crisis will look to spirituality for strength and survival. Spirituality can be a catalyst for the innate self-healing abilities of survivors. Spirituality can manifest through a variety of dimensions and features and is informed by diverse worldviews, cultural factors, religion and faith.

Spiritually informed social workers and other practitioners can enhance care and healing for survivors by strengthening practitioner attributes, incorporating a bio-psychosocial-spiritual assessment and supporting their healing and transformation. By embracing spirituality's connection to overall health and humanity, the human potential for self-healing can be utilised.

References

Agger, I., Igreja, V., Kiehle, R. and Polatin, P. (2012) 'Testimony ceremonies in Asia: integrating spirituality in testimonial therapy for torture survivors in India, Sri Lanka, Cambodia, and the Philippines', *Transcultural Psychiatry*, 49(3–4): 568–89.

Ai, A.L., Peterson, C., and Huang, B. (2003) 'The effect of religious-spiritual coping on positive attitudes of adult Muslim refugees from Kosovo and Bosnia', *The International Journal for the Psychology of Religion*, 13(1): 29–47.

Brunea, M., Haasena, C., Krausza, M., Yagdirana, O., Bustosb, E. and Eisenmanc, D. (2002) 'Belief systems as coping factors for traumatized refugees: a pilot study', *European Psychiatry*, 17(8): 451–8.

Canda, E.R. and Furman, L.D. (2010) *Spiritual Diversity in Social Work Practice*, 2nd edn, New York: Oxford University Press.

Clarke, L.K. and Borders, L.D. (2014) 'You got to apply seriousness: a phenomenological inquiry of Liberian refugees' coping', *Journal of Counseling and Development*, 92(3): 294–303.

Clarkson-Freeman, P.A., Penney, D.S., Bettmann, J.E. and Lecy, N. (2013) 'The intersection of health beliefs and religion among Somali refugees: a qualitative study', *Journal of Religion and Spirituality in Social Work*, 32(1): 1–13.

Clervil, R., Guarino, K., DeCandia, C.J. and Beach, C.A. (2013) *Trauma-Informed Care for Displaced Populations: a guide for community-based service providers*, Waltham, MA: The National Center on Family Homelessness. Online. Available HTTP: www.familyhomelessness.org/media/405.pdf (accessed 6 April 2014).

Crisp, B.R. (2010) *Spirituality and Social Work*, Farnham: Ashgate.

Das, M.M. (2015) *A Critical Exploration of Forces Impacting Mental Health and Psychosocial Wellbeing of Conflict-Induced Displaced Persons in Hong Kong*, Ph.D Thesis, The University of Hong Kong. Online. Available HTTP: http://hub.hku.hk/handle/10722/221171 (accessed 11 November 2015).

Das, M.M. (in press) 'Application of integrative body-mind-spirit approaches within conflict-induced displacement', in C. Chan (ed) *Integrative Body-Mind-Spirit Social Work: an empirically-based approach to assessment and treatment*, 2nd edn, Oxford: Oxford University Press.

Das, M.M. and Chan, C.L.W. (2013) 'Uplifting social support for refugees and asylum seekers', in S. Chen (ed) *Social Support and Health: theory, research, and practice with diverse populations*, New York: Nova Publishers.

Das, M.M., Chui, C.H.K. and Chan, C.L.W. (2013) 'Advocacy', in B.A. Thyer, C.N. Dulmus and K.M. Sowers (eds) *Developing Evidence-Based Generalist Practice Skills*, Hoboken, NJ: John Wiley & Sons.

De Haene, L., Grietens, H., and Verschueren, K. (2010) 'Holding harm: narrative methods in mental health research on refugee trauma', *Qualitative Health Research*, 20(12): 1664–76.

Farmer, B. (2015) *Walking Together: a mental health therapist's guide to working with refugees*, Seattle: Lutheran Community Services Northwest. Online. Available HTTP: http://form.jotform.us/form/51666347065157 (accessed 3 August 2015).

Forced Migration Online [FMO] (2012) *What Is Forced Migration?* Online. Available HTTP: www.forced migration.org/about/whatisfm (accessed 15 January 2014).

George, M. and Ellison, V. (2015) 'Incorporating spirituality into social work practice with migrants', *The British Journal of Social Work*, 45(6): 1717–33.

Gerdes, K.E. and Segal, E.A. (2009) 'A social work model of empathy', *Advances in Social Work*, 10(2): 114–27.

Gozdziak, E.M. (2002) 'Spiritual emergency room: the role of spirituality and religion in the resettlement of Kosovar Albanians', *Journal of Refugee Studies*, 15(2): 136–52.

Grodin, M.A., Piwowarczyk, L., Fulker, D., Bazazi, A.R. and Saper, R.B. (2008) 'Treating survivors of torture and refugee trauma: a preliminary case series using qigong and t'ai chi', *Journal of Alternative and Complementary Medicine*, 14(7): 801–6.

Gulf Coast Jewish Family and Community Services [GCJFCS] *The Role of Spirituality in the Treatment of Torture Survivors*, Florida: National Partnership for Community Training. Online. Available HTTP: http://gulfcoastjewishfamilyandcommunityservices.org/refugee/files/2012/07/Spirituality.pdf (accessed 19 December 2013).

Harvard Program in Refugee Trauma [HPRT] (2011) *Harvard Trauma Questionnaire (HTQ)*. Online. Available HTTP: http://hprt-cambridge.org/screening/harvard-trauma-questionnaire/ (accessed 12 July 2013).

Hollifield, M., Verbillis-Kolp, S., Farmer, B., Toolson, E. C., Woldehaimanot, T., Yamazaki, J., Holland, A., St. Clair, J. and SooHoo, J. (2013) 'The Refugee Health Screener-15 (RHS-15): development and validation of an instrument for anxiety, depression, and PTSD in refugees', *General Hospital Psychiatry*, 35(2): 202–9.

Hussain, D. and Bhushan, B. (2011) 'Cultural factors promoting coping among Tibetan refugees: a qualitative investigation', *Mental Health, Religion and Culture*, 14(6): 575–87.

Jeon, W.T. Yoshioka, M. and Mollica, R.F. (2001) *Science of Refugee Mental Health: new concepts and methods*, Harvard Program in Refugee Trauma. Online. Available HTTP: www.hprt-cambridge.org/wp-content/uploads/2011/01/ScienceofRefugeeMentalHealth.pdf (accessed 13 January 2016).

Lee, M.Y., Ng, S.M., Leung, P.P.Y. and Chan, C.L.W. (2009) *Integrative Body-Mind-Spirit Social Work*, New York: Oxford University Press.

Leung, P., Chan, C.L.W., Ng, S.M.and Lee, M.Y. (2009) 'Towards body-mind-spirit integration: east meets west in clinical social work practice', *Clinical Social Work Journal*, 37(4): 303–11.

MacDuff, S., Grodin, M.A. and Gardiner, P. (2011) 'The use of complementary and alternative medicine among refugees: a systematic review', *Journal of Immigrant Minority Health*, 13(3), 585–99.

McKinney, M.M. (2011) 'Treatment of survivors of torture: Spiritual domain', *Torture*, 21(1): 61–6.

Mollica, R.F. (2006) *Healing Invisible Wounds Paths to Hope and Recovery in a Violent World*, Orlando, FL: Harcourt.

Mollica, R.F. (2008) *Specific Cultural and Evidence Based Practices for the Treatment of Torture Survivors*, Center for Victims of Torture. Online. Available HTTP: http://healtorture.org/sites/healtorture.org/files/PowerPoint%20of%20Specific%20Cultural%20and%20Evidence-based%20Practices%20webinar.pdf (accessed 4 December 2011).

Mollica, R.F. (2013) *Healing a Violent World Manifesto*, Harvard Program for Refugee Trauma. Online. Available HTTP: http://hprt-cambridge.org/wp-content/uploads/2013/01/Manifesto-rev-2013.pdf (accessed 19 November 2014).

Murakami, N. (2015) *Trauma-Informed Care for Refugee Populations: building awareness, skills, and knowledge*, New York: The Center for Refugee Health. Online. Available HTTP: http://centerforrefugeehealth.com/wp-content/uploads/2015/10/Trauma-Informed-Care.pdf (accessed 12 December 2015).

National Association of Social Workers [NASW] (2005) *NASW Standards for Social Work Practice in Health Care Settings*, Washington DC: NASW. Online. Available HTTP: www.socialworkers.org/practice/standards/naswhealthcarestandards.pdf (accessed 10 December 2014).

Oleson, H.E, O'Fallon, A. and Sherwood, N.E. (2012) 'Health and healing: traditional medicine and the Karen experience', *Journal of Cultural Diversity*, 19(2): 44–9.

Park, C.L. and Ai, A.L. (2006) 'Meaning making and growth: new directions for research on survivors of trauma', *Journal of Loss and Trauma*, 11(5): 389–407.

Physicians for Human Rights [PHR] (1999) *Istanbul Protocol Manual on the Effective Investigation and Documentation of Torture and Other Cruel, Inhuman or Degrading Treatment or Punishment*, Geneva: Office of the United Nations High Commissioner for Human Rights. Online. Available HTTP: http://physiciansforhumanrights.org/issues/torture/international-torture.html (accessed 14 November 2011).

Piwowarczyk, L. (2005) 'Torture and spirituality: engaging the sacred in treatment', *Torture*, 15(1): 1–8.

Puvimanasinghe, T., Denson, L.A., Augoustinos, M. and Somasundaram, D. (2014) 'Giving back to society what society gave us: altruism, coping, and meaning making by two refugee communities in South Australia', *Australian Psychologist*, 49(5): 313–21.

Schweitzer, R., Greenslade, J., and Kagee, A. (2007) 'Coping and resilience in refugees from the Sudan: a narrative account', *Australian and New Zealand Journal of Psychiatry*, 41(3): 282–8.

Schweitzer, R., Melville, F., Steel, Z. and Lacharez, P. (2006) 'Trauma, postmigration living difficulties, and social support as predictors of psychological adjustment in resettled Sudanese refugees', *Australian and New Zealand Journal of Psychiatry*, 40(2): 179–87.

Sossou, M.A, Craig, C.D., Ogren, H. and Schnak, M. (2008) 'A qualitative study of resilience factors of Bosnian refugee women resettled in the Southern United States', *Journal of Ethnic and Cultural Diversity in Social Work*, 17(4): 365–85.

Tuskan, J. (2009) *Religion, Spirituality and Faith in the Care of Torture Survivors: part I*, Center for Victims of Torture. Online. Available HTTP: http://healtorture.org/sites/healtorture.org/files/PowerPoint%20Torture%20Spirituality%201%20webinar.pdf (accessed 13 January 2016).

United Nations High Commission for Refugees [UNHCR] (2014) *Partnership Note on Faith-Based Organizations, Local Faith Communities and Faith Leaders*, Geneva: UNHCR. Online. Available HTTP: www.unhcr.org/539ef28b9.html (accessed 8 August 2015).

United Nations High Commission for Refugees [UNHCR] (2015) *UNHCR Mid Year Trends 2015*, Geneva: United Nations High Commissioner for Refugees. Online. Available HTTP: www.unhcr.org/56701b969.html (accessed 12 December 2015).

Vargas, C.M., O'Rourke, D. and Esfandiari, M. (2004) 'Complementary therapies for treating survivors of torture', *Refuge*, 22(1): 129–37.

Vine (2014) *The Vine Community Services, Ltd*. Online. Available HTTP: www.vcsl.org (accessed 8 October 2015).

Whittaker, S., Hardy, G., Lewis, K. and Buchan, L. (2005) 'An exploration of psychological wellbeing with young Somali refugee and asylum-seeker women', *Clinical Child Psychology and Psychiatry*, 10(2): 177–96.

Worland, S. and Vaddhanaphuti, C. (2013) 'Religious expressions of spirituality by displaced Karen from Burma: the need for a spiritually sensitive social work response', *International Social Work*, 56(3): 384–402.

35

Holistic arts-based social work

Diana Coholic

Introduction

While art therapy is usually conducted by graduate-trained professionals with a degree in art therapy, arts-based methods denote the application of art therapy techniques, and are accessible and used by a more diverse group of helping professionals such as social workers. Arts-based methods can include activities such as drawing, painting, creative writing, working with clay and more. I have been studying the benefits of arts-based methods in holistic social group work for almost 10 years. Along with members of my research team, I developed an arts-based mindfulness group programme that facilitates the learning of mindfulness using experiential and arts-based methods such as drawing, painting, making collages, creating with sand, using music, practicing Tai Chi movements, sculpting with clay, listening to guided imageries and creative writing (Coholic 2010). This research was primarily focused on the needs of marginalised children and youth (children involved with child welfare or mental health systems), but we also explored our programme with indigenous women (Coholic *et al.* 2013) and with adults experiencing mental health challenges (Coholic *et al.* 2014). At the beginning of my research career, when I first started exploring the processes and benefits of holistic social group work, our group work was facilitated and studied with women, and teenage girl participants involved with child welfare. Since spirituality and other existential topics are often difficult to articulate in words, it made sense to utilise arts-based methods to explore and express these topics.

Arts-based methods in social work

What do social workers think happens when the arts are applied in practice, research and teaching? This question was considered by Sinding, Warren and Paton (2014), who offered a framework for understanding why social workers utilised arts-based methods. First, these authors explained that arts-informed social work 'gets stuff out' (Sinding *et al.* 2014: 197), which means, in part, that sometimes language cannot capture or express people's experiences but art-making can help a person express their thoughts and feelings. For example, Harley and Hunn (2015) wanted to understand how spirituality was a source of hope and coping for Black adolescents. They used photography in their research as a safer method for the youth to share their personal material; the photographs were symbolic representations of issues, feelings and themes. In fact, using creative methods with youth has long been accepted within helping professions as it is understood that youth often communicate their thoughts and feelings nonverbally through creative activity (Goodman 2005).

Sometimes the point of 'getting stuff out' might be to develop self-awareness and understanding, which certainly reflects one of the goals of the group work that I have studied in my research programme. Indeed, developing both personal and professional self-awareness is often stated as an outcome of arts-based methods (Bartkeviciene 2014). With reference to helping social workers develop therapeutic presence, Jacobs (2015) argued that the art of social work practice resides in the relationship, and contemplative practices are important in helping social workers develop the therapeutic and transitional (transformational) space. To promote contemplative practices, she encouraged social workers to use art, music and poetry, as these activities can evoke emotion, promote empathy and understanding, and provide solace.

Second, art creations and art-making can also help us to understand another's world, encouraging us to see or know things in a different way using our emotions and senses (Sinding *et al.* 2014). Importantly, in this manner, arts-based methods are used not only to help people express themselves but as part of social change and justice activities. For example, in their research with incarcerated Aboriginal women, Walsh, Rutherford and Crough (2013) explained how arts-based methods such as creative writing, photography and digital storytelling enabled participation in research in relevant ways that were inclusive. The research products were egalitarian and ready for social and political action. Foster (2012) used poetry to promote social justice as poetry can promote alternative discourse and challenge dominant ideologies. A poem might impact people on an emotional and spiritual level, and thus, can promote empathy based on these emotional responses. Moxley (2013) argued groups that face oppression can develop personally and contribute to social action through art-making; an avenue of self-expression in which people can individually or with others establish their worldview and construct positions from which they can criticise or illuminate degraded aspects of their lives that others do not notice.

Social work educators have also used arts-based materials such as films to provide an opportunity for students to deconstruct narratives that are understood as a product of communal, socially acquired understandings (Keddell 2011). In this manner, theories can be viewed as fluid metaphors derived from lived experience rather than universal, absolute templates. As Keddell (2011: 410) has stated, 'Arts may encourage a more inductive, interactive, and less rigid use of formal theory'. Walton (2012) also used arts-based methods to encourage breadth and criticality in student reflections on professional communication, which provided a deeper and more detailed level of theoretical analysis. As she noted, there may be a false assumption that the aim of arts work is emotional expression at the expense of analytic understanding.

Walton (2012) also remarked that it is odd that social work remains almost entirely fixed on talk and text when a sustained strand of thinking has characterised the profession as needing intuition and creativity. Similarly, Damianakis (2007: 526) reported that she had found 'no systematic investigation on the ways social workers incorporate the arts … into their knowledge, values, and practices'. There certainly is a lack of arts-based social work intervention research, although perhaps the same could be said in general about intervention research within social work. This being said, earlier writings by social workers such as Goldstein (1992; 1999), Irving (1999) and Siporin (1988) discussed how the arts could help people come to terms with the meaning of life, underscore moral and spiritual issues, endorse diverse ways of understanding marginalised experiences and enhance the quality of the therapeutic relationship (Damianakis 2007). Interestingly, the same has been said about spirituality, in that spiritually-influenced social work can help people address the meaning of life, emphasise moral issues, engage marginalised peoples and non-Western cultures and promote therapeutic presence (Coholic 2016).

Certainly, working with non-Western cultures is a strong rationale for the incorporation of both arts-based methods and spirituality, particularly in social work practice but also in research and education. Moxley (2013) stated that it is puzzling that the arts are not well appreciated in social work, given the centrality of diverse art forms to culture building. Art is a fundamental aspect of culture; art-making may emerge within a group as its principal source of pleasure, interpretation and coping. Huss (2009) used group art-work with Bedouin women, explaining that traditional women living in Westernised cultures do not disclose their problems directly to social workers outside of their own cultural group. Art enabled the women to express themselves in a culturally sanctioned form, with the aim of shifting the understanding of people in power and redirecting interventions. The women's art embodied cultural understandings of problems and solutions.

Similarly, in our work with Aboriginal women, their culture could not be conceived of separately from their spirituality (Coholic *et al.* 2013). Arts-based methods enabled the women to express and develop their cultural/spiritual understandings of their life experiences. For one example, we encouraged the women to draw what they imagined during a guided imagery activity. In describing their drawings, one woman talked about being supported by an 'eagle woman' who gave her a feather and told her that she was her friend, teacher and guide, and that she should not be afraid to ask for help. The woman explained that the eagle woman stated, 'You can do it...you are beautiful and the goodwill is coming'. Another woman who had a similar experience said:

> I headed up towards the sun … I began to feel another presence … the great eagle, he soared with me … He hovered over me, like protection. I felt safe, I felt strong and sacred … the way the eagle flies, so light but with such power, no words, just love.
>
> (Coholic *et al.* 2013: 160)

In harmony with understanding how a particular population and/or culture communicates, one should use methods that are relevant and meaningful for a specific group. For instance, in our experiences, many marginalised and vulnerable children can become easily frustrated and disengaged, have poor listening skills and trouble remaining physically still (Coholic 2011). They are not yet equipped to learn mindfulness from a traditional perspective that relies upon abilities to pay attention, sit still and complete homework outside of the group experience. However, arts-based activities provide an excellent way to assist these youth to develop skills such as paying attention to one's thoughts and feelings (Homeyer 2003), and expressing these aspects of one's life experience to understand them with more depth. This understanding (self-awareness) is crucial for many reasons including the ability to regulate one's emotions as opposed to reacting to them and acting out. Importantly, arts-based and creative methods can help people to express themselves in ways that reflect their capacities and build strengths thereby reflecting a strengths-based approach. They are also great methods of engaging people in helping processes (Leckey 2011; Olson-McBride and Page 2012) and in group work (Haen and Weil 2010).

We have applied arts-based methods for all of these rationales but also because arts-based methods are effective and beneficial. Art therapists have argued for the benefits of art for client change and positive outcomes since the 1970s (Malchiodi 2007). Creative activities have always been evident within mental health, and the arts have an important role to play in improving the health of individuals (Leckey 2011). A critical review of arts-based practices found that these methods are of high benefit especially in the areas of self-discovery and expression (Van Lith *et al.* 2013). Specifically with reference to resilience, arts-based counselling techniques can lead to improvements in this area in addition to wellbeing (Pearson and Wilson 2008), and can improve self-esteem and resilience in adolescents and young adults (Jang and Choi 2012; Roghanchi *et al.* 2013). Macpherson, Hart and Heaver (2016) argued that even short-term visual arts practice interventions can improve youth resilience.

Arts-based methods and spirituality

At the beginning of my research programme, I was interested in learning the benefits of spiritually-influenced group work. We developed a group that had as its overall goal, the development of self-awareness and self-esteem (Coholic 2005). We used a variety of arts-based methods including creative writing, collaging and working with dreams, drawing, working with clay, painting and mindfulness-based activities. Our rationale for using arts-based methods reflected the work of researchers cited earlier in this chapter in that arts-based methods can help people express their thoughts and feelings, and learn about themselves and others. Thus, it seemed an ideal way to assist participants to develop their self-awareness and build group cohesion. Importantly, creative activities are especially relevant methods to use when spirituality is part of the work because spiritual experiences and ideas, which can be embodied and emotional, are often difficult to articulate in words. Similarly, Moxley (2013) argued that art is about emotion and is an important tool for elevating consciousness. Referring specifically to research, Foster (2012) argued that employing art requires a particular ontology; a valuing of experience, feeling, imagination and intuition (often we tend to value logic, numbers and reason more). The same could be said about incorporating spirituality into social work; that we need to be interested in exploring more abstract experiences that may be felt and intuitive.

Mindfulness-based practices and discussions have also been an important part of the group work from the beginning of my research, because mindfulness is a holistic philosophy and a spiritual practice for many people, and it has to do with building self-awareness and self-compassion. Briefly, mindfulness is activity that encourages awareness to emerge through paying attention on purpose, non-judgmentally, in the present moment (Kabat-Zinn 1990). Also, mindfulness has to do with exploring who we are, with questioning our view of the world and with cultivating appreciation for the fullness of life's moments (Gause and Coholic 2010). Indeed, in our early work, we found that mindfulness-based practice was perceived by group participants to help them develop their self-awareness and foster compassion, positive self-esteem and feelings of gratefulness (Coholic 2006). An ability to be mindful can help a person to view negative thoughts as passing events rather than valid reflections of reality (non-judgmental awareness), and it may promote flexible responses as opposed to ruminating about the past (self-regulation of attention). These abilities can assist an individual to build aspects of their resilience through the application of psychological, social, cultural, physical and spiritual resources. Teaching mindfulness by way of arts-based methods has helped us teach this philosophy and practice to vulnerable youth. Mindfulness in social work is a new and growth-area of practice and research, and social workers are taking up mindfulness in creative, strengths-based and holistic ways.

An example of a holistic arts-based activity

We have always incorporated discussions and arts-based activities about dreams into our group work. In an earlier paper, we discussed the connections between dream work and spirituality, pointing out that dreams can provide rich material to work with, and that many cultures believe dreams to be influenced by transcendental forces (Coholic and LeBreton 2007). For instance, some people and/or cultures believe that dreams can contain premonitions or divine messages, or that dreams are a way to communicate with ancestors and others who have died.

Collaging a dream is a particularly effective way to capture and explore it. With a dream in mind, we encouraged participants to look through magazines and cut out any pictures or words that resonated with them, and importantly, not to think too much about this process. Once the collage was constructed, the analysis of it took place. In one group that we studied, Mary produced a dream collage that contained the following words: 'change', 'spirit', 'soothe your soul', 'doors open everywhere', 'that's the way the wind blows', 'taking care of heart and soul', 'air', 'go with your gut' and 'moments matter'. The pictures in the collage included a woman with outstretched arms, a couple canoeing, a wooden path through a forest, butterflies, a woman having a massage, a couple hugging and looking into each other's eyes, and three other lone women looking introspective.

Interestingly, Mary was nervous about discussing her dream collage with the group because she thought the dream signaled that her marriage was in trouble. After processing the dream with the group members, her understanding shifted and a narrative emerged that she was at a moment of critical change in her life but she was not listening to herself; interestingly, she drew in a picture of an ear because she could not find one in the magazines. She concluded that she needed to listen to her spirit/soul and make decisions that were going to be best for her. The dream collage and analysis enabled her to develop self-awareness about her current life situation; a situation that she realised was linked with her spiritual growth.

Within social work, spiritually-influenced practices include topics and processes related to helping people make meaning or sense of significant life events and/or stages, and assisting people to cope. Making-meaning is a process that requires deep reflection (Sheridan 2009). In fact, within social work, spirituality is linked with the human quest for a sense of meaning and purpose (Nelson-Becker and Canda 2008). Thus, as described in the previous example, arts-based methods provide excellent means for engaging in introspective discussions aimed at developing insights about one's life; they help to bring richness and depth into conversations. Additionally, arts-based methods can be used to explicitly facilitate discussions and considerations about spirituality, and may be able to capture some of the person's experiences with spirituality that might be difficult to verbally explain. Simply encouraging participants to draw a picture of what spirituality means to them will usually garner fruitful and interesting discussions.

Thus, arts-based methods do not have to be complicated. For example, 'We are all connected' is an arts-based activity that aims to help group members learn about each other and develop group cohesion. The activity also promotes the idea that while we are all different and diverse, we share commonalities in our experiences, desires, challenges and so on. I have used this activity with adults and it works just as well as with children. Using wooden clothespins and a variety of arts supplies, group participants were encouraged to decorate the clothespin to represent and symbolise themselves. They coloured the clothespins with pastels, glued objects to them, used glitter glue and a variety of other arts supplies. When the group had completed the task, each member shared what their clothespin represented or meant, and then the clothespins were clipped to a string that was hung somewhere in the group room. By hanging the clothespins together, we represented our connection.

The following dialogue was from a group with 12-year-old girls; it very briefly illustrates how the activity can promote personal sharing and discussion about similarities. Also, since the girls introduced a description of their 'soul', one could continue to explore in more depth how they understand their 'soul' and what that means to them opening space in the group for existential and spiritually-influenced discussions.

Sally: I coloured all the bottom pink because everyone says that's the colour of my soul.

Facilitator: Oh, interesting.

Kim: Mine's blue.

Facilitator: So [to Sally] how does pink represent your soul?

Sally: 'Cause apparently, you know how people say pink is a love colour?…Stuff like that. It's because I'm really loveable (laughs).

Facilitator: You girls have talked a lot about feelings related to colours…

Kim: You know what blue meant to me…blue represents caring, and people say that I have a blue soul because I care about others. I care about me…

Steph: I drew music notes 'cause of singing and instruments. And then I wrote dance, and drew a tree because I like nature.

Facilitator: Well that's neat. We both have blue and trees, right? And you've got the music like Sally has. So we can start seeing some connections between us, right?

The enjoyment of arts-based methods

When I began my work in the area of holistic arts-based group work, I did not anticipate how enjoyable and different working with arts-based methods would be for participants in our groups, and since the beginning, this has been a consistent finding in our work with both adults and children (Coholic 2014). For instance, women struggling with substance use explained that the arts-based mindfulness group was different because they had 'fun through it all' and that 'it doesn't have to hurt, at the moment, for you to be able to grow'. One woman stated that she was 'longing for a group' where she could 'deal with my issues in a positive way' (Coholic 2005: 798–9).

More recently, we explored the benefits of our group programme for improving mood and coping in adults seeking mental health services. We found that perceived benefits included the improvement of effective coping strategies, self-awareness, feelings of self-compassion and abilities to focus and pay attention. Importantly, the participants reported on the strength of their group cohesion and the support they felt from the other group members, and they felt very engaged by the methods. Participants commented on the diversity of the group members, stating 'accepting that, embracing that; that was fun, exciting'. Another woman explained that the group enabled her to reconnect with her creativity and to use art as a therapeutic tool for self-expression: 'I wrote so much stuff down. Everything that was in my head. It was like I had an enema or something!' Yet another participant explained that the art-making helped him develop self-awareness: 'It's that whole idea a picture is worth a thousand words and a piece of what we've produced is worth all the feelings and all the subconscious and all the thousand words that could come out of us' (Coholic et al. 2014).

These comments illustrate that arts-based methods can help people develop skills and abilities in an enjoyable and creative manner. Furthermore, the enjoyable nature of arts-based methods engages people in a helping process and helps to build respect and understanding among group members. Consistent with our experience working with marginalised children, we experienced very low attrition from the arts-based mindfulness group with these adults.

In a recent paper, we noted that the average rate of attendance for vulnerable children attending our group programme was 11 out of 12 group sessions (our group programme is 12, two-hour group sessions long) (Coholic and Eys 2016). Clearly, once the children were engaged with the programme, we did not have difficulty keeping them engaged. Indeed, holistic arts-based methods not only engage sometimes difficult to reach children, but the most important element of a programme might be that it involves activity children enjoy so that they will devote effort and time to it (Flook et al. 2010).

Arts-based methods can also facilitate the learning of skills that children can build upon, without focusing on pain-filled experiences (Coholic *et al.* 2009). This is not to say that there will not be pain and suffering in our work but for children (and adults) who experience serious challenges at school, work and home, and feel isolated and alone, the experience of having fun can keep them emotionally receptive so that positive messages can slip through their defenses (James 1989). Currently, we are assessing our arts-based mindfulness group programme with youth attending a short-term in-patient mental health programme. They recently commented on how the arts-based methods are enabling them to connect with one another and discuss issues in a meaningful manner with more depth compared with the rest of their treatment, not to mention that it is a lot of fun.

Summary

Given the difficulty we sometimes experience in engaging people in social work helping and change processes, the attrition rates we suffer in our work, the diverse clientele we work with, and the serious and difficult nature of much of what we do, it begs the question why social workers do not utilise arts-based methods more? To some extent, arts-based methods and spirituality are similar in that, for many of us, these topics and approaches were not part of our social work education and training. That being said, over the past 15 years, this has begun to change. However, a lack of exposure to these topics understandably leaves many social workers unsure of how to proceed. At the same time, social workers are trained to be creative and critical thinkers with open minds, and we have the skills required to use holistic arts-based methods in effective ways. For example, we are trained to assess situations holistically and non-judgmentally. Should someone create something that is of concern (such as a drawing of a death), we have the skills to explore the feelings, thoughts and behaviours that might have led to the creation. Importantly, there is a solid literature and burgeoning research studies to draw on in these fields, which can be used to help develop one's practice and address the need to work from an evidence-informed stance.

Finally, it is important to understand that one does not have to be an artist to utilise arts-based methods. We are not teaching our clients how to make art or art techniques. Arts-based methods and creations should be used as tools for exploration, teaching a concept, exploring an issue, sharing and discussion. The products of these processes should not be 'interpreted' such as some art therapists might do with art produced by a client. The art-based activities can be used as a way to explore the theme of a session, unlike an art class at school where a piece of artwork might be assessed according to the use of a specific technique. Arts-based methods do not have to be complicated or require special supplies or equipment. Finally, engaging with our own creativity can be fulfilling, bringing joy and meaning into our work. This should not be underrated in a profession that demands so much of us.

References

Bartkeviciene, A. (2014) 'Social work students' experiences in "self" and professional "self" awareness by using the art therapy method', *European Scientific Journal*, 10(5): 12–23.

Coholic, D. (2005) 'The helpfulness of spirituality influenced group work in developing self-awareness and self-esteem: a preliminary investigation', *The Scientific World Journal*, 5: 789–802.

Coholic, D. (2006) 'Mindfulness meditation practice in spirituality influenced group work', *Arete*, 30(1): 90–100.

Coholic, D. (2010) *Arts Activities for Children and Young People in Need: helping children to develop mindfulness, spiritual awareness and self-esteem*, London: Jessica Kingsley Publishers.

Coholic, D. (2011) 'Exploring the feasibility and benefits of arts-based mindfulness-based practices with young people in need: aiming to improve aspects of self-awareness and resilience', *Child and Youth Care Forum*, 40(4): 303–17.

Coholic, D. (2014) 'Facilitating mindfulness using arts-based methods and a holistic strengths-based perspective', in M.S. Boone (ed) *Mindfulness and Acceptance in Social Work: evidence-based interventions and emerging applications*, Oakland, CA: Context Press.

Coholic, D. (2016) 'Spirituality, religion, and diversity', in A. Al-Krenawi, J. Graham and N. Habibov (eds) *Diversity and Social Work in Canada*, New York: Oxford University Press.

Coholic, D. and Eys, M. (2016) 'Benefits of an arts-based mindfulness group intervention for vulnerable children', *Child and Adolescent Social Work Journal*, 33(1): 1013.

Coholic, D. and LeBreton, J. (2007) 'Working with dreams in a holistic arts-based group: connections between dream interpretation and spirituality', *Social Work with Groups*, 30(3): 47–64.

Coholic, D., Cote-Meek, S. and Recollet, D (2013) 'Exploring the acceptability and perceived benefits of arts-based group methods for aboriginal women living in an urban community within northeastern Ontario', *Canadian Social Work Review*, 29(2): 149–68.

Coholic, D., Lougheed, S. and Cadell, S. (2009) 'Exploring the helpfulness of arts-based methods with children living in foster care', *Traumatology*, 15(3): 64–71.

Coholic, D., McAlister, H., Smith, D. and Conrad, A. (2014) 'A pilot study exploring the feasibility, suitability, and benefits of an arts-based mindfulness group program for improving mood in adults seeking mental health services', paper presented at the OASW Social Work Provincial Conference, Resilience and Renewal: Envisioning the Future in Social Work Practice, Research, and Education, Toronto, November 2014.

Damianakis, T. (2007) 'Social work's dialogue with the arts: epistemological and practice intersections', *Families in Society*, 88(4): 525–33.

Flook, L., Smalley, S., Kitil, M. J., Galla, B., Kaiser-Greenland, S., Locke, J., Ishijima, E. and Kasari, C. (2010) 'Effects of mindful awareness practices on executive functions in elementary school children', *Journal of Applied School Psychology*, 26(1): 70–95.

Foster, V. (2012) 'What if? The use of poetry to promote social justice', *Social Work Education*, 31(6): 742–55.

Gause, R. and Coholic, D. (2010) 'Mindfulness-based practices as a holistic philosophy and method', *Currents: New Scholarship in the Human Services*, 9(2): 1–23.

Goldstein, H. (1992) 'If social work hasn't made progress as a science, might it be an art?', *Families in Society*, 73(1): 48–55.

Goldstein, H. (1999) 'The limits and art of understanding in social work practice', *Families in Society*, 80(4): 385–95.

Goodman, T. (2005) 'Working with children: beginner's mind', in C. Germer, R. Siegel and P. Fulton (eds) *Mindfulness and Psychotherapy*, New York: The Guilford Press.

Haen, C. and Weil, M. (2010) 'Group therapy on the edge: adolescence, creativity, and group work', *Group*, 34(1): 37–52.

Harley, D. and Hunn, V. (2015) 'Utilization of photovoice to explore hope and spirituality among low-income African American adolescents', *Child and Adolescent Social Work Journal*, 32(1): 3–15.

Homeyer, L. (2003) 'Play therapy: counseling with young children', *Marriage and Family*, 6(2): 163–9.

Huss, E. (2009) 'A case study of Bedouin women's art in social work: a model of social arts intervention with "traditional" women negotiating western cultures', *Social Work Education*, 28(6): 598–616.

Irving, A. (1999) 'Waiting for Foucault: social work and the multitudinous truth(s) of life', in A.S. Chambon, A. Irving and L. Epstein (eds) *Reading Foucault for Social Work*, New York: Columbia University Press.

Jacobs, C. (2015) 'Contemplative spaces in social work practice', *Journal of Pain and Symptom Management*, 49(1): 150–4.

James, B. (1989) *Treating Traumatized Children: new insights and creative interventions*, Massachusetts: Lexington.

Jang, H. and Choi, S. (2012) 'Increasing ego-resilience using clay with low SES (social economic status) adolescents in group art therapy', *The Arts in Psychotherapy*, 39(4): 245–50.

Kabat-Zinn, J. (1990) *Full Catastrophe Living: using the wisdom of your body and mind to face stress, pain and illness*, New York: Delta.

Keddell, E. (2011) 'A constructionist approach to the use of arts-based materials in social work education: making connections between art and life', *Journal of Teaching in Social Work*, 31(4): 400–14.

Leckey, J. (2011) 'The therapeutic effectiveness of creative activities on mental wellbeing: a systematic review of the literature', *Journal of Psychiatric and Mental Health Nursing*, 18(6): 501–9.

Macpherson, H., Hart, A. and Heaver, B. (2016) 'Building resilience through group visual arts activities: findings from a scoping study with young people who experiene mental health complexities and/or learning difficulties', *Journal of Social Work*, 16(5): 541–60.

Malchiodi, C. (2007) *The Art Therapy Sourcebook*, 2nd edn, New York: McGraw-Hill.

Moxley, D. (2013) 'Incoporating art-making into the cultural practice of social work', *Journal of Ethnic and Cultural Diversity in Social Work*, 22(3–4): 235–55.

Nelson-Becker, H. and Canda, E. (2008) 'Spirituality, religion, and aging research in social work: state of the art and future possibilities', *Journal of Religion, Spirituality and Aging*, 20(3): 177–93.

Olson-McBride, L. and Page, T. (2012) 'Song to self: promoting a therapeutic dialogue with high-risk youths through poetry and popular music', *Social Work with Groups*, 35(2): 124–37.

Pearson, M. and Wilson, H. (2008) 'Using expressive counselling tools to enhance emotional literacy, emotional wellbeing and resilience: improving therapeutic outcomes with expressive therapies', *Counselling, Psychotherapy, and Health*, 4(1): 1–19.

Roghanchi, M., Mohamad, A.R., Mey, S.C., Momeni, K.M. and Golmohamadian, M. (2013) 'The effect of integrating rational emotive behavior therapy and art therapy on self-esteem and resilience', *The Arts in Psychotherapy*, 40(2): 179–84.

Sheridan, M. (2009) 'Ethical issues in the use of spiritually based interventions in social work practice: what are we doing and why', *Journal of Religion and Spirituality in Social Work*, 28(1–2): 99–126.

Sinding, C., Warren, R. and Paton, C. (2014) 'Social work and the arts: images at the intersection', *Qualitative Social Work*, 13(2): 187–202.

Siporin, M. (1988) 'Clinical social work as an art form', *Social Casework*, 69(3): 177–83.

Van Lith, T., Schofield, M. and Fenner, P. (2013) 'Identifying the evidence-base for arts-based practices and their potential benefit for mental health recovery: a critical review', *Disability and Rehabilitation*, 35(16): 1309–23.

Walsh, C. A., Rutherford, G. and Crough, M. (2013) 'Arts-based research: creating social change for incarcerated women', *Creative Approaches to Research*, 6(1): 119–39.

Walton, P. (2012) 'Beyond talk and text: an expressive visual arts method for social work education', *Social Work Education*, 31(6): 724–41.

36

Ethical principles for transitioning to a renewable energy economy in an era of climate change

Mishka Lysack

Introduction

Framing an issue as a crossroads is one ethical resource that surfaced in what the German philosopher/historian Karl Jaspers (1953) named the Axial Age. Between the ninth and third centuries BCE, the emergence of several wisdom and faith traditions across multiple cultures signaled a qualitative shift in human social and cultural development: Confucianism and Taoism in East Asia, Buddhism and Hinduism in South Asia, the Hebrew prophets in Judaism in the Ancient Near East and the philosophers in Greece. These ancient wisdom and faith traditions in the Axial Age gave rise to remarkable developments in ethical resources and spiritual perspectives that transformed human culture at that time, and continue to provide an invaluable ethical legacy that still permeates our societies and economies today.

Within this Axial Age, this idea of the decision crossroads emerged in multiple cultures (e.g. Greek philosophy); however, this chapter will highlight how this heuristic tool was refined as one key idea inherited from the Hebrew prophets as they developed the ethical foundation for Judaism. The Jewish prophets took this insight of a crossroads and compressed it into a razor-sharp ethical dilemma of choosing life or death, a leitmotif that arcs over the Hebrew Biblical literature. For the prophets, engaging in social or environmental exploitation or oppressing other members of the community was effectively choosing the way of death. In contrast, to choose life was to align oneself with the moral order and goodness inherent in the natural world, replicating and enacting this ethical posture of compassion and justice in one's relationships with other human and non-human members of the covenant (Habel and Trudinger 2008; Lysack 2015b).

In our time, climate change and environmental decline presents humanity with a similar existential crisis of deciding between two pathways. Scientific research confirms how the planet's ecosystems are already nearing the limits of its carbon budget (Meinshausen *et al.* 2009) and moving beyond their key tipping points (Lenton 2011) into irreversible and dangerous climate change. To minimise the serious consequences, humanity must embark on a pathway of deep decarbonisation eliminating the use of fossil fuels and completely transitioning to renewable energy by no later than 2050. To accomplish this objective, global greenhouse emissions need to peak by 2020, and be on a downward track by 2025, if we are to avoid the worst impacts of climate change (Kolbert 2006).

This decision will not be a single action at one point in time, but rather a choice that needs to be made and re-made over and over again as actions of repeated re-commitment. Governments, decision-makers and the public will be required to re-commit themselves frequently to the challenge of the decarbonisation pathway and transitioning to renewable energy systems and zero-carbon economies. To maintain this trajectory, governments and the public will need to draw on a reservoir of ethical resources.

Among the ethical resources within the spiritual writings of the Hebrew prophetic tradition, this chapter will explore one specific resource that could provide orienting principles for a decarbonised society: the idea of the covenant community. Subsequently, the implications of this metaphor of a covenant community will be examined through the lenses of two leaders from two different sectors (economist Herman Daly and climate advocate Bill McKibben), identifying the key ethical resources and orienting principles arising from this idea of a covenant community that will enable the transition to a renewable energy economy. Finally, this chapter will conclude by highlighting the resources in social work that resonate with these ideas.

The cosmic covenant as template for the zero-carbon, steady-state economy

Hebrew prophets: justice, sustainability and holiness

Recent Biblical scholarship (Habel and Trudinger 2008) has pointed to an alternative worldview to our unsustainable extractive economy embedded in the Hebrew Bible, which provides resources for a position that is spiritually grounded, environmentally informed and politically empowering. In his landmark work, *The Cosmic Covenant*, Murray (1992) maintains that it is the Hebraic notion of a 'cosmic covenant' that offers the most promising framework for a spiritually-grounded environmental and justice ethic. In his nuanced exposition of the key Biblical ideas of the eternal covenant (*Berit olam*) and the covenant of peace (*Berit shalom*), Murray (1992) argues that they offer not only a socio-political perspective, but also a larger frame of the intrinsic moral order of the universe where there is an integrated unity of cosmos, nature and society. Northcott (1996: 168) emphasises that the 'covenant is not simply between humans and God, as anthropocentric exegetes have traditionally held, but is rather a "cosmic covenant" involving all the orders of creation and linking them with the rituals, ethics and society of humans'.

This possibility that there are not two but actually *three partners* in the covenant – 1) God, 2) humanity and 3) all other species and creatures in ecological communities along with the land and the ecosystems – is a startling prospect (Brueggemann 2002). As the model of covenant community is mapped onto the social, political, economic and environmental dimensions of life, covenant is potentially a deeply 'subversive paradigm' that contains rich possibilities of ordering more just and compassionate relationships between people, God and the environment (Brueggemann 1994, 1999). In this framework, humanity and the ecological communities of the earth are covenant-partners with the Divine. Nor is it an option to conceptualise humanity as being in an exclusive covenant relationship with God (the dominant spiritual model), thereby reducing the environment to a source for raw resources for industrial production as well as a sewer for human waste. The health and wellbeing of humanity is inextricably linked with the health of the environment. All develop and flourish together, just as all suffer and deteriorate together. This idea is apparent in the assertion in Job that 'you will be in covenant with the stones of the wild, and the wild beasts will be at peace with you' (Job 5: 23).

Development of covenant community

Historically, the writings of the prophet Hosea are the earliest literary source for the description of the eternal covenant or 'treaty' established by the Divine. This covenant included an environmental dimension 'with the wild animals, with the birds of heaven and the creeping things of the earth' (Hosea 2: 18). Loya (2008) suggests that for the prophet Hosea, the violation of this covenant through spiritual infidelity, ecological destruction and social/economic oppression results in the suffering and grief of the earth. In the same time period, the prophet Amos (about 750 BCE), a farmer himself, criticises the rampant social and economic oppression by using elements of the earth as voices to call the people to return to the covenant relationship (Marlow 2008). Braaten (2008) maintains that in the prophet Joel (about 400 BCE), the natural world is pictured as calling humanity to identify with the covenant community through an environmental disaster of a locust invasion and the resulting devastation of agricultural resources. In the post-exilic period, the prophet Haggai (520 BCE) continued to remind the people of the vision of a sustainable and just society, encouraging reforms of land use and tenure in agricultural economies in harmony with covenant community principles expressed by earlier prophets.

Tension between covenant community and empire: sustainability and justice versus environmental exploitation and social injustice

This vision of the covenant community characterised by ecological sustainability and social justice continued to be expressed through the Hebrew prophets, and was also enacted in certain agricultural practices of the Sabbath of the Land (Exodus 23; Leviticus 25–26). However, this covenant community ideal was also continually resisted by the political and economic elites of the nation. A succession of Jewish kings sought to emulate the imperial tendencies of other countries in the Ancient Near East in the growth of its political economy, military expansion and architectural construction. Over time, these imperial tendencies finally exhausted the social and ecological resources of the country, resulting in a bloated ecological footprint that led finally to collapse through imperial 'overstretch' (Kennedy 1987). Excessive deforestation, agricultural over cropping and overgrazing by animals reduced a great portion of the fertile land to desert. An environmental reading of archaeological findings of cities, such as Jericho, Tyre and Jerusalem in Israel in the eighth century, suggests that an environmental crisis may have caused these cities to be abandoned, precipitated by the abuse that the land suffered during the imperial projects of the Jewish ruling classes (Ponting 1988).

While this ideal of the covenant community and its enactment in social and environmental practice proved to be highly resilient, the great imperial projects of the monarchy, exacerbated by the exploitative practices of the merchant class, not only created increasing economic disparity, but also environmental devastation of the earth community in the created order (Isaiah 5: 8–10). Isaiah sees the ecological degradation of the land and its biotic communities as the result of neglect or intentional resistance to the inherent moral order and goodness of nature (Northcott 1996, 2007).

The most evocative descriptions of this de-creation of creation itself may be found in Isaiah 24 and Jeremiah 4: 23–28, where the wellbeing of the social, political, economic, agricultural and environmental dimensions of life are fundamentally compromised. In these texts, the human community is portrayed as severely threatened. Social disorder and decline in spirituality are related to the 'disruption of the order of nature' (Murray 1992: 60). In our time of climate change and its effects of temperature rise, droughts and crop failures, the images in Isaiah 24: 1–13 are especially chilling:

> Ravaged the earth ... the earth is mourning, withering ... the earth is polluted under the inhabitants feet, for they have ... broken the everlasting covenant ... that is why the inhabitants of the earth are burnt up and few people are left.
>
> (Isaiah 24: 3–6)

A century later than Isaiah, the prophet Jeremiah (about 646–587 BCE) continued to enunciate the vision of the covenant community, and to perceptively denounce environmental devastation, economic exploitation and empty forms of piety. Jeremiah provided provocative critiques and passionate invitations for the nation to return to the values of the covenant community. Jeremiah deftly makes linkages between the religious, environmental and social/economic domains in his analysis of the environmental disturbances of his day, himself being a witness of local climate change and the transformation of the fertile land into lifeless deserts through overcropping, overgrazing and deforestation around 600 BCE (Northcott 2007).

Environmental ethicist Rasmussen (1996: 243) argues that the idea of the covenant community offers an integrated vision of the relationship between God, the environment and humanity that is salient not only to the 'people of the Book' (i.e. Jews, Muslims and Christians), but also 'ethically charged'. As an environmental ethic rooted in ancient wisdom traditions and previous civilizations, the 'covenant' ethic integrates environmental sustainability, social justice and a robust spiritually-grounded ethic that underlines the centrality of environmental justice for the victimised and of healing of the wounded, be they human or non-human members of the earth community.

Ethical principles for a sustainable economy

Drawing on the model of a covenant community in the Hebraic prophetic literature, what ethical resources might be used as building blocks for a sustainable economy in an era of accelerating and irreversible climate destabilisation and environmental degradation? We now examine these ethical resources as developed by McKibben, environmental writer and the founder of 350.org (an advocacy NGO combatting climate change), and Herman Daly, former Senior Economist at the World Bank, and author of several key books in sustainable economics.

1   *The earth's ecological systems and biological communities have intrinsic environmental limits, and the recognition of these limits need to be the reference point for all decisions about energy, society and the economy.* The concept of limits is woven through much of the literature that emerged from the wisdom and faith traditions: limits on the treatment of land, treatment of animals, restrictions on the amount harvested. Similarly, science has elucidated how the 'natural environment places finite limits on our behavior' (McKibben 2005: 8), and climate science research (Meinshausen *et al.* 2009) has demonstrated that the earth has a limit to the amount of carbon that can be burned and released in the atmosphere. As of 2012, the earth had a total carbon budget of 565 gigatons of carbon, beyond which the door closes irreversibly on any prospect of the planet staying below the scientifically-based goal from Conference of the Parties to the UN Framework Convention on Climate Change (COP21) in Paris in December 2015, of maintaining global warming to a level below 1.5°C.

2   *Humanity needs to acknowledge that it has limits,* despite the fact that science and technology has ceded increasing power to humanity, fostering the perception that we have no limits. Hence,

> it is precisely because science and technology has given us such power that the scale of our economy has been able to grow to the point where we must now consciously

face the fundamental limits of creaturehood; finitude, entropy, and ecological dependence.

(Daly 1996: 214)

While it is true that the human species has enjoyed success in thriving in diverse habitats, as a creature, humanity too has an envelope of limits. As Daly (1996) continues:

The hard problem is overcoming our addition to growth as our favored way to assert our creative power, and our idolatrous belief—whether we think in religious terms or not—that our derived creative power is autonomous and unlimited.

(Daly 1996: 224)

3   *There are serious adverse, deadly consequences, when environmental limits are violated.* McKibben (2006: 8) describes violating environmental limits as 'de-creation', an unraveling of the tapestry of creation and the rhythms of nature that give us a sense of stability and home. Similarly, scientists continue to confirm the serious consequences of breaching the planet's environmental limits, mapping out the early warning signs of tipping points (Lenton 2011) that signal the planet shifting into irreversible and dangerous climate change.

4   *An ethic of restraint* is critical if we are to reduce the danger that climate change poses for the human species and the planet as a whole. Hence, 'We *are* different from the rest of the natural order, for the reason that we possess the possibility of self-restraint, of choosing some other way' (McKibben 2006: xx). An ethic of restraint and an envelope of limits are germane to all wisdom and faith traditions that emerged in the Axial Age, and constitute the bridge between wisdom traditions and functional societies and economies. McKibben points out that humanity has exercised the ethic of restraint previously on other issues with some success, such as refraining from the use of nuclear weapons. While humanity has the capacity to extract every molecule of oil, gas and coal and burn it, we also have the capacity to choose not to burn it. In other words, 'Should we so choose, we could exercise our reason to do what no other animal could do: we could limit ourselves voluntarily' (McKibben 2006: 182).

5   *Humanity needs to de-centre itself, and move to where it no longer perceives itself as the centre of the earth.* Both our economy and culture is predicated on the 'assumption that human beings are and should be at the centre of everything' (McKibben 2005: 25). Instead, *humanity needs to reclaim itself as one species among many*, albeit a highly adaptive and intelligent species that now exercises an awesome degree of power over life on the planet. McKibben (2006: 146) perceptively asked, 'What would it mean to our ways of life, … our economics, our output of carbon dioxide and methane, if we began to truly and viscerally to think of ourselves as just one species among many?' In *shifting from an anthropocentric to a biocentric perspective*, humanity can orient itself within a larger web of life, one partner within a cosmic covenant of life, locating the earth rather than humanity in the centre. For the environmental ethicist Aldo Leopold (1966: 240), this new ethical perspective would 'change the role of homo sapiens from conqueror of the land community to plain member and citizen of it', who cares for the health of the land and planet. In so doing, humanity is freed from seeing the land as our 'slave and servant', and now able to experience the natural world as a 'biotic community' (Leopold 1966: 262) or covenant community. As a result, humanity then can shift from extractive and exploitative economics to a sustainable ethic, where something is 'right when it tends to protect the integrity, stability and beauty of the biotic community. It is wrong when it tends otherwise' (Leopold 1966: 262).

6   *Ancient wisdom traditions reveal how humanity also perceived a patterning or order in nature reflected in how it is organised and functions.* For these faith traditions and philosophies, these patterns reflected a *moral order in the universe*, within which humanity could prosper and thrive (Northcott 2007). These insights regarding patterning are reflected in contemporary practices of biomimicry (Benyus 2002) in science and industry, where humanity imitates these patterns and learns how to survive and thrive in diverse environments.

7   *In the cosmic covenant community, nature was not assigned a value by humanity, but perceived as having an inherent value as part of a larger morally ordered cosmos.* In other words, *nature possesses intrinsic worth* as part of a larger cosmic mystery. Daly (1996: 217) argues that all 'living things have both instrumental value for other living things and intrinsic value by virtue of their own sentience and capacity to enjoy their own lives'. Such a perspective is in stark contrast to contemporary economics, where nature is devoid of any worth outside of human use, only having *extrinsic or instrumental value* as an inert resource for extraction, exploitation, consumption and finally disposal (McKibben 2005). Public policy regarding energy, city design and built environment, agriculture and forestry, fisheries and conservation all need to embed this orienting principle of nature possessing intrinsic worth at the heart of their policy development.

8   *Necessity of a shift from short-term to long-term perspectives* as well as *from exclusive to more socially and ecologically inclusive* orientations. The unsustainability of our current economic system is visible 'by its practice of discounting the future, [and] is implicitly willing to say that beyond some point the future is worth nil and might as well end' (Daly 1996: 220). In contrast, the 'steady-state economy' is a 'way of keeping the rich from leaning too heavily on the poor and present generations from leaning too heavily on future generations' (Daly 1996: 215). Not only is it socially inclusive, but it also includes all species in their ecological communities within their environmental support systems in the planet.

9   *Decentring the primacy of the economy.* The dominant economic model currently centres on the understanding that the

> economy is the total system and is unconstrained in its growth by anything. This vision concedes that nature may be finite, but sees it as just a sector of the economy for which other sectors can substitute without limiting overall growth in any important way.
>
> (Daly 1996: 219)

In this understanding, the human economy encompasses everything else, and the environment is a subsystem of the human economy. However, as impacts of climate change multiply and cascade through the planet's living systems and our economy, of necessity, humanity will be forced either to react passively, or to rapidly transition to an economy that is an 'open subsystem of a larger but finite, non-growing, and closed ecosystem on which it is fully dependent' (Daly 1996: 219). Wendell Berry (2010) makes a similar point when he describes the 'Great Economy' (the natural world) as being the envelope within which the human 'small economy' can thrive, rather than the reverse.

10 *Design economies based on oikonomia,* which is Aristotle's term from which we derive the words 'ecology' and 'economy'. Oikonomia is the

> management of the household so as to increase its use value to all members of the household over the long run. If we expand the scope of household to include the larger community of the land, of shared values, resources, biomes, institutions, language, and history, then we have a good definition of "economics for community".
>
> (Daly and Cobb 1994: 138)

The key characteristics of oikonomia are as follows:

> First, it takes the long-run rather than the short-run view. Second, it considers costs and benefits to the whole community, not just to the parties to the transaction. Third, it focuses on concrete use value and the limited accumulation thereof, rather on abstract exchange value and its impetus toward unlimited accumulation.
>
> (Daly and Cobb 1994: 139)

Policy influencing for a sustainable economy and climate/environmental protection: social work resources

These faith and ethical principles have consequences for social work as a profession, while social workers also have an opportunity and responsibility to contribute to the larger shift to a new renewable energy economy and climate protection. What are the contributions that social work could make to this larger transition? John Coates is one of the first scholars to begin writing about ecology and social work, combining his integration of these two fields with a strong political and economic awareness and deep spiritual sensibility. Coates has developed a substantive critique of the dominant economic order of consumerism and the relentless growth that is driving the degradation of the planet's ecological communities, locating the root causes of this deterioration in the current economy and modernity. Coates' (2003a, 2003b) analysis of modernity's beliefs and values is summarised as: 1) primacy of the economic order, 2) industrialism, 3) consumerism, 4) materialism, 5) the myth of progress and 6) individualism. In his analysis of the current economy/society and his exploration of alternatives, Coates articulates principles quite similar to the model of covenant community explored earlier and to the sustainable economy proposed by Daly.

By way of practices, Coates (2007) suggests that through their relational and contextual thinking and their relationship skills, ecosocial workers can mitigate the negative forces of industrialism, consumerism, commodification of the earth's commons and pathological individualism, aiding in the development of intentional communities that regard the earth as sacred. He also insists that an 'important role for social work will be that of *prophet*, of readying individuals and communities to support the transformation in values and lifestyle which will be required if sustainability and social justice are to be attained' (Coates 2000, emphasis added).

With the gap between developed and developing nations, this ethically grounded consciousness also includes a climate and environmental justice mandate that recognises the differential impacts of environmental degradation and climate change on the marginalised peoples of the planet (Coates 2007; Lysack 2008). In describing the political involvement that is necessary to address environmental degradation, Besthorn (2003) proposes both a critical stance of the current political and economic structures, and environmental advocacy as a sustained struggle against the social and economic forces that are the life-support system of environmental deterioration.

Like other social workers who engage in policy influencing to achieve climate protection objectives such as phasing out coal (Lysack 2015a), Dominelli (2011: 430) argues that fighting climate change is not a marginal or fringe activity for social work, but rather a critical imperative, arguing that the profession has an important role to play in 'promoting sustainable energy production and consumption; mobilising people to protect their futures through community social work; and proposing solutions to greenhouse gas emissions'. As community-based social work, Dominelli (2011: 435) lists the practices of 'advocacy and community mobilisation around green technologies to enhance the quality of life in disadvantaged localities and reduce carbon emissions… [by promoting] clean renewable energy'. At the macro-practice level, she encourages the development of skill sets among social workers that include 'lobbying for preventative measure taken at local … national and international levels by advocating policy changes … and dialoguing with policy makers and using the media to change policies' (Dominelli 2011: 437).

Social workers have invaluable conceptual and practice skills for facilitating cross-sector environmental leadership in government, business, civil society, and communities and pressing for environmental, economic and social policy changes that would transition communities and countries from fossil fuel economies to a renewable energy economy and sustainable communities. Many social work skills, such as facilitating group processes in coalitions and networks of professionals and allies (Lysack 2015a) and building capacity for environmental engagement and leadership (Lysack 2012a), are transferable to comparable skill sets of professionals engaged in advocacy and policy influencing for transitioning to a renewable energy economy (Hoefer 2016). Drawing on the strategies and tactics emerging from social movements in history, such as the abolition of slavery movement in England (Lysack 2012b), social workers can also adapt these tools of social change in the current context in order to accelerate the change in our economy and energy systems. In addition, social workers can utilise the conceptual resources from research into the role of emotion and an ethical posture on environmental protection, translating these tools into practices for nurturing the development of committed environmental citizenship (Lysack 2013) as a foundation for transformational change through public engagement.

Scientists have worked hard on solving the difficult scientific problem of climate change, its tipping points and impacts on the earth's systems and ecological communities (Lenton 2011), and the rapidly dwindling carbon budget of the planet (Meinshausen et al. 2009). They remind us with urgency, the time for avoiding the worst of dangerous climate is short, and effective and bold action is required. As McKibben (2013: 255) insists, as he reflects on both the imperative and opportunity for action: 'The old cycle we've always known is very nearly gone, but not quite. It lingers still, and while it does the fight is worth the cost.'

References

Benyus, J. (2002) *Biomimicry: innovation inspired by nature*, New York: HarperCollins Publishers.

Berry, W. (2010) *What Matters? Economics for a renewed commonwealth*, Berkeley: Counterpoint.

Besthorn, F. (2003) 'Radical ecologisms: insights for educating social workers in ecological activism and social justice', *Critical Social Work* 4(1). Online. Available HTTP: www1.uwindsor.ca/criticalsocialwork/radical-ecologisms-insights-for-educating-social-workers-in-ecological-activism-and-social-justice (accessed 15 March 2016).

Braaten, L.J. (2008) 'Earth community in Joel: a call to identify with the rest of creation', in N. Habel and P. Trudinger (eds) *Exploring Ecological Hermeneutics*, Atlanta: Society of Biblical Literature.

Brueggemann, W. (1994) *A Social Reading of the Old Testament*, Minneapolis: Fortress Press.

Brueggemann, W. (1999) *The Covenanted Self: explorations in law and covenant*, Minneapolis: Fortress Press.

Brueggemann, W. (2002) *The Land: place as gift, promise, and challenge in biblical faith*, 2nd edn, Minneapolis: Fortress Press.

Coates, J. (2000) 'From modernism to sustainability: new roles for social work', paper presented at the Joint Conference of the IFSW and the ISASSW, Montreal. Online. Available HTTP: http://ecosocialwork.org/images/pdfs/modtosustainability_jc.pdf (accessed 15 March 2016).

Coates, J. (2003a) *Ecology and Social Work*, Halifax: Fernwood Publishing.

Coates, J. (2003b) 'Exploring the roots of the environmental crisis: opportunity for social transformation', *Critical Social Work*, 4(1). Online. Available HTTP: www1.uwindsor.ca/criticalsocialwork/exploring-the-roots-of-the-environmental-crisis-opportunity-for-social-transformation (accessed 15 March 2016).

Coates, J. (2007) 'From ecology to spirituality and social justice', in J. Coates, J.R. Graham and B. Swartzentruber with B. Ouellette (eds) *Spirituality and Social Work: selected Canadian readings*, Toronto: Canadian Scholars Press.

Daly, H. (1996) *Beyond Growth: the economics of sustainable development*, Boston: Beacon Press.

Daly, H. and Cobb, J. (1994) *For the Common Good: redirecting the economy toward community, the environment, and a sustainable future*, Boston: Beacon Press.

Dominelli, L. (2011) 'Climate change: social workers' roles and contributions to policy debates and interventions', *International Journal of Social Welfare*, 20(4): 430–8.

Habel, N. and Trudinger, P. (2008) *Exploring Ecological Hermeneutics*, Atlanta: Society of Biblical Literature.

Hoefer, R. (2016) *Advocacy Practice for Social Justice*, Chicago: Lyceum Books.

Jaspers, K. (1953) *The Origin and Goal of History*, London: Routledge.

Kennedy, P. (1987) *The Rise and Fall of the Great Powers: economic challenge and military conflict from 1500 to 2000*, New York: Random House.

Kolbert, E. (2006) *Field Notes from a Catastrophe*, London: Bloomsbury.

Lenton, T.M. (2011) 'Early warning of climate tipping points', *Nature Climate Change*, 1: 201–9.

Leopold, A. (1966) *A Sand County Almanac*, New York: Ballantine Books.

Loya, M.T. (2008) '"Therefore the earth mourns": the grievance of Earth in Hosea 4:1–3', in N. Habel and P. Trudinger (eds) *Exploring Ecological Hermeneutics*, Atlanta: Society of Biblical Literature.

Lysack, M. (2008) 'Global warming as a moral issue: ethics and economics of reducing carbon emissions', *Interdisciplinary Environmental Review*, 10(1–2): 95–109.

Lysack, M. (2012a) 'Building capacity for environmental engagement and leadership: an ecosocial work perspective', *International Journal of Social Welfare*, 21(3): 260–9.

Lysack, M. (2012b) 'The abolition of slavery movement as a moral movement: ethical resources, spiritual roots, and strategies for social change', *Journal of Religion and Spirituality in Social Work*, 31(1–2): 150–71.

Lysack, M. (2013) 'Emotion, ethics, and fostering committed environmental citizenship', in M. Gray, J. Coates and T. Hetherington (eds) *Environmental Social Work*, London: Routledge.

Lysack, M. (2015a) 'Effective policy influencing and environmental advocacy: health, climate change, and phasing out coal', *International Social Work*, 58(3): 435–47.

Lysack, M. (2015b) 'The ethical imperative of limits', *Policy Options*, January–February 2015: 23–6. Online. Available HTTP: http://policyoptions.irpp.org/issues/environmental-faith/lysack/ (accessed 16 March 2016).

Marlow, H. (2008) 'The other prophet! The voice of Earth in the book of Amos', in N. Habel and P. Trudinger (eds) *Exploring Ecological Hermeneutics*, Atlanta: Society of Biblical Literature.

McKibben, B. (2005) *The Comforting Whirlwind: God, Job, and the scale of creation*, Cambridge: Cowley Publications.

McKibben, B. (2006) *The End of Nature*, New York: Random House Trade Paperbacks.

McKibben, B. (2013) *Oil and Honey*, New York: Henry Holt and Company.

Meinshausen, M., Meinshausen, N., Hare, W., Raper, S.C.B., Frieler, K., Knutti, R., Frame, D.J. and Allen, M.R. (2009) 'Greenhouse-gas emission targets for limiting global warming to 2°C', *Nature*, 458(7242): 1158–62.

Murray, R. (1992) *The Cosmic Covenant: biblical themes of justice, peace, and the integrity of creation*, London: Sheed & Ward Ltd.

Northcott, M. (1996) *The Environment and Christian Ethics*, Cambridge: Cambridge University Press.

Northcott, M. (2007) *A Moral Climate: the ethics of global warming*, Maryknoll: Orbis Books.

Ponting, C. (1988) *The Green History of the World*, London: Penguin.

Rasmussen, L. (1996) *Earth Community, Earth Ethics*, Maryknoll: Orbis Books.

37

The spiritual dimensions of ecosocial work in the context of global climate change

Fred H. Besthorn and Jon Hudson

Introduction

Global Climate Change (GCC) is the most significant and potentially disastrous natural occurrence to face the human species in the last 10,000 years. Its impact will be experienced by everyone, everywhere for generations to come. Indeed, GCC is the first true planetary emergency requiring a fundamental change in the way humanity comprehends its relationship with the natural world, as well as a change in the modern, economistic value system that has oppressed both human and non-human worlds. The challenges are daunting, but the opportunities are rich in texture and scope. Most interesting is the realisation that GCC is increasingly merging the interests of environmental as well as social, political and economic reform. The climate crisis has the potential to form the basis of 'a powerful mass movement, one that would weave ... a coherent narrative about how to protect humanity from the ravages of both a savagely unjust economic system and a destabilised climate system' (Klein 2014: 8). The question for social work is: what is our role?

This chapter will outline some of the salient features and consequences of Global Climate Change. It will look at the emergence of a relatively new arena of social work theory and practice – increasingly referred to as *ecosocialwork*. It will describe the spiritual dimensions of ecosocialwork and make some observations of how these might assist the profession in contributing to international efforts to understand and address the realities of GCC.

Global climate change: anthropogenic disruption in the anthropocene

The indiscriminate destruction of Earth's ecosystems has grown to such an extent in the last 100 years of the industrial era that human-induced climatic disruption now threatens not only the viability of natural systems but, perhaps, the very survival of the human species. The United Nations Intergovernmental Panel on Climate Change (2014) is unequivocal in its yearly synthesis report, saying that the human species is the single most pervasive cause of accelerated and worsening climate change. This human-caused interference with the global climate or, what many call, *Anthropogenic Climate Disruption* (ACD), has increasingly come to dominate the discourses of political parties, non-government organisations (NGOs), international governing bodies and citizens around the world. As the sobering message – that climate change is real, it is now and it is serious – ripples across the globe, it reiterates the overwhelming international scientific consensus that has existed for well over 30 years that global climate change exists, is human-caused and is already impacting large segments of the world (Davis 2015; Hadley Centre for Meteorological Research 2014; NASA 2015; New Zealand Climate Change Centre 2011; The Climate Institute 2014; US National Academy of Sciences and The Royal Society 2014). Indeed, many in the scientific community suggest that the planet has entered into a new, human-induced geological epoch – often referred to as the *Anthropocene* (Smythe 2014). In other words, this is the first time in the planet's three billion year evolution that human beings and their destructive activities have become the single most significant contributor to fundamental, and likely irreversible, changes in the Earth's biosphere. Without immediate and sustained attention, global climate change may likely become the catalyst for the extinction of the human species. While controversial, a growing number of reputable scholars in a wide variety of natural and social sciences are beginning to acknowledge, at least the possibility, that without immediate action, human beings may be unwittingly in the process of causing their ultimate extinction (Baker and McPherson 2014; Hannah 2011; Hartmann 2013; Jamieson 2014; Kolbert 2014).

Global climate change: rising temperatures, rising tides, rising tensions

The list of deeply troubling ecological and social disturbances associated with Global Climate Change (GCC) encompasses a long inventory of pressing concerns. Several of the most worrying are described as follows.

Temperatures

Average global temperatures are on the rise. Twelve of the last 13 years were among the 12 warmest years ever recorded in terms of average global surface temperature. Worldwide, 2015 is on track to be the hottest year in modern human history (Queally 2015). This is no periodic anomaly given that 2014 was the second hottest year ever recorded. 2013 and 2010 are tied for fourth in the hottest years on record, while 2005 and 2009 rank fifth and sixth respectively (O'Callaghan 2015).

The Intergovernmental Panel on Climate Change (2014) has repeatedly warned that average global temperatures will likely increase by up to 5°C in the next 100 years. Given the self-reinforcing and positive feedback loops associated with runaway greenhouse gas release, especially from the discharge of methane gas long sequestered in permafrost and deep sea beds, atmospheric scientists suggest that this unprecedented temperature rise could happen within the next 40–50 years if not sooner. The Earth's average temperature has already risen by almost 1°C since the beginning of the industrial revolution, much of which is attributed to human industrial activities within the last 60 years (Stronberg 2015). This rate of warming is much higher than that experienced in the past century and is without precedent in the last 10,000 years.

The current 1°C rise in average global temperature is already having a profound impact on climate in terms of the duration and severity of droughts, violent storms, heat waves, snow events, flooding and other erratic weather patterns. There is now mounting evidence that grain and other food crop output would be seriously threatened by rising temperatures, particularly if the global average were to reach 2.5°C above preindustrial levels. Recent research (New *et al.* 2011), published in conjunction with a large international climate conference sponsored by England's prestigious Tyndall Centre for Climate Change Research, strongly suggests that a 4°C rise in temperature is not outside the realm of possibility at the current rate of atmospheric carbon infusion coupled with increases of self-reinforcing positive feedback loops. This would lead to catastrophic social breakdown and is completely 'incompatible with any form of equitable and civilised global community' (Roberts 2011).

Tides

One of the most perilous consequences of Anthropogenic Climate Disruption is the rapid acceleration of risks to the world's oceans and fresh water supplies. Sea levels have been rising twice as fast over the past 10 years than at any time during the previous 100 (Gelspan 2005). At the current rate, global sea-level rises could increase by as much as six metres within the next 100 years, after having already risen by almost 30 centimetres in the past century. This anticipated rise would be enough to submerge major coastal and estuarial areas around the world and would put at risk nearly half a billion people (National Oceanic and Atmospheric Administration 2015). A sea level rise from one to two metres would be a final death blow to most low-lying island nations, already experiencing untold hardship as a result of current sea-level increases (Environmental News Service 2014).

The world's fresh water supplies are also in jeopardy. Only 3 per cent of the world's water is fresh and nearly 70 per cent of this is frozen in the ice of Greenland and the Polar Regions. As global temperatures rise, a steady infusion of fresh water is dumped into the world's ocean basins from melting ice shelves, sea ice and glaciers. Antarctic ice shelves have shrunk by over 40 per cent in just 10 years (Environmental News Service 2005).

Higher temperatures and the corresponding sea-level increases are directly attributable to rising levels of heat-trapping carbon dioxide in the atmosphere. An almost 50 per cent increase in carbon dioxide levels in just the past 150 years reflects an increase that could not occur by natural climatic fluctuation alone (Dunn and Flavin 2002).

Tensions

No serious observer questions that ACD will result in severe droughts, intense storms, heat waves, crop failures and an unremitting cascade of both predictable and yet unpredictable impacts on the world's biotic systems. However, the most immediate threat of global warming is the devastating impacts it has already begun to have on the social and political fabric of organised societies. These include the high probability for economic decline, food and water shortages, mass refugee flows, civil unrest, state collapse and armed conflict (Holthaus 2014). Combine the effects of climate change with already existing problems of global poverty, hunger, corrupt governance, religious/ethnic resentments and growing racial tensions, and the reality of vicious clashes over water, food, land and other survival necessities seems almost inevitable.

The current civil war in Syria and the massive wave of refugees is but one striking example (Femia and Werrell 2012). Climate disruption is implicated as a significant factor creating widespread drought and growing desertification of Syria's once productive agricultural interior (National Oceanic and Atmospheric Administration 2011). This climate-induced agricultural crisis forced millions of rural peoples into the country's urban areas, where long simmering hostilities coupled with overcrowding, unemployment and a general since of desperation lead to ethnic/religious factionalism, social unrest and, eventually, bitter conflict.

Syria's story will likely be repeated over and over again as poor and underdeveloped regions of the world, especially in Africa, Asia and the Middle East, find themselves less able to respond and adapt to new climate realities. Africa, for example, will undoubtedly suffer more than others. Estimates suggest that 75–250 million people will experience moderate to severe water stress as early as 2020 as a consequence of climate change (Intergovernmental Panel on Climate Change 2007). The decline in agricultural yields in this part of the world will also be significant. The consequences of years of record high temperatures, greater drought, greater evaporation and over-usage of freshwater reserves holds the high potential for increased incidents of armed violence. Mali, a country on the southern fringe of the Sahara, is just one of several examples of African countries caught in the chaotic and violent storm occasioned, in part, by precipitous climate change.

The emergence of ecosocialwork

Beginning in the late 1960s and early 1970s, social work began to slowly revitalise its long dormant commitment to analysis and critique of those larger structural/environmental barriers impinging upon individual wellbeing and social stability (Besthorn 2014). A more expansive and holistic kind of environmental metaphor emerged as a counterpoint to an earlier genera-tion of social workers absorbed in individualised and medicalised remedies for intractable social problems. This time, the professional discourse turned not to persons *or* environments but rather in recognition of both persons *and* environments – the interface of persons *in* their unique environmental contexts.

But, despite the rhetoric of persons nested *in* dynamic ecological interaction, the environ-mental construct continued to be narrowly interpreted as either social milieu or, if physical environment was addressed at all, as static background clutter. In the 1980s and 1990s, a small group of international social work scholars began pressing for an extension of the mid-twenti-eth-century version of environmental social work. For this new breed of environmental social worker, the profession's conventional interpretation of its environmental construct prevented it from critically engaging in the emerging discourse of deteriorating global ecosystems. They also asserted that social work could not fully realise its ethical commitments to social and economic justice and service to exploited and oppressed populations until the profession thoroughly con-sidered the inseparable link between human wellbeing and the wellbeing of the planet (Gutheil 1992; Hoff and McNutt 1994; Matsuoka and Kelly 1988; Matthies 1987; Resnick and Jaffee 1982; Soine 1987; Weick 1981).

More recently, a vocal group of international social work scholars from North America, Europe and Australia have begun to advocate for not only incorporating the natural environ-ment into the profession's theoretical formulations, but have been increasingly suggesting that concerns for the natural world must completely transform the way social work is conceived and practiced (Besthorn and Canda 2002; Coates 2003; Jones 2006; Dominelli 2012; West 2007). In many ways, this marked the beginning of a more radical, holistic and transformational ecological social work – simply referred as *ecosocialwork* or *ecosocial work*.

In the last 20 years, there has been a burgeoning of ecosocialwork scholarship on the interrelationship between the natural world and the theory and practice of social work. One ecosocialwork website catalogs nearly 350 conference papers, book chapters and journal articles contributed by social workers or printed in social work publications, between the 1970s and 2011, addressing a variety of topics related to the interface of the natural environment and the practice of social work (Global Alliance for a Deep Ecological Social Work, 2011) Since 2011, the corpus of ecosocialwork literature has continued to expand with an ever-increasing number of books, journal articles, special issues and dedicated conferences held at various loca-tions around the world (Alston and Whittenbury 2013; Besthorn 2014; Coates and Gray 2012; Dominelli, 2012; Gray *et al.* 2013; Hessle 2012; Kwan and Walsh 2015).

The spiritual contours of ecosocialwork

In general, ecosocialworkers are committed to incorporating a deeper, more holistic and trans-formative kind of ecological thinking into social work theory and practice (Besthorn 2014, 2015; Coates and Gray 2012; Dylan and Coates 2012). A review of the ecosocialwork literature suggests a considerable number of thematic areas ranging from supporting grassroots ecological activism, responding to climate disasters, attending to environmentally displaced persons and applying ecosocialwork principles to therapeutic interventions; to name just a few.

An important dimension for many ecosocialworkers is the prominence accorded the inter-relationship between spirituality and its critical role in informing the evolution of a deeper ecological consciousness. As has already been noted elsewhere in this volume, interest in the intersection of spirituality, religious, faith-based institutions and multiple forms of transpersonal experiences and practices have increasingly risen to a place of prominence in the last quarter century in the international social work arena. Similarly, spirituality has also begun to find resonance in this nascent field of ecosocialwork. Dylan and Coates (2012: 142) note that ecoso-cialworkers must understand the spiritual dimensions of the human condition in order 'to link and respond to the interrelated realities of environmental and social challenges'.

In broad relief, the spiritual contours of ecosocialwork are catalysed in the ideas that 1) all species, including the human species, share a common destiny with the Earth; 2) the intercon-nectedness and interdependence of all things is both biological and spiritual and, when properly understood, they help locate a non-anthropocentric place of humankind in the cosmic order of things; and 3) there is no inherent or necessary separation between humanity and nature nor between spirit and temporal – the sacred pervades both in a reciprocal, unending and ubiqui-tous cycle (Besthorn *et al.* 2010; Coates *et al.* 2006). In this regard, Besthorn (2002) notes that humans

> belong, from the very core of our physical bodies to the highest aspiration of our cogni-tive minds, to a constantly emerging cosmic/spiritual process. Humans emerge from, are dependent upon and shall return to an underlying energy or Divine presence pervading all reality. Nothing exists outside of this relationship cycle.
>
> (Besthorn 2002)

In a similar vein, Gray and Coates (2013) have suggested several core assumptions of ecosocial-work's emerging spiritual impulse. These include 1) a commitment to the idea of the Earth as sacred space and place; 2) the essential wholeness of the cosmic order; 3) the fact that everything is emergent – extending from the centre to the periphery of existence in reoccurring cycles; and 4) the interdependence of all things – nothing exists in or of itself, everything is dependent on everything else. Flowing from these is the importance of diversity and inclusivity – the wellbe-ing of Earth systems and humanity is reliant on a diverse and inclusive array of phenomena (biological, genetic, aesthetic, ecological, social, spiritual and historical) in humble engagement. Without diversity, life ceases to exist.

Gray and Coates (2013) also speak to the significance of the individual's co-developmental trajectory. That is, persons develop not as independent, isolated egos, but as individuals linked and embedded – never fully comprehendible except in terms of their nestedness in the com-munity of all beings. It is from the bio-spiritual milieu of our *beingness in the community of all beings* that we begin to transcend our limiting and egocentric worldviews and where creative and transformational action flow toward both the human and the biotic community.

Spiritual dimensions of ecosocialwork in the context of climate change

For those in the international social work community concerned with environmental problems, there is growing recognition that global climate change is fast becoming the defining issue of our time. A recent special edition of *International Social Work* (Drolet 2015) includes a number of important contributions seeking to help the profession better understand and respond to the serious realities of climate change. This adds to a number of previous social work scholarly contributions addressing dimensions of climate change (Alston 2013).

The spiritual dimensions of ecosocialwork can have an influence, in the context of climate change, in a number of different ways. From our perspective, there are several that seem most important – the *transcendence of resistance* and the *transformation of consciousness*. Spirituality can be helpful as people find, or, perhaps better, recover their ability to honestly perceive and to openly acknowledge the stark realities of climate change. Resistance to perceiving the realities of climate change can take many forms – from outright denial to a kind of passive avoidance that minimises the seriousness of climate troubles, while convincing oneself that it's somebody else's issue or someone else's job to do something about it.

This avoidance may also involve holding tightly to a magical hope that some new ecowarrior or some new geoengineering project will arise in the eleventh hour to save us from our collective predicament. Whether a byproduct of fear, grief, helplessness, political or ideological hubris, or some combination of these, many in modern, western societies, still seem paralysed by this personal and collective avoidance response. The future of ecosocialwork's engagement with global climate change issues depends, in part, on its skill in responding to this personal and collective resistance to thinking about and experiencing the overwhelming and seemingly implacable issues associated with global climate change.

Many ecosocialworkers are also convinced that until there is a significant transformation of human consciousness there can be no lasting alteration in the way humanity has come to understand its relationship with the natural world and no enduring action to address the escalating crises of climate. As with many Indigenous, Eastern and Western spiritual traditions, transformation is a key manifestation of the spiritual life and, at some level, spirituality is always about transformation. Indeed, in the absence of a transformational impulse, spirituality tends to become wooden, routinised and doctrinaire.

For many ecosocialworkers, spirituality is a necessary, if not a fully sufficient, condition for affecting personal and collective transformation (Dylan and Coates 2012). The transformational process is both a *transformation from* as well as a *transformation to*. First, it is about the transformation of human consciousness away from a modern Western worldview deeply entrenched in the social, political and ideological values of extraction, consumption, endless growth and incessant profit-making. From here, one finds an opening to an emergent eco-consciousness of connectedness and interdependence. And, from this inner transformation from the old to the new, consciousness flows an outer transformation in action – an active expression of peaceful and just action toward both human and non-human communities.

Conclusion

The United Nations Framework Convention on Climate Change (UNFCCC), the so-called Paris Agreement, issued a 31-page non-binding agreement on action plans to avert global climate disaster. The final wording of the COP21 accord, adopted on 12 December 2015, was endorsed by all 195 participating countries. It has brought renewed hope that the international community has developed a framework that has a chance to meaningfully address the problem of anthropogenic climate disruption.

Unfortunately, in the midst of an enhanced optimism, many critics have said that COP21 does not go far enough. Some point to the non-binding nature of its proposals and the fact that limiting average global temperature increase to 2°C is unrealistic – considering that even if global emissions were to be reduced to zero immediately, global temperature would still likely rise above the 2°C cutoff. In more strident tones, other critics suggest the COP21 accord cannot succeed because it does not address or challenge the underlying assumptions and values of the neo-liberal, capitalist economic system that has been indicted as largely responsible for the calamitous state of the global climate in the first place. They maintain that until global societies, particularly in the rich, Western world, transform their blind belief in the logic of triumphant capitalism, robust response to the climate crisis will never be powerful enough or, under current dire circumstances, fast enough to keep warming below cataclysmic levels.

Ecosocialworkers are convinced that the international social work community must play a larger role in addressing GCC. For many of us, the global climate change predicament is, at important levels, a crisis of spirit that requires a spiritually informed transformation of deeply embedded values, attitudes, beliefs and worldviews glorifying greed, selfish individualism and profit over any other form of collective social organisation and communal association. Change on the outside is never fully possible until there is transformation on the inside. The spiritual contours of ecosocialwork offer one small thread to a larger tapestry of global dissent, protest and lasting change in the context of Global Climate Change.

References

Alston, M. (2013) 'Environmental social work: accounting for gender in climate disasters', *Australian Social Work*, 66(1): 218–33.

Alston, M. and Whittenbury, K. (2013) *Research, Action and Policy: addressing the gendered impacts of climate change*, Sydney: Springer.

Baker, C. and McPherson, G. (2014) *Extinction Dialogs: how to live with death in mind*, Oakland, CA: Tayen Lane Publishers.

Besthorn, F.H. (2002) 'Expanding spiritual diversity in social work: perspectives on the greening of spirituality', *Currents: New Scholarship in the Human Services*, 1(1). Online. Available HTTP: www.ucalgary.ca/currents/files/currents/v1n1_besthorn.pdf (accessed 21 December 2015).

Besthorn, F.H. (2014) 'Ecopsychology meet ecosocialwork: what you might not know. A brief overview and reflective comment', *Journal of Ecopsychology*, 6(4): 199–206.

Besthorn, F.H. (2015) 'Ecological social work: shifting paradigms in environmental practice', in J. Wright (ed) *International Encyclopedia of Social and Behavioral Sciences*, vol. 6, Oxford: Elsevier Press.

Besthorn, F.H. and Canda, E. (2002) 'Revisioning environment: deep ecology for education and teaching in social work', *Journal of Teaching in Social Work*, 22(1–2): 79–102.

Besthorn, F.H., Wulff, D. and St. George, S. (2010) 'Eco-spiritual helping and postmodern therapy: a deeper ecological framework', *Journal of Ecopsychology*, 2(1): 23–32.

Coates, J. (2003). *Ecology and Social Work: toward a new paradigm*, Halifax: Fernwood.

Coates, J. and Gray, M. (2012) 'The environment and social work: an overview and introduction', *International Journal of Social Welfare*, 21(3): 230–8.

Coates, J., Gray, M. and Hetherington, T. (2006) 'An ecospiritual perspective: finally, a place for indigenous approaches', *The British Journal of Social Work*, 36(3): 381–99.

Davis, M. (2015) *Adaption Without Borders? Preparing for indirect climate change impacts*. Online. Available HTTP: www.sei-international.org/news-and-media/3009 (accessed 21 December 2015).

Dominelli, L. (2012). *Green Social Work: from environmental crises to environmental justice*, Malden, MA: Polity Press.

Drolet, J. (2015) 'Editorial', *International Social Work*, 58(3): 351–4.

Dunn, S. and Flavin, C. (2002) 'Moving the climate change agenda forward', in C. Flavin, H. French, G.

Gardner, S. Dunn, R. Engelman, B. Halweil, L. Mastny, A. McGinn, D. Nierenberg, M. Renner and L. Starke (eds) *State of the World 2002*, New York: W.W. Norton.

Dylan, A. and Coates, J. (2012) 'The spirituality of justice: bringing together the eco and the social', *Journal of Religion and Spirituality in Social Work*, 31(1–2): 128–49.

Environmental News Service (2014) *Climate Risk to Island States Focus of World Environment Day*. Online. Available HTTP: http://ens-newswire.com/2014/06/05/climate-risk-to-island-states-focus-of-world-environment-day/ (accessed 21 December 2015).

Fermia, F. and Werrell, C.E. (2012 *Syria: climate change, drought and social unrest*. Online. Available HTTP: https://climateandsecurity.files.wordpress.com/2012/04/syria-climate-change-drought-and-social-unrest_briefer-11.pdf (accessed 5 December 2016).

Gelspan, R. (2005) *Global Denial: Katrina is a portent*. Online. Available HTTP: www.questia.com/magazine/1G1-137403699/global-denial-katrina-is-a-portent-but-will-it-cause (accessed 21 December 2015).

Gray, M., Coates, J. and Hetherington, T. (2013) *Environmental Social Work*, London: Routledge.

Gutheil, I. (1992) 'Considering the physical environment: an essential component of good practice', *Social Work*, 37(5): 391–6.

Hadley Centre for Meteorological Research (2014) *Too Hot, Too Cold, Too Wet, Too Dry: drivers and impacts of seasonal weather in the UK*. Online. Available HTTP: www.metoffice.gov.uk/media/pdf/h/9/Drivers_and_impacts_of_seasonal_weather_in_the_UK_archive_CS01_Tagged.pdf (accessed 18 September 2015).

Hannah, L. (ed) (2011) *Saving a Million Species: extinction risk from climate change*, Washington, DC: Island Press.

Hartmann, T. (2013) *The Last Hours of Humanity: warming the world to extinction*, Cardiff, CA: Waterfront Digital Press.

Hessle, S. (2011) 'Editorial', *International Journal of Social Welfare*, 21(3): 229.

Hoff, M.D. and McNutt, J.G. (eds). (1994) *The Global Environmental Crisis: implications for social welfare and social work*, Brookfield, VT: Ashgate Publishing.

Holthaus, E. (2014) *New U.N. Report: climate change risks destabilizing human society*. Online. Available HTTP: www.slate.com/blogs/future_tense/2014/03/30/ipcc_2014_u_n_climate_change_report_warns_of_dire_consequences.html (accessed 21 December 2015).

Intergovernmental Panel on Climate Change (2007) *Climate Change 2007: synthesis report*. Online. Available HTTP: www.ipcc.ch/pdf/assessment-report/ar4/syr/ar4_syr.pdf (accessed 2 February 2015).

Intergovernmental Panel on Climate Change (2014) *Climate Change 2014: impacts, adaptation and vulnerability. Summary for policymakers*. Online. Available HTTP: www.ipcc.ch/pdf/assessment-report/ar5/wg2/ar5_wgII_spm_en.pdf (accessed 2 February 2015).

Jamieson, D. (2014) *Reason in a Dark Time: why the struggle against climate change failed and what it means for our future*, New York: Oxford University Press.

Jones, P. (2006) 'Considering the environment in social work education: transformations for eco-social justice', *Australian Journal of Adult Learning*, 46(3): 364–82.

Klein, N. (2014) *This Changes Everything*, New York: Simon and Schuster.

Kwan, C. and Walsh, C. (2015) 'Climate change adaptation in low-resource countries: insights gained from an eco-social work and feminist gerontological lens', *International Social Work*, 58(3): 385–400.

Kolbert, E. (2014) *The Sixth Extinction: an unnatural history*, New York: Picador Press.

Matsuoka, J. and Kelly, T. (1988) 'The environmental, economic, and social impacts of resort development and tourism on native Hawaiians', *Journal of Sociology and Social Welfare*, 15(4): 29–44.

Matthies, A. (1987) 'Ekologinen sosiaalityo' [Ecological social work], *Sosiaaliviesti*, 2(1), 32–7.

Närhi, K. (2004) *The Eco-social Approach in Social Work and the Challenges to the Expertise of Social Work*, Jyväskylä: University of Jyväskylä. Online. Available HTTP: https://jyx.jyu.fi/dspace/bitstream/handle/123456789/13326/9513918343.pdf?sequence=1 (accessed 21 December 2015).

New, M., Liverman, D., Betts, R., Anderson, K. and West, C. (eds) (2011) 'Four degrees and beyond: the potential for a global temperature increase of four degrees and its implications', *Philosophical Transactions of the Royal Society A*, 369(1934).

New Zealand Climate Change Centre (2011) *The Challenge of Limiting Warming to Two Degrees*. Online. Available HTTP: www.nzclimatechangecentre.org/sites/nzclimatechangecentre.org/files/images/research/NZCCC_Climate_Brief_1_%28November_2011%29%20V2.pdf (accessed 14 August 2015).

National Aeronautical and Space Administration [NASA] (2015) *Global Climate Change. Vital signs of the planet: How do we know?* Online. Available HTTP: http://climate.nasa.gov/evidence/ (accessed 25 January 2015).

National Oceanic and Atmospheric Administration (2011) *NOAA Study: human-caused climate change a major factor in more frequent Mediterranean droughts.* Online. Available HTTP: www.noaanews.noaa.gov/stories2011/20111027_drought.html (accessed 21 December 2015).

National Oceanic and Atmospheric Administration (2015) *State of the Climate Reports: global analysis September, 2015.* Online. Available HTTP: www.ncdc.noaa.gov/sotc/global/201509 (accessed 4 October 2015).

O'Callaghan, J. (2015) *It's Official: 2014 was the hottest year on record-and 10 of the warmest have been since 1998.* Online. Available HTTP: www.dailymail.co.uk/sciencetech/article-2901776/It-s-official-2014-hottest-year-record-10-warmest-1998.html (accessed 8 January 2015).

Queally, J. (2015) *Never Seen Anything Like This Before as 2015 Set to Be Hottest Year on Record.* Online. Available HTTP: www.commondreams.org/news/2015/10/22/never-seen-anything-2015-set-be-hottest-year-record (accessed 21 December 2015).

Resnick, H. and Jaffee, B. (1982) 'The physical environment and social welfare', *Social Casework*, 63(6): 354–62.

Roberts, D. (2011) *The Brutal Logic of Climate Change.* Online. Available HTTP: http://grist.org/climate-change/2011-12-05-the-brutal-logic-of-climate-change/ (accessed 21 December 2015).

Smythe, K. (2014) 'Rethinking humanity in the anthropocene: the long view of humans and nature', *Sustainability*, 7(3): 146–53.

Soine, L. (1987) 'Expanding the environment in social work: the case for including environmental hazards content', *Journal of Social Work Education*, 23(2): 40–6.

Stronberg, J. (2015) 'Greenhouse gas increases are leading to a faster rate of global warming', in L. Starke (ed) *Vital Signs: the trends that are shaping our future, vol. 22*, Washington, DC: Worldwatch Institute.

The Climate Institute (2014) *Climate Risks around Australia: what the latest report of the Intergovernmental Panel on Climate Change means for Australians.* Online. Available HTTP: www.climateinstitute.org.au/verve/_resources/TCI_MediaBrief_IPCC_March2014.pdf (accessed 4 June 2015).

US National Academy of Sciences and The Royal Society (2014) *Climate Change: evidence and causes.* Online. Available HTTP: http://dels.nas.edu/resources/static-assets/exec-office-other/climate-change-full.pdf (accessed 21 December 2015).

Weick, A. (1981) 'Reframing the person-in-environment perspective', *Social Work*, 26(2): 140–3.

West, D.S. (2007) 'Building a holistic environmental model for global social work', *International Journal of Interdisciplinary Social Sciences*, 2(4): 61–5.

38

Ultimate concerns and human rights

How can practice sensitive to spirituality and religion expand and sharpen social work capacity to challenge social injustice?

Fran Gale and Michael Dudley

Introduction

Spirituality and religion are among the very last human rights to be implemented in social work. However, there is a difference between a right in the Conventions and Codes of Ethics and grounding that right in social work praxis. Understood as a human right possessed by individuals, spirituality and religion are, nonetheless, increasingly esteemed as important aspects of culturally competent social work practice, i.e. that social workers are cognisant of diverse ethnic groups' religious affiliations and practice. Consequently, an intention to progress and deepen anti-oppressive and anti-racist practice is a key motivation for including spirituality and religion in social work literature and practice.

Social work is now facing unprecedented challenges in a post-secular (Habermas 2006), globalised world, where the impact of globalisation on those individuals, groups and communities who are most disadvantaged and vulnerable leaves social work to pick up the pieces (Dominelli 2010). This chapter argues that social work practice that is alive to spirituality and religion can construct a critical practice that expands its capacity to galvanise social justice. Spirituality and religion, through their potential to bring together 'situated' contextual knowledge of people's 'glocal' needs, ultimate concerns, oppression and forms of resistance, can be a significant catalyst in social work practice for inspiring and motivating social justice. Nevertheless, the claim that religion and spirituality can challenge oppression and disadvantage arising from social processes including globalisation remains at the level of the romantic unless the 'knowledge from the margins', which this chapter argues they can deliver, has a conduit for practice.

An established discourse in social work practice, human rights, offers an important conduit for the application of such 'glocalised' knowledge in progressing social justice. Human rights' key characteristics of universality (rights belong to everyone) and indivisibility (i.e. rights come as a package; no one right 'trumps' another) (Ife 2012: 10–11) enable it to address universalised, globalising discourses. At the same time, religion and spirituality as contextualised knowledge takes account of 'syncretic practice of cultures and religions and the ways in which people are located at the intersection of multiple axes' (Dhaliwal, 2012: 317), enabling 'glocal' differences to enrich the human rights frame. This concurrence can enliven social work to be powerfully instrumental in its contemporary practice context: that of a globalised, post-secular world.

Religion or spirituality: implications for social justice

Spirituality and/or religion are sculpted by a lens of history, cultures, life circumstances, society and power relations: they are significant for understanding intersectionality and accessing 'knowledge from the margins' (D'Amico 2007: 38). However, the way spirituality and religion are often constructed and addressed in social work literature and practice reveals itself as insufficient and problematic for critical social work. This next section of the chapter argues that a broader, more inclusive definition than that often used in social work literature is more consistent with a critical social work approach.

Much social work literature on spirituality and religion converges in emphasising 'spirituality'; distinguishing it from religion (Wong and Vinsky 2009). Spirituality is generally depicted as the search for ultimate meaning and purpose 'which is individualistic in nature' (Henery 2003: 1111); as a universal quality of human experience; 'transcending all historical, cultural and ideological discourses and practices' (Wong and Vinsky 2009: 1349) and sometimes as inclusive of 'many eras and traditions and containing elements common to all religions' (Wong and Vinsky 2009: 1346). Spirituality has been taken for granted as 'transcending ... religious beliefs' although able to be expressed within those beliefs (Wong and Vinsky 2009: 1345). Spirituality, however, supposedly transcends religion's limitations by severing its cultural, historical and ideological roots, and foregrounding fundamental values and precepts without negative associations or local, archaic or incomprehensible references (Mercadante 2014; Thomas 2006).

Religion on the other hand is seen as an institutional context for spiritual beliefs, customs, tradition, scripture and rituals (Wong and Vinsky 2009). In social work education and practice, religion is often constructed as a 'communal phenomenon' (Henery 2003: 1111). Yet the concept of 'religion' as stable and precise is a Western folk category (Fountain 2015); as in different traditions the intuitions that support fullness of life may vary (Hense 2014); and the global meaning and expression of 'religion' is diverse, dynamic and fluid (Hefferan 2015; Tomalin 2015).

When scrutinising social work texts, Henery finds, it is spirituality they urge should be incorporated in social work education and practice. Thus, spirituality becomes the 'favoured half of the [spirituality/religion] binary' in social work (Henery 2003: 1109). Elevating spirituality sets up a hierarchy in which spirituality is favoured and religion often assumed to be more conservative than spirituality. While acknowledging a focus on the spirituality half of the binary may be done with the intention of being inclusive, Wong and Vinsky have questioned:

> What ordering of social relations is produced in a discourse of spirituality that is dismissive of history and traditions and what is being asked of people of marginalised and racialized communities who must fight to have their traditions and histories recognised within the dominant culture?'
>
> (Wong and Vinsky 2009: 1155)

Accordingly, Henery warns that a spiritual/religion binary can mask and block recognition of significant social and political issues and thus 'complement rather than counteract dominant social arrangements' (Henery 2003: 1112). Consequently, elevating spirituality can undermine key elements of critical social work practice and what critical social work stands for. Drawing on Carrette and King (2004), Wong and Vinsky (2009) reveal the term 'spirituality' to be a Euro-Christian construct. Rather than being universal, spirituality is an historical construct, which embodies a specific ordering of social relations.

Thus, the apparent cultural inclusiveness the umbrella use of the term 'spirituality' in social work literature is generally intended to offer may actually provide, as Henery (2003) argues, a new expression of Western racism. For many peoples of diverse historical and cultural contexts, the history and tradition of their religious and spiritual experiences and practices are indivisibly grounded in the history of their community for which their religion and spirituality can be a source of support and a source of resistance. Religious and spiritual experiences, beliefs and concerns represent 'situated knowledge', 'knowledge from the margins', which can offer not only different ways of knowing, but different ways to challenge oppression and disadvantage. In their work advancing social justice and wellbeing of Pakeha, Māori and Pacific Island peoples, the Family Centre of New Zealand are explicit about integrating spirituality and religion, since spirituality and religion are relevant and significant in defining community and culture. Sole parents participating in research at the centre, for example, describe their spirituality and religion as co-existing in symbiotic relationship with their culture (Waldegrave *et al.* 2011).

Arguments against a 'spiritual/religion' binary are further reinforced from critiques of neo-liberalism and interrelated constructs of consumerism and individualism. This line of critique draws on Giddens' (1991) and Bauman's work (1997) on late modernity: 'Commodities for western spiritual consumers' is the way these critics describe how practices from historically rich and complex Indigenous traditions and Eastern religions are becoming separated from their roots and being commodified in the West into techniques and methods (Gray 2008; Wong and Vinsky 2009). Again, spirituality is frequently presented as consumerist, about individual self-expression and comprising personal experiences and sensations (Gray 2008; Henery 2003). Disengaged from deliberation about public goods, spirituality risks accommodating dominant culture and power relationships rather than being oppositional to them and to structural inequalities (Mercadante 2014).

Ethnic minorities, asserts Henery (2003: 1111), are 'generally characterized as first religious and only then spiritual', observing they are often placed in the disfavoured half of the spirituality/religion binary. Wong and Vinsky (2009) agree, observing that minority racialised groups are often represented as more religious than spiritual in social work literature. This binary resonates with what has been described as a revival of 'civilizational discourse' where cultures and religions are ordered in hierarchical fashion (Brown 2008). As part of this process, minority groups become stigmatised and 'contained'. Butler (2008: 14) critiques this process as a cultural assault on minorities.

While religion can be emancipatory or oppressive (e.g. it is sometimes perceived as operating against individuality, suppressing self-expression and placing people in positions of vulnerability to sexual, mental and/or physical abuse (Hennery 2003), spirituality can also be oppressive and/or emancipatory (D'Amico 2007: 8). Rather than avoid both, this recognition underscores the need for human rights-based practice, and including, as in any social work practice, a critique of power relations.

Crucially, this does not mean that spirituality and religion should not ever be separated as it can be important to do so, nor, as Wong and Vinsky (2009) hasten to point out, should moves to separate them always be seen as practices of neo-liberal individualism and Euro-Christian ethnocentrism. Rather, the argument is that 'the spiritual but not religious' position in social work should not be the dominant and defining discourse, and that it is essential for critical practice to 'remain … open to the experience of spirituality and/or religion' in the cultural, historical context as well as local circumstances in the lived experience of service users (Wong and Vinsky 2009: 1356).

This kind of framing of spirituality and religion follows Crisp's lead (Crisp 2010), avoiding prescription, yet brings together the varied discourses on spirituality and religion through framing discussion around understanding what spirituality and religion means in lived experience.

This, as Crisp points out, allows for shifts that may occur in the kinds of spiritual and religious issues that arise at different points in time for any one person, group or community as well as in different locations. For many, their religion and/or spirituality is sensitive to their social locations and can be influenced by factors including legacies of colonial relations; differentially racialised discourses and social treatment at a national state level and local cartographies of power including the multiple interactions within local urban spaces/neighbourhoods with national and trans-national networks and politics (Dhaliwal 2012). Such a multiplicity of influences articulate with each other to create a dynamic rich 'glocal' register (Dhaliwal 2012: 16–17), one expression of which coheres in spiritual and religious commitments and identifications registering a range of global and local concerns and needs.

Spirituality, religion and human rights discourse: an emancipatory conduit

Human rights discourse, now expanded beyond its original individual focus, incorporates collective realisation of rights (Twiss 2004). Strongly influenced by a theology of liberation, womanism, a black feminist perspective, for example, emphasises the right to health of people and their communities as the absence of oppression (Musgrave *et al.* 2002). Human rights, by their nature, Ife (2012) advocates, present a challenge to and combat oppression. Rights, such as the practice of spirituality and religion, understood at a social group level and collectively realised, can challenge those structures and discourses of oppression that position some groups as 'lesser' than others.

Children as a group, for example, are often seen as 'lesser' than adults, and because of this they frequently have their spirituality unacknowledged or denied. In social work with children, Crompton (2000) argues that supporting children's rights to spiritual wellbeing is not an optional extra, a fairy tale or a nuisance; rather it is about taking children seriously. Children's rights not being taken seriously also exemplifies the way genuine universalism has often been absent from customary understandings of human rights: in Ife's words, 'not everyone has been thought of as "human"' (Ife 2012:7); some are viewed as 'different' or 'lesser' than others.

While achievement of spiritual and religious rights can lead to greater social justice for disadvantaged social groups, at the same time, spirituality and religion can be powerfully instrumental in realising other human rights. Women in Morocco have successfully used Islamic scriptures to argue for and develop a new approach to poverty, which integrates rights to education, improved sanitation and housing (Sadiqi 2006). This is a significant example of where spirituality and religion brought about change: these rights are held by all people everywhere, but needed action to realise and exercise in practice. This action involved constructing spaces for discussion and debate in a public community context. Examples such as this underline the frequently intimate connection between rights and spiritual and religious traditions: as Ife affirms, 'concepts of human rights are embedded in all major religious traditions and can be found in many different cultural forms' (Ife 2012: 2). Given the diverse, dynamic nature of many religious traditions, religious communities have summoned and adjusted international human rights frameworks to local and national situations, or have invoked different parts of their religious traditions to further human rights (Peach 2000). Disenfranchised groups may work, in local contexts, to secure greater 'human rights' by reinterpreting religious or spiritual frameworks from within, in the interests of social justice (Tomalin 2015). In Egypt, for example, women used the Qur'an to argue against female genital mutilation, maintaining it is not an Islamic practice (Piecha 2016).

While spiritual and religious beliefs may provide an alternative reference point in affirming values of humanity, they may not alone be enough to bring about change (D'Amico 2007). They can, however, not only stimulate engagement with social issues but religious and spiritual discourses can construct frameworks for creating positive change (Dhaliwal 2012). Gandhi built the campaign against poverty and freedom from colonial rule, for example, on Hindu teachings of ahimsa (Mische 2007).

Locating spiritual and religion sensitive social work practice in a globalised, post-secular context

Globalisation definitions generally describe rapidly growing interconnections and interdependence 'such that the world is … becoming a single place' (Mittelman 2000: 5) through increasingly swift exchange of ideas, finances, resources and people (Gamble 2012). This is achieved via new information technologies enabling virtual dimensions, affiliations and communities as well as swift, accessible modes of transport that have 'collapsed time and space' (Dominelli 2010: 26). The nub for critical social work is that these conventional definitions of globalisation are silent about hierarchies of power (Mittelman 2000). Yet these power hierarchies present critical social work practice with unprecedented challenges.

Experienced at a 'grass roots level' the dominant form of globalisation, i.e. economic neo-liberalism, has led to a 'widening gap between rich and poor and deterioration of public social policy that neo-liberalism' (in the heightened integration of markets in the global economy) has brought and continues to bring about (Mittelman 2000: 4) as well as 'a loss in the degree of control exercised locally' (Mittelman 2000: 6). Explicit about the resulting range of consequences, Dominelli (2010: 26) specifies 'unemployment and reduced service provision' as well as 'widespread uneven economic growth, large scale migrations of people, spread of organised crime such as the arms and drug trade and human trafficking and increasing levels of poverty' that bring distress to individuals, groups and communities. This leaves social work involved, as previously noted, and as Dominelli (2010: 20) points out, in 'picking up the pieces'.

Resistance to these processes can come in the shape of some spiritual and religious groups taking extremist political and/or fundamentalist forms with closed communitarian characteristics, as they develop in 'an ever expanding ideological void, as alternatives, in large part to (global) market and consumer led neo-liberalism' (Dhaliwal 2012: 34). Racism and persecution of minorities including religious persecution and discrimination continue to be frequent reasons for claiming asylum internationally (Fox 2015; The Association of Religion Data Archives and Bar-Ilan University 2016). Social work, in response, can find itself more involved in work in communities to work against immersion 'in intolerance and exclusion' (Ife 2012: 20).

At the same time, spirituality and religion can and do act as progressive counterforces to problems associated with globalisation, providing an alternative reference point through affirming an ethics of care; a valuing of humanity and contesting the neo-liberal emphasis on profits. For example, at the inception of Citizens UK, a multi-faith organisation originating from Christian groups, social workers along with researchers and spiritual and religious leaders were funded by the Cadbury Trust to go on training programmes to build the group based on a democratic, multi-faith collaborative approach that also includes secular organisations. The group's aims are to mobilise local initiatives addressing issues reflecting local and global concerns such as welfare, drug problems, employment and housing scarcities (Jamoul and Wills 2008).

Globalisation has also amplified the 'post-secularisation' of society. Increasing spiritual and religious pluralism and new transnational spiritual and religious dynamics are linked, in large part, to large scale movements of people as well as other processes of globalisation (Thomas 2005). This increasing movement of peoples around the globe heightens the relevance of spirituality and religion in social work practice for all social workers (Martin and Martin 2003). Commitment to critical social work practice, Wong (2004) observes, involves commitment to diversity and difference and the many different ways of knowing: this is important in challenging the status quo. Fook (2012: 41) similarly argues that critical social work is open to new ways of 'seeing what knowledge is, how it is generated and expressed and whose perspectives count'.

Alternative ways of knowing can open up consideration of alternative ways of challenging oppression (D'Amico 2007). Post-secularity deconstructs and disrupts secularisation; it imagines the dynamic co-existence of spiritual, religious and secular viewpoints in dialogue (Habermas 2008; Stoeckl 2011). This is significant in post-secular globalised societies where the interfaces between state and civil society represent a dynamic zone where 'subjectivities, representation and claims making and are highly contested' (Dhaliwal 2012: 25). Religion and spirituality are central in systems of representation and different groups such as Sikhs, Muslims, Christians, Buddhists and Hindus are often differently racialised at national levels and within dominant discourses (Dhaliwal 2012).

The state's acknowledgement of the rights of minority communities to self-govern may, in some cases, allow structural racism and women's intra-communal oppressions to occur; for example, occurrences of gender- and honour-based violence and forced marriage in Britain (Patel 2013; Siddiqui 2014). Controversy has ignited around state accommodation of parallel religious laws, which some powerful religious leaders support and some women may effectively utilise, but many survivors and feminists oppose (Patel 2013; Siddiqui 2014). Feminist concerns, for example, may then get discarded on grounds of 'inauthenticity' or 'westernisation' (Dhaliwal 2012: 27). As Reichert (2011) points out, however, the defining of values and norms is often done by those in power.

Feminists such as Dhaliwal (2012), Patel (2013) and Siddiqui (2014) are wary of this trend in relations between the state and civil society where co-existence can be premised on crude systems of representation and where the position of community leaders can correspond with reification of particular norms and homogenisation of communities, and as a consequence state acknowledged religious and cultural practices can erase the combination of different religious, cultural beliefs and practices or lived reality. Homogenisation tendencies can be further reinforced by 'glocal' pressures on minority communities including pressures 'to assert themselves as alternatives to (global) market and consumer led neo-liberalism'. Such factors can impel 'religious communitarianists' to push for strong boundaries and sealed spaces of governance over which they exercise influence and control and become more or less self-managing units (Dhaliwal 2012). Observing that religious and spiritually-based organisations are increasingly 'acting as a buffer against the welfare state deficit' (Dhaliwal 2012: 320) as a result of neo-liberal policies and subsequent public funding cuts to welfare services, Dhaliwal (2012: 35) expresses concern that in the UK, for example, some fundamentalist 'closed' groups, in making 'religious incursions into social welfare provision' could have the effect of access to services becoming based on 'categorical religious affiliation' with real consequences for the ability of those that do not subscribe to their definitions to be able to access limited community based public services. Dhaliwal (2012: 29) concludes, 'It is vital that the range of differences within minority communities are not devalued and undermined by those forces that may promote absolutist, sealed identities'. Similarly, Blakey, Pearce and Chesters (2006) argue that there are many different minorities with conflicting interests and values, and it is important the membership of religious and spiritual groups and organisations also speak for themselves.

Social work practice has involvement in safeguarding the rights of minorities within minorities, for example, women's rights, LGBT peoples in communities that may be seen as 'absolutist' while also, at the same time, ensuring that specialist ethnic and culturally sensitive services and advocacy groups are preserved with equitable access to services. A human rights lens assists the move away from stereotyped, reified religious and spiritual groups' 'mono' identities. Ife and

Morley (2002) quote the Dalai Lama's (1993) comment, 'Rights assume basic human needs common to all humanity', observing how this understanding undermines hardened stereotypes, moving us away from 'perceptions of the 'other' that exist at national and international levels – while respecting and not denying difference (Ife and Morley 2002).

Undeniably, a majority of spiritual and religious organisations provide services not only for those who share their religious and spiritual traditions, but without proselytising, to all in need, whatever their beliefs. When the Sydney home of a local non-Muslim family was destroyed, for example, and the crisis accommodation offered by state-based welfare too limited, the Muslim Women's Association (MWA) in Australia provided the family with longer-term housing. The MWA and its Executive Director, a social worker, like a multitude of similar groups, see service provision as not based solely on religious and spiritual identity but, rather, that the fundamental basis for their service is need (Krayem and Moussa 2015).

Rather than simply 'pick up the pieces', how can social work initiate social justice inspired change?

Concern with disadvantage and injustice that affects day-to-day lives is integral to both beliefs and practices of many spiritualties and religions (D'Amico 2007). This cannot be reduced to a matter of simply filling in the gaps in the limitations of, for example, state-based welfare provisions, but rather is also about fostering alternative imagined futures, providing hope for achieving something different. As D'Amico explains, one step to dismantling oppression is to be able to envision alternatives (2007); alternatives that, in the context of globalisation, could make the productive potential of globalisation serve the goal of equity (Ife 2012).

Nancy Fraser's tripartite model of social justice proposes the fundamental question of social justice oriented interventions: 'is this going to promote participatory parity?' (Fraser 1996). Benhabib (2002) appeals for a dynamic discussion process between civil society and state institutions, and joins Fraser in calling for decisions affecting the wellbeing of a collectivity to be the outcome of a procedure of free and reasoned deliberation among all people concerned.

Responding to Reichert's (2006: 29) calls for social work to ask questions such as 'whose voices are being heard?' and 'how can all voices be heard?', social workers can initiate practices that support and enable the construction of cooperative spaces for active democratic participation from which all concerned can participate on an equal basis (Benhabib 2002). This is crucial, since potential limits of this approach include a tendency to assume 'the space is flat' and not recognise that 'local cartographies of power' may influence who participates in the debate (Dhaliwal 2012: 258). Such spaces need to offer the opportunity for genuine 'recognition' (Fraser 1996) and that all voices, those of minorities as well as those of minorities within minorities, are not muted but have engagement. Consequently, constructing spaces that afford maximum democratic participation and where debate can be guided by an ethics of care that encompass differences (Dhaliwal 2012) is essential for social justice inspired change.

Dhaliwal (2012: 322) observes that spirituality and religion along with 'secular humanism …' flow in the same direction as a commitment to … social justice, towards the collective improvement of people's lives'. Spiritual, religious and secular alliances exemplify Habermas' account registering the post-secular nature of our society, and describing the need to respond, in order to progress social justice, through constructing public space that enables parity of participation for all:

> The expression post-secular does more than give public recognition to religious fellowships in view of the fundamental contribution they make to the reproduction of motivations

and attitudes that are socially desirable. The public awareness of a post secular society also reflects the normative insight that has consequences for the political dealings of unbelieving citizens with believing citizens.

(Habermas 2006: 46)

Habermas goes on to point out that in post-secular society there is increasing consensus that 'modernisation of the public consciousness' involves assimilation and reflexive transformation of both religious and secular mentalities, observing that if all understand this as 'a complementary learning process', then they have reasons to take seriously each other's contributions in public debate (Habermas 2006: 46–7).

This is the context in which social work now practices, and social work has a major stake in both process and outcome.

Conclusion

This chapter has argued that social work engages with a social justice-inspired conception of spirituality and religion, and that this potential relationship with spirituality and religion can contribute to transformative social work practice.

Spirituality and religion do not constitute a unified coherent discourse. Yet as a source of people's desires and meaning-making, spirituality and religion share recurrent understandings of human dignity and solidarity with human rights. Like human rights, they are enduringly occupied with human flourishing and social justice. By incorporating knowledge that is 'grass-roots', 'glocal' (global and local) and 'from the margins', they inform and embrace humanity and critique globalisation's miseries. Retrieving people's ultimate concerns, they assist the transformation of traditional power relations. Moreover, in a post-secular world, with religion acknowledged as an organising principle in state governance and civil society, spirituality and religion exert major influence in the way governments respond and resources are invested. They share in a reflexive post-secular dialogue (Habermas 2008).

Spirituality and religion thus engage social work. Not only are they mandated, being fundamental to culturally sensitive social work practice, but they allow local and cultural differences to be acknowledged, thus fulfilling social work's brief of re-presenting people's 'situated' needs, oppressions, resistances and ultimate concerns and their claims to 'glocal' social justice. Spirituality and religion complement social work's diverse interests and practices, support its inevitably different construction in different locations (Ife 2012) and broaden its relevance to diverse groups outside dominant European and North American cultures.

Social work activities at different levels are characterised by rights (Ife 2012) and social work's inevitably different construction in different locations accommodates diverse interests and practices, thus benefitting the profession.

Human rights frameworks that act as a conduit for such contextual, 'situated' knowledges may tackle the injustices of oppression and disadvantage arising from globalisation, particularly dominant neo-liberal economic globalisation. Furthermore, a universal human rights framework that supports religious and spiritual expression affords opportunities for local and cultural differences to be expressed and heard. Such a human rights framework may provide an institutionalised channel for these local expressions of spiritualities, which in turn can inform the application of human rights principles.

Social work practice exemplifies the potential applications of these processes of discovery. Being informed by universal human rights conceptions and discourses, it explores and anchors these in local contexts, cultures and communities (Ife 2012), and in so doing, it may also avail itself of religious and spiritual, situated, 'glocal' knowledge. Thus allied with the quest for genuine recognition, representation and re-distribution that is central to achieving social justice (Fraser 1996), social work may construct itself a more locally and globally relevant transformative role, that is powerfully instrumental in its contemporary context, practising in a globalised, post-secular world.

References

Bauman, Z. (1997) *Post Modernity and Its Discontents*, Oxford: Polity Press.
Benhabib, S. (2002) *The Claims of Culture: equality and diversity in the global era*, Princeton: Princeton University Press.
Blakey, H., Pearce, J. and Chesters, G. (2006) *Minorities Within Minorities: beneath the surface of community participation*, York: Joseph Rowntree Foundation. Online. Available HTTP: www.jrf.org.uk/report/minorities-within-minorities-beneath-surface-community-participation (accessed 4 July 2016).
Brown, W. (2008) *Regulating Aversion: tolerance in the age of identity and empire*, Princeton: Princeton University Press.
Butler, J. (2008) 'Sexual politics, torture and secular time', *The British Journal of Sociology*, 59(1): 1–23.
Carrette, J. and King, R. (2004) *Selling Spirituality: the silent takeover of religion*, New York: Routledge.
Crisp, B.R. (2010) *Spirituality and Social Work,* Farnham: Ashgate.
Crompton, M. (2000) *Who am I? Promoting children's spiritual wellbeing in everyday life: a guide for all who care for children.* Online. Available HTTP: www.barnardos.org.uk/resources (accessed 17 August 2016).
The XIV Dalai Lama Of Tibet (1993) 'Human rights and universal responsibility', presented at Non-governmental Organizations: The United Nations World Conference on Human Rights, 15 June 1993, Vienna, Austria. Online. Available HTTP: http://home.primusonline.com.au/peony/dalai_lama_statement.htm (accessed 18 August 2016).
D'Amico, M. (2007) 'Critical postmodern social work and spirituality'. Unpublished Master of Social Work thesis, RMIT University. Online. Available HTTP: http://researchbank.rmit.edu.au/eserv/rmit:6645/Damico.pdf (accessed 4 July 2016).
Dhaliwal, S. (2012) 'Religion, moral hegemony and local cartographies of power: feminist reflections on religion in local politics'. Unpublished Doctor of Philosophy Thesis, Goldsmiths, University of London. Online. Available HTTP: https://research.gold.ac.uk/7802/1/SOC_thesis_Dhaliwal_2011.pdf (accessed 13 July 2016).
Dominelli, L. (2010) *Social Work in a Globalizing World*, Cambridge: Polity.
Fook, J. (2012) *Social Work: a critical approach to practice*, 2nd edn, London: Sage.
Fountain, P. (2015) 'Proselytising development', in E. Tomalin (ed) *The Routledge Handbook of Religions and Global Development*, London: Routledge.
Fox, J. (2015) *Equal Opportunity Persecution*. Online. Available HTTP: www.foreignaffairs.com/articles/2015-08-31/equal-opportunity-oppression (accessed 1 February 2016).
Fraser, N. (1996) 'Social justice in the age of identity politics: redistribution, recognition, and participation', *Nancy Fraser: The Tanner Lectures on Human Values*, delivered at Stanford University 30 April 30–2 May 1996. Online. Available HTTP: http://tannerlectures.utah.edu/_documents/a-to-z/f/Fraser98.pdf (accessed 4 July 2016).
Gamble, D. (2012) 'Wellbeing in a globalized world: does social work know how to make it happen?' *Journal of Social Work Education*, 48(2): 669–89.
Giddens, A. (1991) *Modernity and Self Identity: self and society in the late modern age*, Cambridge: Polity Press.
Gray, M. (2008) 'Viewing spirituality in social work through the lens of contemporary social theory', *The British Journal of Social Work*, 38 (1): 175–96.
Habermas, J. (2006) 'Pre-political foundations of the democratic constitutional state?', in F. Schuller (ed) *Dialectics of Secularization: on reason and religion*, San Francisco: Ignatius Press.
Habermas, J. (2008) 'Notes on post-secular society', *New Perspectives Quarterly*, 25(4): 17–29.
Hefferan, T. (2015) 'Researching religions and development', in E. Tomalin (ed) *The Routledge Handbook of Religions and Global Development*, London: Routledge.
Henery, N. (2003) 'The reality of vision: contemporary theories of spirituality in social work', *The British Journal of Social Work*, 33(8): 1105–13.
Hense, E. (2014) 'Introduction: present-day spiritualities in confessional, popular, professional and aesthetic

contexts: contrasts or overlap?', in E. Hense, F. Jespers and P. Nissen (eds) *Present-Day Spiritualities: contrasts and overlaps*, Leiden: Brill.

Ife, J. (2012) *Human Rights and Social Work: towards rights-based practice*, 3rd edn, Cambridge: Cambridge University Press.

Ife, J. and Morley, L. (2002) 'Integrating local and global practice using a human rights framework', paper presented at the International Schools of Social Work [IASSW] Conference, Montpellier, July 2002.

Jamoul, L. and Wills, J. (2008) 'Faith in politics', *Urban Studies*, 45(10): 2035–56.

Krayem, M. and Moussa, I. (2015), Muslim Women's Association, Sydney, NSW, personal communication.

Martin, E. and Martin, J. (2003) *Spirituality and the Black Helping Tradition in Social Work*, Washington, DC: NASW Press.

Mercadante, L.A. (2014) *Belief Without Borders: inside the minds of the spiritual but not religious*, New York: Oxford University Press.

Mittelman, J.H. (2000) *The Globalization Syndrome: transformation and resistance*, Princeton: Princeton University Press.

Mische, P. (2007) 'The significance of religions for social justice and a culture of peace', *Journal of Religion, Conflict and Peace*, 1(1). Online. Available HTTP: www.religionconflictpeace.org/volume-1-issue-1-fall-2007/significance-religions-social-justice-and-culture-peace (accessed 4 July 2016).

Musgrave, F., Allen, E.C. and Allen, G.J. (2002) 'Spirituality and health for women of color', *American Journal of Public Health*, 92(4): 557–60.

Parekh, B. (2002) *Re-thinking Multi-culturalism: cultural diversity and political theory*, Cambridge: Harvard University Press.

Patel, P. (2013) *The Use and Abuse of Honour Based Violence in the UK*. Online. Available HTTP: www. opendemocracy.net/5050/pragna-patel/use-and-abuse-of-honour-based-violence-in-uk (accessed 13 July 2016).

Peach, L.J. (2000) 'Human rights, religion and (sexual) slavery', *Annual of the Society of Christian Ethics*, 20: 65–87.

Piecha, O.M. (2016) *Stop FGM: also in the Middle East*. Online. Available HTTP: http://en.wadi-online. de/index.php?option=com_content&view=article&id=1067:stop-fgm-also-in-the-middle-east&catid= 11:analyse&Itemid=108 (accessed 29 July 2016).

Reichert, E. (2006) 'Human rights: an examination of universalism and cultural relativism', *Journal of Comparative Social Welfare*, 22(1): 23–36.

Reichert, E. (2011) *Social Work and Human Rights: a foundation for policy and practice*, 2nd edn, New York: Columbia University Press.

Sadiqi, F. (2006) *Morocco's Veiled Feminists*. Online. Available HTTP: www.project-syndicate.org/commentary/morocco-s-veiled-feminists (accessed 2 February 2016).

Siddiqi, H. (2014) 'Violence against minority women: tackling domestic violence, forced marriage and honour-based violence.' Covering documents for Doctor of Philosophy thesis, University of Warwick, United Kingdom. Online. Available HTTP: http://wrap.warwick.ac.uk/64295/1/WRAP_THESIS_Siddiqui_2014.pdf (accessed 13 July 2016).

Stoeckl, K. (2011) 'Defining the post secular', paper presented at the seminar of Professor Khoruzhij, Academy of Sciences, Moscow, February 2011. Online. Available HTTP: http://synergia-isa.ru/wp-content/uploads/2012/02/stoeckl_en.pdf (accessed 15 February 2016).

The Association of Religion Data Archives and Bar-Ilan University (2016) *The Religion and State project*. Online. Available HTTP: www.religionandstate.org (accessed 1 February 2016).

Thomas, O. (2006) 'Spiritual but not religious: the influence of the current romantic movement', *Anglican Theological Review*, 88(3): 397–415.

Thomas, S.M. (2005) *The Global Resurgence of Religion and the Transformation of International Relations: the struggle for the soul of the twenty-first century*, Basingstoke: Palgrave Macmillan.

Tomalin, E. (2015) 'Introduction', in E. Tomalin (ed) *The Routledge Handbook of Religions and Global Development*, London: Routledge.

Twiss, S B (2004) 'History, human rights, and globalization', *Journal of Religious Ethics*, 32(1): 39–70.

Waldegrave, C., King, P., Maniapoto, M., Tamasese, T.K, Parsons, T.L. and Sullivan, G. (2011) *Resilience in Sole Parent Families: a qualitative study of relational resilience in Māori, Pacific and Pakeha sole parent families*. A Report by The Family Centre Social Policy Research Unit for The Foundation for Research Science and Technology Funded Resilience in Vulnerable Sole Parent Families Research Programme (Family Centre NZ). Online. Available HTTP: www.familycentre.org.nz/Publications/PDF's/Resilience%20Sole%20Parents%20Final%20Report%20MSD.pdf (accessed 13 July 2016).

Wong, Y.R. (2004) 'Knowing through discomfort: a mindfulness-based critical social work pedagogy', *Critical Social Work*, 4(1). Online. Available HTTP: www1.uwindsor.ca/criticalsocialwork/knowing-through-discomfort-a-mindfulness-based-critical-social-work-pedagogy (accessed 13 July 2016).

Wong, Y-L.R. and Vinsky, J. (2009) 'Speaking from the margins: a critical reflection on the "spiritual-but-not-religious" discourse in social work', *The British Journal of Social Work*, 39(7): 1343–59.

39

Addressing spiritual bypassing

Issues and guidelines for spiritually sensitive practice

Michael J. Sheridan

Introduction

The relationship between spirituality and social work has had a long history in the United States, with five broad phases as outlined by Canda and Furman (2010). Preceded by thousands of years of *Indigenous* ways of helping, the profession's *sectarian origins* at the turn of the twentieth century were based primarily on Judeo-Christian understandings of charity and communal service. A period of *professionalism and secularisation* emerged from the 1920s to the 1970s, during which secular humanistic and scientific understandings of the human condition were viewed as a more valid base for the profession. From 1980 to 1995, the profession witnessed a *resurgence of interest in spirituality,* which yielded tremendous growth in both knowledge dissemination and organisational efforts dedicated to promoting the integration of spirituality and social work while being firmly positioned within the profession's core values and ethics.

Canda and Furman (2010) propose that we are currently in a fifth phase, where all previous developments are coalescing and accelerating with a particular emphasis on *transcending boundaries* – whether these boundaries are religious, spiritual, disciplinary, or national in nature. They point to similar developmental stages regarding spirituality and social work in other countries, but hasten to point out that specific Indigenous, sectarian, secular and socio-cultural influences and histories have created unique trajectories within each nation. For example, other world religions such as Buddhism, Confucianism, Islam, Shamanism and Daoism; post-colonial responses to the suppression of Indigenous spiritual teachings; and non-sectarian perspectives, such as humanism, deep ecology and transpersonalism, have all had varying impacts on the profession in different regions of the globe (Canda 2009).

While it is apparent that the topic of spirituality is achieving legitimacy in varying degrees within the profession worldwide, this accomplishment has generally occurred by highlighting its relevance and positive role in clients' lives. Over the past 20 years, the social work literature has exploded with both conceptual articles and empirical studies on integrating spirituality within fields of practice (Canda 2009). The evolution of this knowledge base has been vital for the on-going development of effective and ethical spiritually sensitive practice.

However, it is important to recognise what Pargament (2007) observed in his book on spiritually integrated psychotherapy: spirituality can be a source of problems as well as solutions. This chapter explores a particular aspect of this critical observation known as *spiritual bypassing*.

Defining spiritual bypassing

The term *spiritual bypassing* was first coined by John Welwood (1984) to describe avoidance (or 'bypassing') of psychological work by focusing solely on the spiritual. This bypassed work may include issues at the physical, cognitive, emotional, or interpersonal levels (Cashwell *et al.* 2007) and often involves unfinished developmental tasks (Welwood 2000). Spiritual bypassing is also referred to as *premature transcendence* (Harris 1994; Welwood 2000), as it represents an attempt to rise above the complex and often messy nature of being human. It occurs when 'spiritual' concerns are elevated, while 'human' issues are deemed unimportant, often resulting in neglect of significant aspects of daily life.

Masters (2010) describes spiritual bypassing as a kind of spiritual tranquiliser that results in avoidance of the problem at hand. He further points out that our current day societies don't provide much guidance for facing painful realities at either the individual or collective level: 'spiritual bypassing fits almost seamlessly into our collective habit of turning away from what is painful, as a kind of higher analgesic with seemingly minimal side effects' (2010: 1). Indeed, many of our modern solutions to problems seem to be about numbing pain rather than confronting it, whether through pharmaceuticals, denial, or distractions of all kinds, including spiritually related activities.

Spiritual bypassing is indeed harmful for both psychosocial development and spiritual growth (Welwood 2000). From a psychological perspective, such bypassing cuts off the opportunity to address and resolve important intra- and interpersonal issues. Although initially used to compensate for various challenges, such as low self-esteem, depression, anxiety, or dependency issues, bypassing creates new problems as the person attempts to live out a spiritual persona that is not grounded in reality. For example, someone may try to avoid fears of intimacy by practicing detachment and renunciation in search of higher spiritual goals. Rather than addressing underlying relational wounds, the person is simply borrowing the cloak of spiritual truths to feel less vulnerable in human relationships.

Concurrently, spiritual bypassing also produces impediments to authentic spiritual growth. First, it truncates the process of spiritual development by trying to jump over key stages to a higher plane, leaving development incomplete (Masters, 2010). Strikingly described by Clarke *et al.* (2013: 88), 'clients in spiritual bypass are figuratively trying to stand on the top rung of a ladder with broken, incomplete, and unstable lower rungs'. This often occurs when spiritual beliefs and practices are used in the service of denial or defence against real-life human issues. As a result, spirituality becomes compartmentalised and remains un-integrated within overall functioning (Welwood 2000). Second, spiritual bypassing can also lead to an unbalanced spirituality where one aspect of a polarity is favoured over others: 'Absolute truth is favoured over relative truth, the impersonal over the personal, emptiness over form, transcendence over embodiment, and detachment over feeling' (Welwood 2011: 1). The result is 'an ungrounded, partial, and lopsided version of spiritual awareness' (Caplan 2009: 122). Thus, contrary to the intended outcome, spiritual bypassing can derail or even undo strides that have been achieved as a result of deeply committed spiritual practice.

Eight faces of spiritual bypassing

Spiritually sensitive social work facilitates healing and growth within a holistic and integrated approach (Canda and Furman 2010). This approach often requires direct, yet sensitive exploration of spiritual bypassing in its various guises in order to support overall healthy development and functioning. The following provides descriptions of eight manifestations of spiritual bypassing.

Quest for perfection or compulsive goodness

One 'face' of spiritual bypassing is a striving for perfection or unrealistic goodness. All religious and spiritual traditions point to virtues that followers strive to develop within themselves (e.g. the mercy of Jesus Christ, the compassion of the Buddha, the integrity and sincerity of the Prophet Muhammad). While providing important models for life, turning spiritual ideals into rigid prescriptions can be an indicator of spiritual bypassing. Welwood (2011) refers to this as 'the spiritual superego' – a harsh inner voice telling the individual how they should always think, speak or feel and what they should always (or never) do. Welwood explains that when the singular goal of spiritual practice is to 'be good', it is being used as a defence against an underlying sense of deficiency or unworthiness and represents a kind of inner violence. That which is not seen as part of the ideal is deemed unacceptable and relegated, in Jungian terms, to the 'Shadow' (Cashwell *et al.* 2004). A false spiritual persona is shown to the world, while the true self is denied (Caplan, 2009).

Avoidance/repression of undesirable or painful thoughts/emotions

Closely related to striving for perfection and goodness is the second face of spiritual bypassing: avoidance or repression of difficult or unwanted thoughts and emotions (Cashwell *et al.* 2004; Masters 2010; Welwood 2000). When these don't align with the spiritual persona that is being cultivated, they are not acknowledged or allowed to exist. Compassion, forgiveness and generosity are allowed; anger, jealousy and fear are denied. When this splitting of 'good' and 'bad' cognitions or affects occur, the person loses the opportunity to use them for work on developmental tasks, unresolved emotional issues, or guides to deeper truths (Welwood 2011). Unacknowledged thoughts and emotions cannot be worked through, leading most often to unconscious, reactive behaviour versus mindful, constructive responses to life.

Fear of individuation and avoidance of responsibility/accountability

Individuation, or the process of becoming a differentiated human being with one's own beliefs and ideals separate from those of parents and society, is required for both personal development and spiritual growth (Welwood 2000). When spiritual practices or beliefs are used to avoid the fear of becoming one's own person and sidestep responsibility or accountability for one's actions, it represents a bypassing of important developmental tasks. This is different than turning to prayer, contemplation, or spiritual advice as a positive use of spirituality. Rather, it is an abdicating of one's role in decision-making and discounting the necessary collaborative nature of relationship with a divine source. As one Alcoholics Anonymous slogan reminds us, 'It's fine to pray to God for potatoes, but you also need to get out a hoe'. This kind of spiritual bypassing can also lead to what Caplan (2009) calls *mutual complicity*, a kind of spiritual co-dependence with religious leaders or spiritual teachers that relieves us from taking responsibility for our own lives.

Fear of intimacy, closeness, vulnerability

The fourth manifestation of spiritual bypassing focuses on avoiding challenges or difficulties in relationships. Welwood (2000, 2011) states that this is because most of our unresolved psychological wounds are relational and generally initially formed through our relationships with early caregivers. A basic human need is to be loved and to know that we are lovable. When we experience inadequate or harmful love as a child, our ability to value our self and others is damaged – what Welwood calls a 'relational wound' or 'wound of the heart' (2011: 2). Misappropriation of spiritual teachings is used during spiritual bypassing to avoid dealing with this wound or feeling the pain of it. Sometimes there is flight into spiritualised detachment, protecting the person from the openness and vulnerability that real intimacy requires. Other times there is a rush toward fusion, or spiritualised communion, in order to deny the separateness and differences that are an inherent part of any relationship. Although seemingly different when viewed from the outside, both strategies are an attempt to provide a buffer against additional relational wounding while parading as a spiritual virtue or experience. And both serve to circumvent the personal work on capacities needed for healthy relationships (e.g. maintaining appropriate boundaries, negotiating closeness and distance, honest communicating of needs and wants).

Spiritual obsession/addiction

The fifth face of spiritual bypassing can be described as obsession or addiction to spiritual pursuits as a way to avoid facing the challenges of everyday life (Cashwell *et al.* 2007). The behaviours displayed by this type of bypassing are many. It may be constant engagement with religious or spiritual books, tapes or videos; essentially spending one's life in conceptual or virtual space while seldom emerging into real life. It may involve constantly chasing a spiritual high from one spiritual workshop or talk to the next while failing to integrate learning into new perspectives and behaviour. Or it might include continually ramping up spiritual practices as if training for a marathon while ignoring responsibilities in other areas of life. Rather than engaging in spiritually-based behaviours to advance understanding and spiritual growth, these kinds of activities are used as a way out of facing uncomfortable realities or engaging in difficult change. As with all addictions, spiritual bypassing activities are used to self-medicate versus working through issues.

Blind faith in charismatic leaders/teachers

The sixth form of spiritual bypassing is perhaps the best known, as we are generally aware of stories where followers have been deceived and harmed by unscrupulous charismatic leaders or teachers (Caplan 2009). Welwood (2000) points out that sometimes followers with unresolved family issues will project onto spiritual teachers the qualities they wished their own parents had possessed. In such cases, there is the attempt to heal earlier wounds or trauma through winning the approval or love of the spiritual leader. Spiritual bypassing in these instances abdicates the believer's responsibility for reflection and discernment of both the teachings and the teacher. In the worst-case scenario, a tragedy occurs, like that of Jonestown and cult leader, Jim Jones, where hundreds of people lost their lives in a mass murder–suicide. At the very least, this form of spiritual bypassing stunts psychosocial development and hinders authentic spiritual growth.

Spiritual narcissism or ego inflation

Using spiritual practices or beliefs to elevate oneself, especially in comparison to others, is a type of spiritual bypassing known as spiritual narcissism or ego inflation. It is perhaps best described as a kind of 'I'm enlightened [or saved] and you're not' syndrome (Cashwell *et al.* 2010: 163). This ego-centred spiritual elitism is an attempt to shore up a shaky sense of self (Welwood 2000). While displaying a façade of high religious or spiritual attainment, the internal reality is often a fear-based sense of inadequacy or unworthiness. As with other forms of spiritual bypassing, there are negative consequences to the person due to avoidance of necessary work in other areas. But this face of spiritual bypassing is also particularly dangerous to others in the orbit of the person engaged in the bypassing. Spiritual narcissism and ego inflation is often one of the major dynamics at play when clergy or spiritual teachers violate their sacred authority and engage in physical, sexual and psychological abuse or coercion of their parishioners or followers (Caplan, 2009). In these cases, the unaddressed wound of the religious or spiritual leader leads to the egregious wounding of others.

Flight into humanitarian causes

One of the hallmarks of mature religious faith or spirituality is attention to the suffering of humankind and other beings (Fowler 1981). But commitments of this kind can also be used to avoid personal challenges and situations as well as enhance the wellbeing of others. Flight into humanitarian causes, the final face of spiritual bypassing, can be difficult to discern because by its very nature it appears to be highly virtuous (Welwood 2000). This can occur on a relatively small stage, as the woman who takes care of everyone else in the neighbourhood to avoid facing her own unmet needs. Or it can operate within a much larger sphere, as with the social justice leader who mounts heroic actions against injustice affecting thousands, while ignoring the plight of his own children. Similar to the other seven forms of spiritual bypassing, the dividing line between healthy and unhealthy use of spirituality here is more about the underlying function and consequences of the avoidant behaviour than the particular action itself.

Case examples

The following composite cases are offered here for the purpose of illustrating the various faces of spiritual bypassing described previously. As composite cases, the names and identifying information do not represent any one particular individual.

The Dutiful Daughter

Helen was the oldest of three children born to a Methodist minister, Thomas, and his schoolteacher wife, Sarah. Both parents emphasised devotion to God and excellence in education. Helen strived for perfection in both areas and was generally rewarded for her efforts both within and outside of the family. She was often praised for giving help to others, from caring for her mother during her migraine headaches, to keeping her younger siblings quiet while her father prepared his sermons, to helping her teachers during Sunday school. Teachers, neighbours and members of the church all remarked on what a good and dutiful daughter she was, sometimes saying 'she was too good to be real'.

While the external picture of the family was one of harmony and happiness, the internal, day-to-day reality was quite different. Sarah had initially been drawn to Thomas because of his clarity about how to live a good, Christian life. But early in their marriage, she found herself chafing at Thomas's insistence that he knew what was best about everything – from handling finances to raising children to managing their marital relationship. After a brief period when she fought to have her own views and needs heard, Sarah acquiesced to her husband's dictates, given that he was 'a man of God'. She eventually withdrew from genuine interaction and intimacy with Thomas, often citing the need to recover from her frequent headaches. By the time Helen was three, her parents marriage was one of strained co-existence, covering up a myriad of intense emotions and disappointments. She learned to bring home 'blue ribbons' (e.g. gold stars on school papers, perfectly memorised Biblical passages) in an attempt to make her parents happy and alleviate the sadness and unease that was the underlying climate of the household. She also learned to tamp down any thoughts, emotions, or behaviours that did not fit the image of a good and dutiful daughter.

Helen's childhood survival strategies of hyper-vigilance, people-pleasing and denial of her own self were carried into her own marriage and family, as she, too, worked to create a home life that was well-ordered and guided by religious tenets. She concentrated on taking care of the needs of others and continued to deny or push away thoughts and emotions that did not align with her picture of herself as a good wife and mother. This self-view was threatened, however, when she learned that her husband was having an affair. Unable to handle the intense feelings of betrayal and anger she felt toward both her husband and God, Helen turned to her minister for guidance. As her husband had ended the affair and was pleading for forgiveness, this religious leader instructed her to pray for the ability to forgive and focus on mending her marriage. Although she diligently tried to follow this advice, and told her husband that she forgave him, she was deeply troubled by vindictive thoughts and feelings of rage that she could not seem to dispel, chiding herself that if she were 'a better servant of God' she would not be having these reactions. She eventually found relief by busily engaging in church activities, which took up more and more of her time. As time went on, she found herself estranged from her husband, emotionally detached from her children and plagued with physical problems – repeating the same dynamics of her family-of-origin.

Helen's story illustrates several faces of spiritual bypassing. Although her early experiences with religion provided structure, security and clear guidance for living, her parents' inability to deal with their own or their children's emotional needs contributed to Helen's development of a false spiritual self, or the tendency to act as one imagines a spiritual person would (Caplan 2009). Helen's efforts at being the perfect daughter reflect the first type of spiritual bypassing, the *quest for perfection and compulsive goodness*. She cultivated this persona in order to cover up other unwanted aspects of herself. This persona was supported by her *avoidance and repression of undesirable or painful emotions*, the second face of spiritual bypassing. When she could not deny the intense feelings she had as a result of her husband's affair, it created much suffering for Helen, which led to engagement in another aspect of spiritual bypassing: *fear of intimacy, closeness and vulnerability*. Really confronting her feelings about the affair would have required Helen to be open and honest with herself and her husband about its impact. Additionally, Helen's increasing busyness in church activities as an avoidant coping strategy reflects a fourth face of spiritual bypassing: *fear of individuation and avoidance of responsibility/accountability*. Rather than do the hard work of discerning what she really thought and felt about the affair and what she truly wanted in her marriage, these activities served as a distraction and way to avoid this work. With the support of a spiritually sensitive social worker, helping her face these challenges while respecting her faith, Helen may have come to a deeper understanding and perhaps a more solid commitment to both her marriage and her religion. Unfortunately, the guidance from her minister unwittingly diverted her from the spiritual and psychological growth that may have resulted from a more holistic approach.

The Ceaseless Seeker

Marcus grew up the only child of a mother, Louise, who struggled with depression and abuse of prescribed medications. When his father left when Marcus was two years old, he became his mother's sole confidant and reason for living. When his mother was in a good emotional space, they had many great times together, but when she was in a depressed state, life was very difficult. She would alternately demand attention from Marcus and then order him to leave her alone, leaving the boy confused and fearful. When Louise was high on medication, she could be very expansive and flattering of Marcus, telling him he was the most wonderful son in the world. During times when she abstained from taking pills, she became harshly critical, telling him that he was no good and would never amount to anything. His own sense of wellbeing ricocheted between glorious highs and despairing lows, all dependent on how his mother was treating him. He learned to wear a mask with her, closely reading her cues as to what his responses should be at any given moment.

Early on, Marcus found respite in books, walks in nearby woods and drawing in scores of notepads he kept hidden under his bed. He was drawn to tales of heroic adventures and other worlds, picturing himself as the lone voyager overcoming evildoers and harsh surroundings. By adolescence he found books on spiritual journeys and mysticism, which bolstered his sense that there was more to life than what the world was telling him. He eventually found one friend, Darius, who shared his passion for the mystical, with whom he spent many hours in deep conversation and debate. He felt these interactions were the only times he felt 'real' and felt truly lost when Darius and his family moved away.

Marcus eventually left for college and really enjoyed his courses in philosophy and religious studies. He tried to make new friends, but he found interacting with others his age difficult. His peers seemed superficial and frivolous, and he couldn't seem to connect with girls that caught his interest. In his sophomore year, he decided that the conventional path of college and career was not for him and he began his spiritual search in earnest. Drawn to Buddhism, Marcus spent the next several years exploring various paths in this tradition and developing a set of daily spiritual practices. He frequently changed course, however, as various teachers failed to yield what he was looking for. After many attempts to find the right path, he finally found a teacher that seemed to hold the key to what he was seeking. This teacher required celibacy and detachment from worldly pursuits, which Marcus agreed to readily. He vowed to turn his life over to supporting this teacher and his teachings. He became a trusted confidant and was given more and more responsibilities for the spiritual community. Marcus felt that he had found his true home at last.

This peace was challenged whenever Marcus had contact with his mother, who had many health issues and was imploring him to come home and take care of her. At times, he felt guilty for what he thought was a lack of compassion for his mother, but told himself he had a higher calling. He finally cut off all ties with his mother with the support of his teacher. Marcus decided that his life purpose was to help lead others to enlightenment and that attachment to any one person was a renunciation of this purpose. He ignored whispers and concerns about his teacher's harsh treatment and financial demands of devotees and chose to believe that those who were critical must be at a lower level of spiritual development than he was. Whenever doubts about his teacher arose, he increased his spiritual practices.

Marcus's story reveals aspects of the same faces of spiritual bypassing that is evident in Helen's story, including attempts at perfection; avoidance of painful thoughts and emotions; apprehensions about engaging in real human intimacy; and fears of individuation and personal responsibility. But his narrative also contains elements of other manifestations of bypassing, as well. The solace that his early spiritual leanings provided for Marcus as a child became *spiritual obsession and addiction* later in his life. Rather than supporting his life purpose, his spiritual seeking became a substitute for living. We also see elements of *blind faith in charismatic leaders/teachers* as Marcus eschewed undertaking a discerning look at his teacher's behaviour and avoided determining his own core values and framework for living. There are also features of *spiritual narcissism or ego inflation* in Marcus's reaction to others' concerns about his teacher's shortcomings. By holding himself as more 'spiritually evolved' than others, he was able to feel special and important while repressing feelings of inadequacy or unworthiness – as well as deny uncomfortable truths about his teacher. Finally, while his goal of assisting others on their spiritual path was a virtuous one, it could be viewed as a *flight into humanitarian causes*. By focusing on the development of others, he was able to circumvent taking full responsibility for his own growth. It is unlikely that Marcus would seek professional help unless some facet of his carefully constructed life shatters, but if and when he does, a spiritually sensitive social worker could help him face the realities of his past and current circumstances while supporting a fuller and more balanced integration of spiritual principles and practices into his daily life.

Preliminary guidelines for addressing spiritual bypassing

Both of the cases described highlight the need to address the negative as well as positive use of spirituality in clients' lives. A review of 26 studies of social workers suggests that practitioners struggle with this area: 'in terms of assessing clients' particular support systems, beliefs, and/or practices, social workers appear to be more comfortable helping clients consider how these are *helpful* rather than *harmful*' (Sheridan 2009: 118). Although this discomfort is understandable, social workers must not turn away from their responsibility to address these issues as part of ethical practice. Being a spiritually sensitive social worker does not mean ignoring the potential negative or harmful aspects of spirituality. We must determine how to address such issues while affirming the relevance and positive role of spirituality in clients' lives. The following three practice principles are offered as possible guidelines for how we can begin to meet this challenge.

Understand the role of spirituality in clients' lives

Acknowledgement of the relevance of spirituality in clients' lives is central to spiritually sensitive social work. In the context of addressing spiritual bypassing, it reminds the practitioner to be mindful of the multi-faceted function of spirituality in clients' lives – to remember and honour the positive even while exploring the negative. For example, if a caregiver of an elderly parent uses their faith to provide meaning and positive coping strategies in their caregiving situation, it would be a mistake to dismiss these important functions and focus only on the use of spirituality to avoid painful feelings. Likewise, it would also be detrimental to the client to sidestep explora-tion of this type of spiritual bypassing. The practitioner should find ways to support the positive functions while broaching the negative aspects with sensitivity and respect, which may require careful timing. It would be undoubtedly unhelpful to address the bypassing of difficult emotions at a particularly intense period of caregiving when the client is relying on spirituality to maintain functioning. Instead, the practitioner can address this issue at a later point or when the client provides an opening for discussion of this area. Keeping issues of timing in mind, a truly holistic approach to practice means addressing both helpful and harmful aspects.

Be aware of possible bias in determining spiritual bypassing

Continually reflecting on one's own bias is an essential element of spiritually sensitive practice. In the area of spiritual bypassing, it requires the practitioner to discern whether identifying a particular belief or practice as 'bypassing' is taking into account the cultural context of the client or whether it is based on their own bias. For example, repeating a particular prayer several times a day could be seen as an avoidant strategy if the practitioner had a negative or uninformed view about this spiritual practice. In assessing whether an activity is reflective of spiritual bypassing or not, the practitioner must consider the effects of the activity versus their own unfamiliarity or discomfort with the practice. Is it allowing the person to function within the rest of their life or is it getting in the way of functioning? Is it helping them face a particular situation or is it helping them avoid it? Awareness of potential bias is particularly important when working with clients who have a different cultural or national background than the practitioner. Consultation with others, including religious or spiritual leaders, who are grounded in the client's lived experience is warranted in instances where the practitioner lacks relevant knowledge.

Upholding the value of self-determination

Self-determination is a core value of social work practice that often presents challenges to practitioners. When addressing spiritual bypassing, the task is the same as in any circumstance when a social worker needs to uphold the right of clients to make their own choices even when that choice may not seem optimal in the eyes of the practitioner. For example, a practitioner may view a client's decision to join a religious group or follow a spiritual teacher as evidence of a type of spiritual bypassing known as 'blind faith' or 'avoiding personal responsibility'. In this situation, the practitioner may wish to adamantly point out that this is an unwise decision. Conversely, it may be tempting to avoid discussion with the client even though the practitioner is concerned about it. Upholding the value of self-determination while addressing the possibility of spiritual bypassing requires a mid-way response; one that involves exploration of the practitioner's concerns while ultimately affirming the client's right to make life decisions. Of course, determination of harm to self or others must be part of the practitioner's deliberation here as it would be in any other practice situation.

In closing, it should be noted that the majority of social workers report they receive little or no instruction on any aspect of spirituality and practice within their educational programmes (Sheridan 2009). It is hoped that this chapter will spur discussion and dialogue about the need to include content on spiritual bypassing as the profession attempts to rectify this deficit in social work education. Thorough and balanced attention to the role of spirituality in clients' lives – including the negative as well as the positive aspects – is needed in order to support ethical, effective and spiritually sensitive social work practice.

References

Canda, E.R. (2009) 'Spiritually sensitive social work: an overview of American and international trends', paper presented at International Conference on Social Work and Counseling Practice, Hong Kong, June, 2009.

Canda, E.R. and Furman, L.D. (2010) *Spiritual Diversity in Social Work Practice: the heart of helping*, 2nd edn, Oxford: Oxford University Press.

Caplan, M. (2009) *Eyes Wide Open: cultivating discernment on the spiritual path*, Boulder: Sounds True.

Cashwell, C.S., Bentley, P.B. and Yarborough, J.P. (2007) 'The only way out is through: the peril of spiritual bypass', *Counseling and Values,* 51(2): 139–48.

Cashwell, C.S., Glosoff, H.L. and Hammond, C. (2010) 'Spiritual bypass: a preliminary investigation', *Counseling and Values,* 54(2): 162–74.

Cashwell, C.S., Myers, J. E. and Shurts, W. M. (2004) 'Using the developmental counseling and therapy mode to work with a client in spiritual bypass: some preliminary considerations', *Journal of Counseling & Development,* 82(4): 403–9.

Clarke, P.B., Giordano, A.M., Cashwell, C.S. and Lewis, T.F (2013) 'The straight path to healing: using motivational interviewing to address spiritual bypass, *Journal of Counseling and Development,* 91(1): 87–94.

Fowler, J. (1981) *Stages of Faith: the psychology of human development and the quest for meaning,* New York: Harper & Row.

Harris, B. (1994) 'Kundalini and healing in the West', *Journal of Near-Death Studies,* 13(2): 75–9.

Masters, R.A. (2010) *Spiritual Bypassing: when spirituality disconnects us from what really matters,* Berkeley: North Atlantic Books.

Pargament, K.I. (2007) *Spiritually Integrated Psychotherapy: understanding and addressing the sacred,* New York: The Guilford Press.

Sheridan, M.J. (2009) 'Ethical issues in the use of spiritually based interventions in social work practice: what we are doing and why', *Journal of Religion and Spirituality in Social Work,* 28(1): 99–126.

Welwood, J. (1984) 'Principles of inner work: psychological and spiritual', *Journal of Transpersonal Psychology,* 16(1): 63–73.

Welwood, J. (2000) *Toward a Psychology of Awakening,* Boston: Shambhala.

Welwood, J. (2011) 'Human nature, Buddha nature: on spiritual bypassing, relationship and the dharma', *Tricycle,* 20. Online: Available HTTP: www.tricycle.com/interview/human-nature-buddha-nature (accessed 14 February 2016).

Part VII
Conclusion

Developing the agenda for religion and spirituality in social work

Beth R. Crisp

Introduction

This volume has sought to examine and discuss the place of religion and spirituality in social work with the aim of stimulating and provoking the social work community to further develop its thinking and practice regarding religion and spirituality. It has done so by maintaining an emphasis on examining new perspectives and cutting-edge issues, and by including a mix of well-known contributors and emerging scholars in this field. Any single book or project has its limitations, and some of these were identified back in Chapter 1. Nevertheless, this volume is testimony to the burgeoning growth of scholarship and practice in this field over the last two decades. There remain, however, some challenges and opportunities for developing the agenda for religion and spirituality in social work. In particular, these relate to the perceived legitimacy of religion and spirituality within social work practice, and the need to further develop scholarship in this field.

Establishing legitimacy in social work practice

In the early 1990s, Michael Sheridan and colleagues proposed that as many as one-third of all service users in the United States presented to social workers with issues in which religion or spirituality was potentially an issue (Sheridan *et al.* 1992). While the proportion of service users this applies to in other countries is unknown and may vary, contributors to this volume from a range of countries would all concur that religion and spirituality are important concerns for many service users.

While there are many areas of social work in which social workers may get away with little or no understanding of the place of religion in the lives of the people they work with, this is unlikely to be so for those working with refugees. For many refugees, the persecution they have fled is directly associated with their religious beliefs (Hodge 2007a). For example, within living memory there were Jews fleeing the Holocaust in Europe and Muslims, Hindus and Sikhs all displaced after the partitioning of the Indian sub-Continent. In other conflicts, religion has been entwined with culture and/or ethnicity, such as the civil war in the former Yugoslavia. Wherever they come from and whatever their religion, the lives of many refugees attest to the notion that:

religion in a civil society cannot be ignored, nor can it be privatised, and nor can it be relegated to the margins. Religious groups contribute to the spiritual and social wealth of the nation. But religion can also be divisive ...

(Bouma *et al.* 2011: 80)

In particular, there are numerous instances in history when religious beliefs and/or spiritual practices have been used as justification for violence and abuse:

We live still in a world where religious values are used to justify violence and to impose life limiting expectations on individuals and communities. This happens at many levels: continuing warfare in many parts of the world, tensions within communities where there is religious intolerance; an expectation, for example, that women remain married in spite of domestic violence; at policy and program levels such as whether funding should be provided for condoms in AIDS prone areas.

(Gardner 2011: 20)

Arrival in a new country can bring an end to some difficulties, but new ones may emerge in the form of barriers to religious and spiritual practice:

Voices from minority communities revealed that they were acutely aware of the difficulties they face in being heard and in practising their religion at times, particularly the difficulties in building schools and places of worship in the face of concerted local opposition, and reactions to the physical expression of their faith through clothes and appearance. ... members of minority communities indicated that religious minorities' perception of "accommodation" is not that accommodations challenge core values but rather they allow for different religious expressions; for example, permitting Sikh boys to have long hair at school or Muslim girls to wear the hijab.

(Bouma *et al.* 2011: 24)

However, apart from groups such as refugees where issues associated with religion and spirituality may be impossible to avoid, social workers often fail to consider religion and spirituality as relevant factors in people's lives (Askeland and Døhlie 2015) or as potentially rich resources for both individuals and communities (Furness and Gilligan 2010). Furthermore, it is not unheard of for social workers who advocate anti-oppressive practice to have no hesitation in denigrating persons of faith (Crisp 2011; Thyer and Myers 2009). Yet such a position is arguably at odds with the definition of social work approved by the International Federation of Social Workers (IFSW) and the International Association of Schools of Social Work (IASSW) in July 2014:

Social work is a practice-based profession and an academic discipline that promotes social change and development, social cohesion, and the empowerment and liberation of people. Principles of social justice, human rights, collective responsibility and respect for diversities are central to social work. Underpinned by theories of social work, social sciences, humanities and indigenous knowledge, social work engages people and structures to address life challenges and enhance wellbeing.

(IFSW and IASSW 2014)

Such theories and knowledge are key to the curriculum in social work education, but practitioners often feel inadequately prepared to explore the significance of religion or spirituality

(Horwath and Lees 2010). Nor does holding religious or spiritual beliefs and/or engaging in practices associated with a religion or spirituality necessarily result in social workers having relevant knowledge about religion and spirituality as might be required in their professional work with service users (Rizer and McColley 1996). Recognising this as an issue, the *Global Standards for the Education and Training of the Social Work Profession* have, for more than a decade, acknowledged the need for social work education to promote respect for different religions and for social workers to have some knowledge as to the roles that religion and spirituality play in the lives of the users of social work services (IASSW and IFSW 2004). Such guidance, however, may have little or no influence on regulations guiding social work education in different countries. For example, the recent Croisdale-Appleby (2014) report *Re-visioning Social Work Education: An Independent Review* (Croisdale-Appleby 2014), which made recommendations as to what is required in social work education in England, made no mention of religion or spirituality as areas of knowledge social workers should have. However, the lack of content about religion and spirituality is certainly not confined to England (Crisp 2011).

One suggestion that has been made is that specific teaching on religion and spirituality be taught as an elective to social work students (Sheridan *et al.* 1994). However, such offerings are most likely to attract students who are sympathetic to, or have an interest in, religion (Crisp 2011) and fail to tackle the broader issue of social workers needing to be able to recognise the complexities of religious beliefs, identities and practices (Anderson-Nathe *et al.* 2013). Another proposal is that teaching on religion and spirituality be included as part of cultural competence training (Crook-Lyon *et al.* 2012). While this may ensure that issues of religion and spirituality are recognised for minority groups or groups with special needs such as immigrants or refugees, religion and spirituality as a legitimate aspect in the lives of cultural majority service users may be overlooked. Arguably a more encompassing approach is that proposed by Fiona Gardner in her chapter in this volume, which recognises religion and spirituality as some of the many factors that warrant a social worker's consideration. As Gardner demonstrates, generic skills such as the ability to engage in critical reflection, along with an openness to considering the impact of religion and spirituality, can enable social workers to work effectively with service users from diverse religious and spiritual viewpoints. Furthermore, as Fran Gale and Michael Dudley have pointed out, having one's religion or spiritual viewpoint recognised is a human right but this is not necessarily straightforward and there may be many tensions to be negotiated:

> Inevitably, there will always be inherent tensions in balancing human rights, religious beliefs and religious practice, such as the freedom of religion and belief versus freedom of expression ... the conflicts between individual rights and community rights and conflicts between particular groups. These frictions can be deep.
>
> (Bouma *et al.* 2011: 30)

However, silencing any discussion of religion may play a role in 'creating and re-creating patterns of exclusion' (Taket *et al.* 2009: 183). On the other hand, it is also important that social workers be able to distinguish between religion and other forms of oppression such as race, ethnicity and language, which are often conflated (Ashencaen Crabtree and Wong 2013).

Establishing the legitimacy of religion and spirituality in social work practice cannot be left solely to individual social workers. Organisations can legitimise the place of religion and spirituality for service users by recognising these factors in their policies and procedures. For example, including information about religion and spirituality on an assessment protocol indicates to staff that this is necessary for a holistic assessment (Furness and Gilligan 2010). There is also a growing recognition of the need for community leaders and organisations to have sufficient knowledge and skills to handle the complexities of religious and spiritual beliefs and practices (Dinham 2011). Consequently:

> Within service providing organisations, a major challenge is that of designing and implementing policies, systems and practices that are inclusive, that respond to diversity rather than creating a limited understanding of majority or "normal" needs, against which other groups are constructed as deviant with "abnormal" needs, attracting shame or stigma. It is important to re-orient the mainstream towards inclusivity rather than creating a variety of special case responses that are highly limited in funding and scope.
>
> (Taket *et al.* 2009: 183)

As to how this occurs in practice will undoubtedly reflect the different roles that religion and spirituality play in the civic life in countries as well as varying political contexts, cultural values and historical developments that have influenced the development of social work practice (Appleton 2005; McDonald *et al.* 2003). This might explain the rising popularity of mindfulness in Western social work settings, albeit typically presented in a form divorced from its Buddhist roots (e.g. Beckett and Dickens 2014; Foulk *et al.* 2014). Moreover, 'social policy ambitions and social needs differ, and the economic conditions to address them also vary widely' (Trygged and Eriksson 2012: 656). Hence, this volume has presented a range of ways in which religion and spirituality are recognised and/or incorporated into organisational practices, some of which will have more application for individual readers than others.

Developing social work scholarship in religion and spirituality

One of the strengths of this volume has been the inclusion of perspectives from a broad range of places. Consequently, it is perhaps unsurprising that this has revealed a wide range of theoretical and methodological paradigms being utilised by social work researchers concerned with religion and spirituality. There are nevertheless some paradigms that tend to have local associations, which impact on the development of research agendas. For example, when asked to compare research from the US and UK in the area of spirituality and mental health, John Swinton, whose professional backgrounds are nursing and theology, noted:

> There is therefore an interesting difference in approach and style with UK-based studies tending to focus on research that is primarily aimed at practice which, at times reacts strongly against the methods and assumptions of science, and the US where the emphasis is on credibility and importance of science for helping us to understand the health benefits of religion.
>
> (Swinton 2007: 302)

Such methodological differences are not only apparent in social work research and practice more generally but particularly in social work scholarship associated with religion and spirituality. For example, articles outlining the development of quantitative measures such as those produced by Chamiec-Case (2009), Hodge (2007b) and Oxhandler and Parrish (2016) not only hardly included any mention of literature originating from outside the United States, but are consistent with Swinton's (2007) contention that much US research was concerned with measurement of religious participation or of the health benefits of religion and spirituality on individuals. Such research is not unproblematic. While the following statement was written in Australia, it well describes much of the US research:

In the past, religiosity has been measured by how often one attends church, or observes other aspects of a faith. Many measures that are currently used rest on Christian and Protestant assumptions about religion. However, … new measures are needed as many identify with a religion culturally, not necessarily practising that faith in its organised and official contexts.

(Bouma *et al.* 2011: 81)

By way of contrast, Swinton suggested that much of the UK research around religion and spirituality was concerned with concepts, the meaning of the care provided for service users and practice issues. While these questions are important, the use of other theoretical and methodological paradigms is broadening the scope of social work scholarship associated with religion and spirituality. Contributors to this volume have utilised approaches including adopting a critical theoretical paradigm (John Fox and Mark Henrickson), historical research (Mark Smith), narrative approaches (Laura Béres and Irene Renzenbrink), socio-legal research (Janet Melville-Wiseman) and organisational case studies (Eva Jeppsson Grassman).

Rather than arguing as to the relative merits of such approaches, the strengths of these and other approaches must be considered as social work scholarship in religion and spirituality continues to evolve. Extending the range of methodologies enables new questions to be asked, which is important if we are to keep developing the *breadth* of scholarly canon of social work research on religion and spirituality and not just the quantum of publications.

At the beginning of this project, I had somewhat naïvely hoped that one of the outcomes of this volume might be the development of an international research agenda concerning religion and spirituality in social work. However, differences in the way that welfare services are administered and provided, differential understandings of what social work is and the mandate of social workers, differences as to expectations about the place of religion and spirituality, and what are considered acceptable methodologies for researching religion and spirituality, all vary considerably between countries and make the development of a single research agenda almost impossible. Nevertheless, such differences should not be taken as a rationale for limiting ourselves to the research and practice questions and paradigms that have already found favour in our home contexts. Rather, being open to foreign ideas from our colleagues working in different countries or from different methodological paradigms is a scholarly necessity.

Some of the chapters are likely to expose readers to ideas and knowledge for which they have no apparent need. For example, Nehami Baum's chapter, about the issues for a group of Haredi women in Israel studying social work, is at one level very specific. However, social work educators in many countries face questions about what adaptations are possible in order to meet the needs of students of particular religions and not compromise professional requirements. Employers and civic authorities also regularly face questions as to what allowances can be made to enable people to meet their religious beliefs or obligations (Maddox 2011). Furthermore, the Haredi are just one of many examples of religious groups whose members seek to limit their contact as far as is possible with those outside their religion (Doherty 2012).

Although each of the chapters in this volume raises its own questions, either explicitly or implicitly, reading across chapters can enable seemingly idiosyncratic events in individual countries to be theorised and contextualised. For example, Malta joining the European Union, and the Church of Sweden being disestablished and no longer being a state church, could readily be understood as unrelated events. However, both involve political decisions, which have led to the opening up of new conversations as to the potential contribution of religion and spirituality in social work practice. Undoubtedly there will be differences as to how these issues play out and are resolved in different countries, but a starting assumption of uniqueness breeds insularity and limits the likelihood of engaging in potentially fruitful dialogue with colleagues elsewhere. Conversely, assumptions of homogeneity may also be scrutinised.

Utilising a comparative lens when reading apparently disparate contributions different countries or different fields of practice can enable questions to emerge, which may not be so apparent from a single chapter. Some of the questions which emerged for me as editor were as follows:

- Does the local religious/spiritual culture have implications for social work practice, and if so, how?
- Has religion been associated with the establishment and maintenance of social and political elites, and if so, how?
- What role can religion and spirituality play in assisting individuals and communities that have been affected by war and civil unrest?
- Is there a role for religious and spiritual organisations in supporting the development of professional social work services in direct service provision and/or social work education and scholarship?
- Should the state or philanthropists pay for services provided by religious or spiritual organisations?
- How do we best equip social workers to provide religiously/spiritually sensitive practice?
- Is it appropriate to consider the tenets of a particular religion or spirituality, when establishing what is appropriate and ethical professional social work practice?
- Is religion and spirituality relevant throughout the lifetime or more particularly at certain points?
- What are the obligations of social welfare organisations in promoting and protecting the religious and spiritual beliefs of service users?
- How do social workers take seriously the religious and spiritual needs of those they work with, particularly when there is an apparent clash with other needs or values?
- How can arts-based or other non-traditional ways of working benefit service users?
- How can religious or spiritual beliefs/value systems inform macro practice, such as policy development?

This is far from an exhaustive list, and hopefully the contributions in this volume will stimulate readers to ask further questions, and even lead to scholarly research to answer these. However, consideration by readers as to *why* they consider particular questions to be those most salient and worthy of their attention, is also necessary given the limited resources available to most scholars to engage in their intellectual endeavours.

Conclusion

This volume provides glimpses into the overlapping domains of social work practice and scholarly research as they respond to very real issues and conundrums that emerge when religion and spirituality are taken seriously and regarded as integral to humanity. In grappling with these realities, there are often no easy answers and the ways forward suggested by some authors may even be distasteful to some readers. But rather than simply dismissing these authors and/or their solutions to the 'problems' associated with religion and spirituality, readers are invited to 1) consider the conditions that led to authors proposing what they have; 2) identify and explore other solutions that might be both more appropriate but also feasible; and 3) share these new ways of thinking with colleagues locally, nationally and internationally. It is only as we develop new insights and share these within the social work profession that our practice and scholarship can continue to develop and evolve.

References

Anderson-Nathe, B., Gringer, C. and Wahab, S. (2013) 'Nurturing "critical hope" in teaching feminist social work research', *Journal of Social Work Education*, 49(2): 277–91.

Appleton, L. (2005) 'The role of non-profit organizations in the delivery of family services in 11 EU member and applicant states', *International Social Work*, 48(3): 251–62.

Ashencaen Crabtree, S. and Wong, H. (2013) '"Ah Cha"! The racial discrimination of Pakistani minority communities in Hong Kong: an analysis of multiple, intersecting oppressions', *The British Journal of Social Work*, 43(5): 945–63.

Askeland, G.A. and Døhlie, E. (2015) 'Contextualizing international social work: religion as a relevant factor', *International Social Work*, 58(2): 261–9.

Beckett, C. and Dickens, J. (2014) 'Delay and anxiety in care proceedings: grounds for hope?', *Journal of Social Work Practice*, 28(3): 371–82.

Bouma, G., Cahill, D., Dellal, H. and Zwartz, A. (2011) *Freedom of Religion and Belief in 21st Century Australia*, Sydney: Australian Human Rights Commission. Online. Available HTTP: www.humanrights.gov.au/sites/default/files/content/frb/Report_2011.pdf (accessed 3 August 2016).

Chamiec-Case, R. (2009) 'Developing a scale to measure social workers' integration of spirituality in the workplace', *Journal of Religion and Spirituality in Social Work*, 28(3): 284–305.

Crisp, B.R. (2011) 'If a holistic approach to social work requires acknowledgement of religion, what does this mean for social work education?', *Social Work Education*, 30(6): 657–68.

Croisdale-Appleby, D. (2014) *Re-visioning Social Work Education: an independent review*, London: Department of Health. Online. Available HTTP: www.gov.uk/government/uploads/system/uploads/attachment_data/file/285788/DCA_Accessible.pdf (accessed 3 May 2015).

Crook-Lyon, R., O'Grady, K., Smith, T., Jensen, D., Golightly, T. and Potkar, K. (2012) 'Addressing religious and spiritual diversity in graduate training and multi-cultural education for professional psychologists', *Psychology of Religion and Spirituality*, 4(3): 169–81.

Dinham, A. (2011) 'A public role for religion: on needing a discourse of religious literacy', *International Journal of Religion and Spirituality*, 2(4): 291–302.

Doherty, B. (2012) 'Quirky neighbors or the cult next-door? An analysis of public perceptions of the Exclusive Brethren in Australia', *International Journal for the Study of New Religions*, 3(2): 163–211.

Foulk, M.A., Ingersoll-Dayton, B., Kavanagh, J., Robinson, E. and Kales, H.C. (2014) 'Mindfulness-based cognitive therapy with older adults: an exploratory study', *Journal of Gerontological Social Work*, 57(5): 498–520.

Furness, S. and Gilligan, P. (2010) *Religion, Belief and Social Work: making a difference*, Bristol: Policy Press.

Gardner, F. (2011) *Critical Spirituality: a holistic approach to community practice*, Farnham: Ashgate.

Hodge, D.R. (2007a) 'Advocating for persecuted people of faith: a social justice imperative', *Families in Society*, 88(2): 255–62.

Hodge, D.R. (2007b) 'The spiritual competence scale: a new instrument for assessing spiritual competence at the programmatic level', *Research on Social Work Practice*, 17(2): 287–94.

Horwath, J. and Lees, J. (2010) 'Assessing the influence of religious beliefs and practices on parenting capacity: the challenges for social work practitioners', *The British Journal of Social Work*, 40(1): 82–99.

International Association of Schools of Social Work [IASSW] and International Federation of Social Work [IFSW], (2004) *Global Standards for the Education and Training of the Social Work Profession*. Online. Available HTTP: http://cdn.ifsw.org/assets/ifsw_65044-3.pdf (accessed 3 August 2016).

International Federation of Social Workers [IFSW] and International Association of Schools of Social Work [IAASW] (2014) *Global Definition of Social Work*. Online. Available HTTP: http://ifsw.org/get-involved/global-definition-of-social-work/ (accessed 3 August 2016).

McDonald, C., Harris, J. and Wintersteen, R. (2003) 'Contingent on context? Social work and the state in Australia, Britain and the USA', *The British Journal of Social Work*, 33(2): 191–208.

Maddox, M. (2011) 'Are religious schools socially inclusive or exclusive? An Australian conundrum', *International Journal of Cultural Policy*, 17(2): 170–86.

Oxhandler, H.K. and Parrish, D.E. (2016) 'The development and validation of the Religious/Spiritually Integrated Practice Assessment Scale', *Research on Social Work Practice*, 26(3): 295–307.

Rizer, J.M. and McColley, K.J. (1996) 'Attitudes and practices regarding spirituality and religion held by graduate social work students', *Social Work and Christianity*, 23(1): 53–65.

Sheridan, M.J., Bullis, R.K., Adcock, C.R., Berlin, S.D. and Miller, P.C. (1992) 'Practitioners' personal and professional attitudes and behavior toward religion and spirituality: issues for education and practice', *Journal of Social Work Education*, 28(2): 190–203.

Sheridan, M.J., Wilmer, C.M. and Atcheson, L. (1994) 'Inclusion of religion and spirituality in the social work curriculum: a study of faculty views', *Journal of Social Work Education*, 30(3): 363–76.

Swinton, J. (2007) 'Researching spirituality and mental health: a perspective from the research', in M.E. Coyte, P. Gilbert and V. Nicholls (eds) *Spirituality, Values and Mental Health: jewels for the journey*, London: Jessica Kingsley Publishers.

Taket, A., Foster, N. and Cook K. (2009) 'Understanding processes of social exclusion: silence, silencing and shame' in A. Taket, B.R. Crisp, A. Nevill, G. Lamaro, M. Graham and S. Barter-Godfrey (eds) *Theorising Social Exclusion*, London: Routledge.

Thyer, B.A. and Myers, L.L. (2009) 'Religious discrimination in social work academic programs: whither social justice?', *Journal of Religion and Spirituality in Social Work*, 28(1–2), 144–60.

Trygged, S. and Eriksson, B. (2012) 'How do students perceive the international dimension in social work education: an enquiry among Swedish and German students', *Journal of Social Work Education*, 48(4): 655–7.

Index